International Healthcare Professionals' Handbook

International Healthcare Professionals' Handbook

A Success Guide to Working in the UK for Nurses, Midwives and Allied Health Professionals

ANNESHA ARCHYANGELIO, MSc IPC, Msc Management & Leadership, Bsc Health Studies, Mary Seacole Leadership Award, RGN

Regional Director of Nursing
Commissioning and Transformation
NHS England
England, United Kingdom

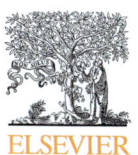

ELSEVIER

ISBN: 978-0-323-93261-5

Content Strategist: Robert Edwards
Content Project Manager: Tapajyoti Chaudhuri
Cover Design: Greg Harris
Marketing Manager: Deborah J. Watkins

Printed in India

Last digit is the print number: 9 8 7 6 5 4 3 2 1

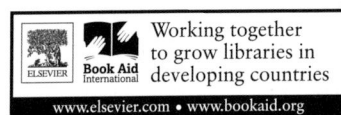

Working together to grow libraries in developing countries

www.elsevier.com • www.bookaid.org

CONTENTS

International nurses (IRs), midwives, allied health professionals (AHPs) and health-care support staff are vital to the sustainability of the healthcare system in the United Kingdom (UK). They are essential in supporting patients, carers and families to ensure they receive the best care possible and bring diversity to the health and care workforce. This book was authored by Annesha Archyangelio to support and educate IRs, mid-wives, AHPs and other staff in new cultures, who bring equality, diversity and inclusion (EDI) to the workplace. Undeniably, international staff contribute significantly to fill-ing the staffing gaps in the UK healthcare system; this book supports their recruitment and retention, which contributes to the delivery of high-quality and safe care across the health and care system.

Many IRs, midwives, AHPs, and healthcare support staff dream of working abroad in countries such as the UK, and others are recruited and invited to work in the UK to meet the workforce demands. Whatever the process used to recruit international staff to enter the UK, this book helps newly recruited staff to navigate the new systems, flour-ish, thrive and succeed in their healthcare roles. Whether the goal is promotion into senior roles; competent and effective service and care delivery; or health and well-being (HWB), happiness and long-term job satisfaction in a career they love, this book pro-vides support for all internationally recruited staff, and the managers and leaders who support them in their role.

This is the opportune time for this book, given that it weaves in the learnings from the global COVID-19 pandemic that disproportionately affected individuals from a black and minority ethnic (global majority staff) background (Public Health England, 2020c). Utilising the guidance and strategies in this book will help those from an inter-national and diverse background to achieve better outcomes while working through the post-COVID-19 pandemic recovery period and other similar future events that may occur.

The broad themes of this book include preparing internationally recruited nurses (IRNs) and other healthcare staff for successful completion of the recruitment process, including exams and Nursing and Midwifery Council (NMC) competencies. There is information on the history of nursing and the wider National Health Service (NHS), and a basic guide to the NHS structure and the wider health and social care service. The book includes details on the organisation and regulation of healthcare; nursing and other healthcare processes; and models of nursing, healthcare and service delivery in the UK. Details on professional organisations, trade unions and healthcare registration bod-ies are also included in this book.

Regarding cultural competency, communication challenges including professional issues related to communication are discussed, along with solutions such as the use of everyday healthcare-related terminologies to communicate in the healthcare setting, as well as documentation and recording in nursing.

To support IRNs and other healthcare staff, the book includes strategies for coping and flourishing in their role, and information on career and study pathways in the UK healthcare system. This includes professional leadership in healthcare, career conversations and options, working in multiprofessional teams and dealing with daily and longer-term challenges. There is a chapter on accelerating staff development and progression in the workplace to support staff in achieving career promotions.

The final chapters and sections of this book include reflections from the author, including hints and tips on navigating barriers and challenges; the languages used in the UK; competencies and tools used in healthcare; units of measurements; abbreviations; and further resources, reading, links and other sources of information.

To all IRs, midwives, AHPs and healthcare support staff, we welcome you and wish you great success, satisfaction and happiness in your work and social life in the UK.

This book serves as a success guide for you, providing strategies, tips and tricks to navigate life and work as healthcare staff in the UK, contributing to diverse senior leadership in healthcare.

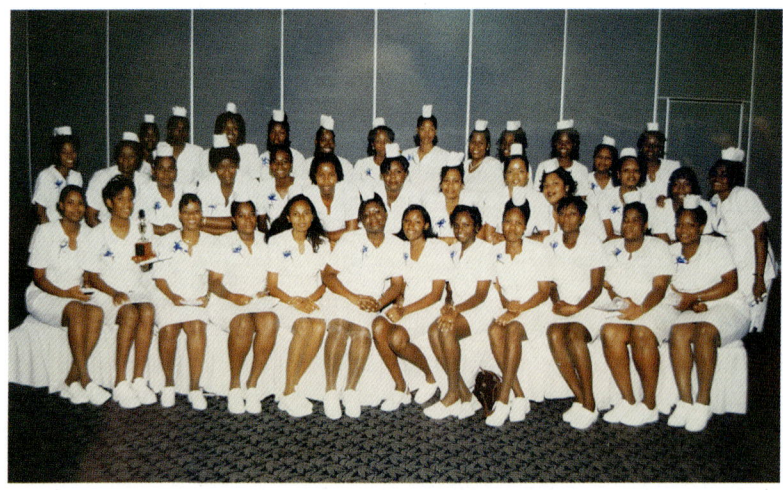

School of Nursing Graduates, Jamaica 2001.

Annesha Archyangelio

This book has been written to help internationally recruited staff who enter the UK to live, work and thrive in their new environment. It recounts an abundance of lived experience and provides support to guide staff through the various processes. The author, Annesha Archyangelio, is a director of nursing and healthcare leader with over 20 years' experience in the National Health Service (NHS) and private sector. She has held several challenging senior roles at the regional and national level, including as part of the response to the COVID-19 pandemic. She aspires to holding an executive-level position within the NHS.

Her senior roles include being a Regional Director of Nursing Professional and System Leadership within NHS England, where she works as part of the regional leadership team and leads multiple complex portfolios to deliver safe and high-quality care to the population. She was also Regional Director of Nursing at NHS England, overseeing the commissioning of healthcare and ensuring the quality and safety of services across regional geographies. She was Director of Infection Prevention and Control (IPC) and led on IPC and the COVID-19 response at all levels across organisations, hospitals and systems to ensure pandemic requirements were met.

Annesha started her nursing career in Jamaica, where she studied general nursing, including midwifery, mental health and paediatric nursing, and she worked as a nurse at Kingston Public Hospital. She also previously worked in education, teaching the sciences.

Annesha immigrated to the UK as an internationally trained and recruited nurse. In the UK, she has held various positions across the NHS, including at acute trusts; NHS England, where she was working with the Integrated Care Systems (ICSs); within clinical commissioning groups (CCGs) and the community; in the fields of mental health and learning disability and autism (LDA); in the independent sector; in the health and justice sector; and as an independent consultant.

Annesha was a Chief Nursing Officer (CNO) Nurse Fellow in professional leadership at NHS England in the CNO's team, where she authored The Matron's Handbook (https://www.england.nhs.uk/wp-content/uploads/2020/08/Matrons_Handbook.pdf).

She created the @MatronNetwork in her national role and continues to implement The Matron's Handbook today. She was a Health Service Journal (HSJ) Award finalist and won the HSJ Highly Commended Award for The Matron's Handbook, national engagement and implementation work.

Annesha is a Registered General Nurse (RGN) and holds a BSc in Heath Studies, an MSc in IPC, an MSc in Management/Leadership and a Ponsonby Travel Scholarship; she also won a Mary Seacole Award. She was an honorary researcher at Imperial College London and an honorary lecturer at University College London (ULC), and has been a Florence Nightingale Foundation (FNF) Leadership Scholar Mentor and Mary Seacole Programme Mentor.

Annesha is an ambassador for Black and Ethnic Minority (BAME) staff development and created the NHS BAME Leadership Talent national network @nhsbame and the BAME Leadership Talent resources to support staff. She was the Regional CNO and Chief Midwifery Officer (CMidO) BAME Strategic Advisory Group Lead. She served on the Infection Prevention Society (IPS) Board and Royal College of Nursing (RCN) Board, and as a trustee and board member of Peace Hospice Care.

ACKNOWLEDGEMENTS

I would like to thank my family, friends and colleagues for their support. Thanks go to my mother Ena, my sons Aiden and Nathaniel, my sisters Faith and Natoya and the rest of my family, who provide inspiration, motivation and drive. I would like to thank the staff at Elsevier who are involved with this book, including Robert Edwards and Tapajyoti Chaudhuri, for their flexibility and support in completing the book.

Annesha Archyangelio

Introduction

1.1 The Broad Themes

The broad themes of this book include (1) preparing internationally recruited (IR) staff for successful completion of the recruitment process; (2) strategies for coping with and flourishing in their role; (3) cultural competency and communication challenges and solutions; and (4) accelerating staff development and progression in the workplace. These are presented in the next few chapters of this book.

Regarding the preparation of internationally recruited healthcare staff (IRCS) for successful completion of the recruitment process, preparing for and sitting exams, as well as subsequent progression, are key success criteria.

This book provides an introduction to professional organisations, healthcare registration bodies and trade unions, including the Nursing and Midwifery Council (NMC), Royal College of Nursing (RCN), Health and Care Professions Council (HCPC) and other professional bodies. Moreover, it provides a guide to the structure of the National Health Service (NHS), including an introduction to NHS England, the Care Quality Commission (CQC) and other regulatory organisations and bodies.

The book provides information on and an introduction to the structure of the NHS and the wider health and social care service.

This book also includes information on the organisation and regulation of healthcare in the United Kingdom (UK), including for nurses, midwives, allied health professionals (AHPs) and healthcare support staff.

There are also elements regarding nursing and other healthcare processes, which are required to ensure delivery of best practice.

This book includes information on nursing, midwifery and AHPs adaptation and assessment programmes, and career support and development.

This book includes information on the history and milestone of the wider NHS. It also includes information on current models of nursing, healthcare and service delivery.

Strategies for working and flourishing as IR staff are outlined, including advice on the pathways of development into senior roles and information on where to access funded, non-funded and free training and development resources.

Processes for accelerating development and progression in the workplace for IR staff are detailed, along with any additional study or training that may be needed to 'top-up' original programmes of study, including to convert some qualifications to UK awards. This is then followed by any additional development required for progression in the workplace.

The section on cultural competency, which highlights strategies to address communication challenges and general cultural competency, is aimed at all nurses, midwives, AHPs and care staff in the workplace.

Communication challenges and solutions are also discussed, including everyday healthcare-related terminologies commonly used to communicate (including via emails and formal letters) with staff, patients, families and carers, and which are often unfamiliar to individuals from other countries. This covers communication specific to nursing and related to wider healthcare practice.

There are also elements regarding documentation and recording in nursing, which are required to ensure delivery of best practice.

The final chapters and sections of this book include useful information, including reflections from the author, languages used in the UK, competencies and tools used in healthcare, applying for jobs, units of measurement, abbreviations and further information including reading material, resources, links and other resources.

1.2 History of Nursing

This book includes information on the history of nursing in the UK and further afield. Nursing has come a long way from the routine task of cleaning and feeding another person to having access to hospital treatment, thanks to the advent of anaesthetics and antiseptic for surgery and advanced medical techniques, and finally to the introduction of nursing schools to train and educate nurses to work in hospitals. The profile of the nursing profession has rapidly gained momentum since then, with advances being seen in nursing education and medical care.

Today, nursing in the UK is a highly technical profession that requires formal training at a university or other higher education institution and graduation with a Bachelor of Science (BSc) degree in nursing. Florence Nightingale and Mary Seacole are key historic figures who championed nursing and the nursing profession throughout their lives. Thomas (2016) outlines the key timeline of the profession of nursing, nurse education and medical advances, which ranged from as far back as 1796 detailing the smallpox vaccine discovery by Edward Jenner, ranging through the Mary Seacole in 1855, and the Nightingale Training School opens at St Thomas' Hospital in London in 1860. This timeline progressed through the establishment of nursing associations and professional bodies to the present day with advances in nursing and midwifery.

1.2.1 THE HISTORY OF NURSING

With all nurses requiring a degree from 2009, the professionalisation of nursing became increasingly evident, with nurses gaining an extended knowledge base, including in research. Nurses and midwives also needed to register with the NMC to comply with the code of practice and be offered a job by employers, where they work to a specified job description (JD) that outlines their roles and responsibilities.

The expansion of newly available treatments and specialities enables nurses to acquire enhanced knowledge and advanced professional decision-making skills, underpinned by the higher academic standards of nursing education.

There have been significant and further advances in the nursing professional since the nurse training programme became a degree programme in 2009. Table 1.1 shows the milestones (NHS England, 2023a) and history of the NHS from 2010 onwards.

Nursing in the UK is now a more culturally diverse profession with the increase in nurses entering the UK from across the world. Therefore it is important for all staff to be advocates of inclusivity, equality and diversity, including supporting international staff to grow and thrive. Nursing in the UK is a well-respected profession and nurses are members of a discipline with strict codes of conduct. Professional satisfaction and remuneration are paramount in nursing and midwifery, with the aim of delivering high-quality care to patients even in the most challenging and adverse circumstances. There have been narratives in recent years describing our nurses and doctors as heroes in the face of the COVID-19 pandemic; they certainly are heroic, going above and beyond to administer care to the UK population. The COVID-19 pandemic emphasised the personal and professional challenges faced by nurses and other healthcare professionals, who the public looked on as 'masked heroes', but many felt they were just doing their job. This pandemic, like others before it, highlighted the risks taken by nursing professionals at work. The effects of the pandemic were not equal among healthcare workers, some of whom died after contracting COVID-19. Some staff were impacted more than others, particularly those from Black, Asian and minority ethnic backgrounds (Public Health England (PHE), 2020c. This indicates the importance of paying special attention to supporting staff from international, Black, Asian and minority ethnic backgrounds. Elements of infection prevention and control (IPC) are included to this end in sections 4.3.5 on IPC and 4.3.4 on COVID-19 in the UK.

Nursing, midwifery and wider healthcare staff deliver vital services every day, from the bottom of our hearts, and represent the future of healthcare in the UK. For these reasons, everyone is thankful, grateful and proud of everything that healthcare staff do.

This is also important for the sustainability of the NHS, as *'The NHS will last as long as there are folks left with the faith to fight for it.'* (Aneurin 'Nye' Bevan) (Bailey, 2022).

Nurses, midwives and related professionals have come a long way, with degrees now covering all areas of theory and practice including the everyday challenges faced in the healthcare setting. Moreover, there are many specialist, practice and professional areas that staff can enter into. These include nursing for adults, children and those with learning disabilities or mental health needs, as well as psychiatric and community nursing. There are also specialities in midwifery, health play specialists, health visitors, high-intensity therapists, paramedics and physician associates. Moreover, there are many other specialist areas such as emergencies, assisted living, care homes, cardiovascular nursing and neonatal and obstetric nursing. Finally, there are excellent career paths (see Figs 5.1–5.4 and 6.1) through which nurses can progress to become directors of nursing, chief nurses and even chief executives.

TABLE 1.1 ■ Milestones and History of the NHS

Year	Event
1948	The NHS is born, providing healthcare services that are free for all at the point of delivery.
1949	The Ministries of Health and Labour, along with the Colonial Office, the General Nursing Council and the Royal College of Nursing, begin a massive recruitment drive throughout the West Indies for staff for the NHS.
1953	DNA's structure is discovered by two Cambridge University scientists, James D Watson and Francis Crick, revolutionising the study of disease caused by defective genes. The discovery included vital work from Rosalind Franklin.
1956	Polio immunisation programme begins.
1956	The first kidney dialysis is performed by Frank Parsons at Leeds General Infirmary, marking the opening of the first artificial kidney unit in the UK.
1957	The whooping cough immunisation programme begins.
1958	Polio and diphtheria vaccination programmes ensure that everyone under 15 years of age is vaccinated.
1958	The first successful cardiopulmonary bypass programme in the UK begins at Hammersmith Hospital, London.
1960	The first kidney transplant takes place at the Edinburgh Royal Infirmary, involving identical twins.
1960	The first implantable heart pacemaker is used.
1962	The first full hip replacement is carried out by Prof. John Charnley at Wrightington Hospital in Wigan.
1967	The first successful treatment is achieved for rhesus disease of the newborn, which causes serious health problems including deafness and blindness.
1968	The measles vaccine is introduced.
1968	The first heart transplant is carried out by South African-born surgeon Donald Ross at the National Heart Hospital in London.
1968	Europe's first liver transplant is performed by Prof. Sir Roy Calne at Addenbrooke's Hospital in Cambridge.
1972	Computerised tomography (CT) scans revolutionise the way doctors examine the body, allowing three-dimensional images to be produced from a large series of two-dimensional X-rays.
1973	The number of cases of whooping cough falls to nearly zero due to an immunisation programme.
1978	The world's first test-tube baby, Louise Brown, is born via in vitro fertilisation (IVF), developed by Dr. Patrick Steptoe.
1979	The first successful bone marrow transplant in a child is carried out by Prof. Roland Levinsky at Great Ormond Street Hospital, London.
1979	A UK heart transplant programme begins at Papworth Hospital, Cambridgeshire, carried out by the surgeon Sir Terence English.
1980	Magnetic resonance imaging (MRI) scans are introduced.
1980	Keyhole surgery is used successfully for the first time to carry out the removal of a gall bladder.
1983	A UK liver transplant programme begins.
1983	The first combined heart and lung transplant in the UK is performed by Prof. Sir Magdi Yacoub at Harefield Hospital, Middlesex.

TABLE 1.1 ▪ Milestones and History of the NHS—cont'd

Year	Event
1986	An artificial heart programme begins at Harefield Hospital, Middlesex.
1986	The first lung-only transplant in Europe is carried out by Prof. John Dark at Freeman Hospital, Newcastle.
1987	The world's first heart, lung and liver transplants are carried out by Prof. Sir Roy Calne and Prof. John Wallwork at Papworth Hospital in Cambridge.
1987	Britain's first-ever purpose-built AIDS ward is opened at Middlesex Hospital by Princess Diana.
1987	Britain's first successful heart transplant baby is operated on at Freeman Hospital in Newcastle.
1988	Free breast screening is introduced to reduce breast cancer deaths in women aged over 50 years, the first of its kind in the world.
1992	A vaccine against *Haemophilus influenzae* type B (Hib), a cause of childhood meningitis, is introduced as part of a vaccination programme.
1992	The world's first laser surgery on babies in the womb takes place at King's College Hospital, London to treat potentially fatal twin-to-twin transfusion syndrome.
1994	The NHS Organ Donor Register is set up for people wishing to donate their organs.
1999	The UK becomes first country in the world to use a vaccine against Group C meningococcal disease.
2000	NHS walk-in centres are introduced to offer easy access to a range of services.
2002	The first successful treatment of a child in the UK via gene therapy is achieved at Great Ormond Street Hospital, London.
2006	The NHS Bowel Cancer Screening Programme is launched for those aged 60–69 years, the first-ever screening programme targeting both men and women.
2007	The introduction of the robotic arm leads to groundbreaking heart operations for patients with fast or irregular heartbeats.
2007	The first living donor in the UK is reported at St James' Hospital in Leeds when David Lomas, aged 20 years, donated part of his liver to his father Stephen, aged 50 years, who had advanced liver disease.
2007	St James's Institute of Oncology, the largest cancer centre in Europe, opens in Leeds.
2008	A vaccine to prevent cervical cancer (human papillomavirus vaccine (HPV)) is made available to all girls aged 12 years.
2010	The UK's first cochlear implant operation is performed to provide hearing in both ears.
2011	Successful trial of an artificial pancreas.
2011	The UK's first selective dorsal rhizotomy (SDR) operation is performed – Beau Britton, aged 7 years, from Cornwall is the first child to be funded by a local NHS trust for this neurological procedure.
2012	Announcement of deoxyribonucleic acid (DNA) mapping for patients with cancer and rare diseases (100,000 Genomes Project).
2012	The first UK hand transplant is carried out by a surgical team at Leeds General Infirmary.
2013	The Cancer Drugs Fund is established, creating a national list of approved fast-track drugs and giving uniform access to treatment across the country.
2016	The first double hand transplant is performed at Leeds Teaching Hospital NHS Trust.

(Continued)

TABLE 1.1 ■ Milestones and History of the NHS—cont'd

Year	Event
2016	NHS England funds bionic eye surgery.
2017	Rollout of mechanical thrombectomy enabling patients with stroke in England to receive this revolutionary new treatment.
2017	NHS England announces the world's largest single pre-exposure prophylaxis (PrEP) implementation trial to prevent human immunodeficiency virus (HIV) infection.
2018	NHS England announces that children in England will be the first in Europe able to access chimeric antigen receptor T-cell therapy (CAR-T), marking the beginning of a new era of personalised cancer medicine.
2019	NHS England strikes a world-leading deal to enable everyone with hepatitis C to receive curative treatment at a cost-effective price, which will enable England to eliminate the virus before 2030.
2019	NHS England funds the first-ever treatment for children with spinal muscular atrophy.
2019	NHS England strikes a deal for a first in a new generation of gene therapies that can cure blindness in children.
2019	Patients in England living with cystic fibrosis are given access to all three licensed treatments.
2020	The NHS calls for NHS Volunteer Responders.
2020	The first known case of COVID-19 is reported in the UK—in December. The COVID-19 vaccination campaign starts with 90-year-old grandmother Margaret Keenan from the UK, who became the first person in the world to receive the Pfizer COVID-19 vaccine following its clinical approval.
2020	The NHS becomes the first health system in the world to commit to becoming carbon net zero.
2021	The first new treatment for sickle cell disease in over 20 years is rolled out to patients in England, with life-saving benefits.
2021	Dexamethasone, discovered as an effective treatment for COVID-19 in a clinical trial in the NHS, saves 1 million lives worldwide.
2021	The first climate-friendly baby is born in Newcastle Hospitals NHS Trust.
2022	NHS England strikes a deal for the 'world's most expensive drug (**Libmeldy**)', which can offer babies and young children with metachromatic leukodystrophy (MLD) the prospect of a normal life.
2022	The NHS conducts the first net zero operation at Solihull Hospital.
2022	The Innovative Medicines Fund, which enables faster patient access to promising new drugs, is launched.
2022	The 100th cancer drug is fast tracked to patients through the Cancer Drugs Fund.
2022	For the first time, the NHS treats patients with sickle cell disease using a life-changing drug.
2022	NHS staff are honoured with the George Cross by Her Majesty The Queen at Windsor Castle.

With permission from NHS England; NHS England (2023). NHS History: Milestones of the NHS. https://www.england.nhs.uk/nhsbirthday/about-the-nhs-birthday/nhs-history/. Accessed 18 May 2023.

1.3 History of the NHS and Health and Social Care Services

The history and milestones of the NHS and health and social care services are outlined in Table 1.1. These track the story of the organisation, including how it was set up and how it has improved and changed over time (Nuffield Trust, 2023). The timeline covers healthcare before the NHS as well as the following periods: 1948–1957: establishment of the NHS; 1958–1967: the renaissance of general practice and hospitals; 1968–1977: rethinking the NHS; 1978–1987: clinical advances and financial crisis; 1988–1997: new influences and pathways; 1998–2007: Labour's decade; 2008–2017: an uncertain path ahead; and a 70-year perspective on the NHS (Nuffield Trust, 2023).

The NHS was established on 5 July 1948, which Aneurin 'Nye' Bevan described as 'a great and novel undertaking'. Many people contribute to the NHS, including those who are professionally involved and those receiving care, and it is important to maintain a chronological framework of the main clinical and organisational events (Nuffield Trust, 2023).

1.4 Guide to Success for International Staff

This book fulfils the needs of international nurses, midwives, AHPs and other healthcare staff working in the UK and its healthcare system, covering the topics of international recruitment, retention, support and development, as well as cultural aspects. The book details the programme that international nurses, at home and abroad, need in order to develop and succeed in the healthcare system in the UK. It includes an updated version of 'Everyday English for International Nurses' (Parkinson & Brooker, 2004) among other elements from that publication, which provided a dictionary of key terms and colloquialisms that are useful for nurses, midwives, AHPs and care staff coming from abroad to work in the NHS and healthcare services in the UK.

The needs of IR staff nurses, midwives, AHPs and care staff, who train abroad and come to work in the UK, are addressed by this book, which covers health and wellbeing, development and career progression in the workplace; it is also relevant to staff with an international background training in the UK. Advice regarding the process of recruitment from abroad is included, where there are various processes that staff need to complete including registering with the NMC or the HCPC (for AHPs). This book will support the increasing number of international registered nurses, midwives, AHPs and care staff who are rapidly recruited from abroad and come to live and work in the UK, thus helping to address the staffing gaps in the UK's healthcare system. Key to this process is supporting newly arriving IR staff and giving them the chance to adapt and learn how to navigate UK healthcare systems and processes easily. This book provides comprehensive advice and useful information to enable international nurses, midwives and AHPs to thrive in the UK. Moreover, it supports the needs of this growing population of international staff, who are eager to develop and desire support from those who have already succeeded in the healthcare system. Working in a new country and healthcare system can be daunting and challenging, and adapting to new ways of working in the UK, the

NHS and the wider healthcare system can take a long time. Comprehensive information regarding the type of support that nurses, midwives, AHPs and carers from the UK and abroad require is provided in the following chapters. This book will help to significantly shorten the time required for adaptation by introducing staff to the UK, the NHS and the wider healthcare system, as well as other sectors, in a smooth and supportive manner. This is achieved by going in depth into the practical steps required to succeed as international staff in the UK. This involves the provision of step-by-step information where required, including signposting to key resources. The NHS employs millions of staff, standing as one of the largest single healthcare systems in the world.

This book is unique in describing the lived experience of nurses, midwives, AHPs and care staff, and drawing on the experience of other international nurses. It encompasses the lessons of the COVID-19 pandemic, as the author is a former Director of Infection Prevention and Control (DIPC) who worked on the frontline during the pandemic. Information on the COVID-19 pandemic (section 4.3.4) and IPC (sections 4.3.5) is provided, including first-hand experience of the author pertinent to coping during challenging situations.

Another unique facet of this book is that at the time of writing, the author was a practising Director of Nursing who had worked in all areas of healthcare. Therefore while current approaches to nursing and midwifery are detailed in the book, the author's own experience as an IR nurse is at the heart of the book.

The audience for this book includes international nurses, midwives, AHPs and other healthcare workers of all bands, both UK based and those from abroad. This includes nonregistered staff such as healthcare support workers, care staff, porters and domestic staff who will benefit from the sections regarding life in the UK and the UK healthcare system. The book will also be a useful resource for directors of nursing and chief nurses, across the UK and abroad, who would like to support the recruitment, retention, development, and progression of their NHS staff, who number more than 1.2 million. Additionally, we expect that those in the social care, private and independent sectors, as well as social enterprises in the UK and the thousands of international nurses and other staff who come to the country every year from regions such as the Caribbean, Europe, Australia, Asia, Africa and even the United States, will enjoy this book. It can be used by staff from across the globe as part of their early preparation, making their transition to a new work setting and a new life a little easier.

This book can serve as essential or supplementary reading material for those completing nursing, midwifery or AHP courses, as well as for those enrolled in other healthcare programmes or formal training or instructional courses, providing guidance that will help them with their studies and subsequent careers.

This book aligns with the requirements of the NHS 10-year Long-Term Plan, helping international staff coming to work in the UK play their part in contributing as nurses, midwives, AHPs, healthcare managers and leaders.

The NHS (2023b) 'Quick Guide: Code of Practice for International Recruitment' outlines the code of practice for international recruitment, highlighting and explaining important guiding principles employers should follow when recruiting from overseas.

1.4.1 BENEFITS, REWARDS AND RECOGNITION OF WORKING IN THE UK HEALTHCARE SYSTEM

There are many benefits, rewards and forms of recognition associated with working in the UK healthcare system, as detailed throughout this book. Some specific benefits, rewards, forms of recognitions and perks of working in the UK Healthcare system include:

- Working across broad areas of healthcare practice.
- A standard 37.5-hour working week.
- A pension contributed to by employers and free NHS pension scheme seminars (NHS Business Services Authority, 2023). These provide information on the basics of the NHS pension scheme (NHSPS), pension reforms and flexible working, the 'McCloud remedy' (merging all public service pensions into one entity), and special class (SC)/mental health officer (MHO) status.
- Developmental support and training that is sponsored, paid for or subsidised by employers, including university courses, coaching and mentoring, among other types of support.
- Alumni membership after course completion.
- A minimum of 27 days of annual leave.
- Paid sick leave.
- Flexible working patterns.
- Retire and return option.
- NHS discounts on many brands.
- Health insurance from some private organisations.
- Support with health and wellbeing.

In the NHS, there is free access to healthcare for all at the point of care (NHS 2023a).

1.5 Summary

This introductory chapter covers the history of nursing, the NHS and the wider health and social care service, and the broad themes of this book including (1) preparing IR staff for successful completion of the international recruitment process; (2) strategies for coping with and flourishing in their role; (3) cultural competency and communication solutions and (4) accelerating staff development and progression in the workplace. This chapter detailed milestones in the history of the NHS and health and social care services (Table 1.1). A guide to success for international staff is presented in the following chapters, comprising the bulk of the book.

CHAPTER 2

Preparing Internationally Recruited Staff for Successful Completion of the International Recruitment Process

2.1 Introduction

This chapter includes content on how to enter the United Kingdom (UK) health and care system from abroad; Nursing and Midwifery Council (NMC) registration, competencies and exams, such as the International English Language Testing System (IELTS) exam and objective structured clinical examination (OSCE); NMC revalidation; and other elements that are required for compliance with the NMC code of practice. It also makes reference to professional organisations, healthcare registration bodies and trade unions.

2.2 How to Enter the UK Healthcare System From Abroad

2.2.1 MOVING TO THE UK FROM OUTSIDE THE EUROPEAN ECONOMIC AREA

Most National Health Service (NHS) services operate a residence-based healthcare system, making the majority of NHS services free to people who are usually resident in the UK. This is not based on nationality, tax payment, National Insurance (NI) contributions, being registered with a general practitioner (GP) (NHS, 2023b), having an NHS number (NHS, 2023c) or being a property owner in the UK. Ordinary resident means that the individual is living in the UK on a legal and fully settled basis, which requires evidence such as resident identification (ID), a passport and a utility bill for verification (NHS, 2023d).

2.2.2 INDEFINITE LEAVE TO REMAIN

The immigration status of indefinite leave to remain (ILR), granting the right to live in the UK on a permanent basis, is one of the official 'ordinary resident' statuses for individuals subject to immigration control.

Family members of an European Economic Area (EEA) national who are resident in the UK may not be subject to immigration control, regardless of being from outside the EEA, and can apply to join family living permanently in the UK (GOV.UK, 2023c).

Family members of people from Northern Ireland who live in the UK may be able to join that person without paying the immigration health surcharge, provided they meet the definition of an eligible person from Northern Ireland (GOV.UK, 2023d).

Otherwise, an individual may be eligible to apply for presettled or settled status under the European Union (EU) Settlement Scheme based on that relationship with UK family members, to join family living permanently in the UK. Once individuals have obtained either presettled or settled status, they will not be charged for their healthcare providing they have lived in the UK on an officially settled basis for some time (GOV.UK, 2023c).

2.2.3 HOW CAN INDIVIDUALS WORK IN THE NHS AS HEALTH PROFESSIONALS FROM OVERSEAS?

Individuals from outside the UK, except those from the Republic of Ireland, require permission from UK Visas and Immigration (UKVI). UKVI is responsible for managing migration for overseas health professionals to work in the UK, who ordinarily require entry clearance prior to travelling to the UK (NHS, 2023e).

2.2.4 OVERSEAS HEALTH PROFESSIONALS (NHS, 2023e)

For qualified overseas healthcare professionals who are thinking about working in healthcare and living in the UK, this section provides useful information, including professional registration and immigration requirements (NHS, 2023f).

International recruitment (IR) is used by many employers in the UK and across the world as one of the means of filling vacancies in specific areas and professions in the UK where there are significant skills and staff shortages, including in the NHS and wider healthcare sector.

Employers are constantly actively recruiting from overseas to fill a wide range of professional vacancies and key checks and tests that need to be completed are in place. Great emphasis is placed on increasing the supply of overseas nurses and other healthcare staff into the UK, which has almost unlimited working opportunities across the country.

Individuals who would like to work in the NHS and wider healthcare sector as an overseas health professional (excluding from the Republic of Ireland) should seek permission from UKVI to work in the UK, as well as entry clearance to travel to the country. Individuals can obtain a visa and entry clearance by demonstrating that they meet key requirements to work in the UK, which uses a points-based immigration system; this can be done via the EU settlement scheme or by acquiring a biometric residence permit (BRP) (GOV.UK, 2023f).

2.2.5 POINTS-BASED IMMIGRATION SYSTEM

The Home Office, which includes UKVI, manages and governs the way individuals from outside the EEA can work, train or study in the UK. This involves the use of the points-based immigration system, which was fully introduced in 2021 and provides a route for both EEA and non-EEA nationals to work, train or study in the UK providing they meet the requirements. This applies to all individuals from outside the country who would like to live and work in the UK, excluding individuals from the Republic of Ireland and people who are already in the UK (GOV.UK, 2023g).

An unlimited number of skilled UK migrants are allowed to enter the UK providing they meet the skilled worker criteria to live and work in the country (GOV.UK, 2023g). A Health and Care Worker visa (GOV.UK, 2023h) grants permission to health and care professionals to travel to or stay in the UK and take a job within the NHS for which they are eligible or to work as an NHS supplier or in adult social care. Applications are assessed using a points system that is intended to only allow entry to those whose skills will benefit the UK. The number of points required and the way the points are awarded depend on the category under which individuals apply, which reflects job offers, skill level, language competence, qualifications and other specific criteria.

Some occupations are recognised by UKVI as 'shortage occupations' and are on the national shortage occupation list, which is reserved for occupations for which there are not enough suitably qualified and skilled workers from the resident labour market to fill the available vacancies. A full list of the shortage occupations can be found on the gov.uk website (GOV.UK, 2023i) and includes key jobs such as all types of health services and public health; residential, day and domiciliary care; care workers and home carers; and healthcare roles. Individuals are advised to check the website to establish which route of entry they are eligible to apply for.

The EU settlement scheme provides EU nationals with a route to residency in the UK; more information can be found online, including how to apply to the scheme (GOV.UK, 2023j). EU, EEA or Swiss citizens who do not already have temporary or permanent leave to remain can apply to the EU Settlement Scheme to continue living in the UK with either presettled or settled status. Further information for EU citizens and families can be found on the gov.uk website (GOV.UK, 2023i).

A BRP card (GOV.UK, 2023k) is issued to foreign nationals automatically when they apply for a visa or immigration; it holds their biographic details, including name and date and place of birth, as well as biometric information including fingerprints and a digital facial image. It also shows their immigration status and entitlements while they are in the UK. As part of recruitment practice in the NHS, identity checks are used to verify that an individual's identity is genuine.

BRP cards can be used to verify identity and individuals can also sign up to the Home Office's online portal (GOV.UK, 2023l) to view or prove their immigration status and obtain a code to share their right to work with an employer. The code is sent to employers to confirm their immigration status. Further information about the BRP and its application can be found on the gov.uk website (GOV.UK, 2023k).

Further information is also available regarding specific healthcare professionals from overseas, including allied health professionals (AHPs) (NHS, 2023h) such as radiographers, podiatrists, paramedics and physiotherapists; dentists (NHS, 2023i); doctors (NHS, 2023j); healthcare scientists (NHS, 2023k) such as biomedical scientists and audiologists; midwives (NHS, 2023l); nurses (NHS, 2023m); and pharmacists NHS (2023n). International medical graduates or doctors from outside the EEA can apply for and accept employment in training posts that may qualify for sponsorship under a skilled worker visa (GOV.UK, 2023g). Further information regarding these employment opportunities can be found on the NHS Jobs website (NHS Jobs, 2023).

2.2.6 POSTGRADUATE VISA TO WORK IN THE UK AFTER INTERNATIONAL STUDY

International students who have completed a UK bachelor's degree, postgraduate degree or other eligible course can apply for a graduate visa (GOV.UK, 2023m), which gives them time to settle in the UK and find permanent jobs.

2.2.7 APPLYING FROM OVERSEAS TO WORK IN THE UK

The NHS is the largest single employer in the UK; it employs over 1.2 million people, which represents approximately 5% of the UK's working population. The workforce is diverse and multicultural, like the patient population, but more efforts are needed to ensure a diverse workforce at senior levels and initiatives such as this book will contribute to that. Employers are looking beyond the UK and Europe to attract the best talent to the NHS and healthcare workforce and more actions are being taken to increase diversity in senior roles.

Professionally qualified healthcare staff from outside the UK are particularly welcome to apply from overseas through the NHS Jobs website (2023). The main things that applicants need to be aware of are detailed later in this chapter.

The requirements for the role being applied for can be found in the job description (JD) and person specification (PS), which is provided for all jobs advertised on the NHS Jobs website. Individuals need to have the relevant experience and qualifications prior to applying for each job. They must demonstrate clearly in the application form that they meet the essential criteria for the post to be considered for interview. For very popular posts, employers may only consider those applicants who also meet the desired criteria outlined in the PS (NHS Jobs, 2023).

IR of healthcare professionals via NHS Jobs complies with the code of practice for IR, which promotes the best possible standards in IR and discourages any inappropriate practices that could impact on other countries' healthcare systems or the interests of those who apply for posts.

Individuals need to register with the appropriate regulatory body where the post being applied for requires professional registration; some NHS employers may be able to help with this, including in cases where the registration process has already commenced in the individual's home country prior to arriving in the UK. Further information regarding the system for assessing immigration applications to the UK can be found on the Health Careers website (NHS, 2023e).

The right to work in the UK for individuals from outside the UK and Ireland is determined using a points-based immigration system (GOV.UK, 2023f).

Health and social care professionals trained overseas who come to work in the health and social care sector in the UK can apply for health and social care jobs at gov.uk (Department of Health and Social Care, 2023a) (Box 2.1).

For further information on applying for health and social care jobs in the UK, refer to gov.uk (Department of Health and Social Care, 2023a), which provides details on the following:

- Introduction to the health and social care system.
- IR agencies and how to avoid scams.
- Employment offers and contracts.
- Finances and the cost of living in the UK.
- Immigration and regulatory processes.
- Pastoral support, induction and beyond.

BOX 2.1   Moving to the UK From Abroad: Personal Testimony

The author herself moved to the UK from abroad, as an internationally recruited (IR) nurse who was trained in Jamaica. Hence, she is speaking from a personal point of view, reflecting on her learnings and experience in this book. The contents of this book include real situations and examples that helped her to successfully progress to director level as an IR nurse.

- What to do if you think you are being exploited.
- Contract checklist including guidance on repayment clauses.
- Principles around repayment clauses.
- List of professional regulatory bodies.
- List of diaspora associations and support organisations.

(Department of Health and Social Care, 2023a)

2.2.8 LIFE IN THE UK TEST

Once you have settled in the country, you can apply to take the Life in the UK Test as part of your application for British citizenship or settlement in the UK (GOV.UK, 2023a).

2.2.9 BRITISH CITIZENSHIP APPLICATION

As an internationally recruited staff member, you can apply for British citizenship if you have ILR or settled status in the UK (GOV.UK, 2023b).

2.3 Professional Organisations and Healthcare Registration Bodies

Professional organisations and healthcare registration bodies include the NMC and the Health and Care Professions Council (HCPC). There are also trade unions, including the Royal College of Nursing (RCN) and the Royal College of Midwives (RCM), which support and regulate healthcare delivery in the UK, as detailed in the following sections.

2.4 The Nursing and Midwifery Council

NMC registration, competencies, and associated exams and processes, such as the IELTS exam and OSCE, are outlined next, along with NMC revalidation and other elements required for compliance with the NMC code (NMC, 2023c) to ensure safe healthcare practices.

2.5 NMC Exams and Processes: IELTS Exam and OSCE

2.5.1 NMC REGISTRATION

The NMC is the independent regulator for nurses and midwives in the UK, as well as nursing associates in England (NMC, 2023a), ensuring safe, effective and kind nursing and midwifery practice that improves health and wellbeing for all. To enquire or register with the NMC, search the register for more information (NMC, 2023d).

2.5.2 NMC COMPETENCIES

The NMC competencies detail the requirements for nurses, midwives and nursing associates after they qualify, i.e. the standards that they must meet consistently (NMC, 2023e) during their careers. These include competencies for entry onto the register for adult nursing, mental health nursing, learning disabilities nursing and children's nursing. Further information on the NMC competencies can be found by reviewing the standards for competence for registered nurses (NMC, 2023e).

2.5.3 INTERNATIONAL ENGLISH LANGUAGE TESTING SYSTEM

IELTS is an accepted English language test for study, migration or work. Information, processes and other elements required for this exam can be accessed by reviewing the NMC English language requirements (NMC, 2023f).

2.5.4 ACCEPTED ENGLISH LANGUAGE TESTS

For those who require one, it is important to undertake the correct English test to enter the UK and practice as a healthcare professional. The two language tests that are accepted as evidence of staff's ability to communicate effectively in English are the IELTS exam and the Academic and the Occupational English Test (OET). These are reviewed and updated regularly to take account of new legal requirements. The required scores must be achieved in the four areas of reading, writing, listening and speaking, and the test scores are valid for 2 years (NMC, 2023f).

2.5.5 USING SUPPORTING INFORMATION FROM EMPLOYERS

There may be an option to use Supporting Information From Employers (SIFE) from the UK employer to support the application, as supplementary evidence of clinical competence in English in this language domain. This may be possible if the required score is narrowly missed in one language domain (by no more than 0.5 in IELTS or half a grade in OET) and test-combining options are exhausted (if there is an attempt to combine test scores).

To do this, staff must have:

- Worked in the UK with the same employer for least 12 months (or full-time equivalent) at the point of application in a nonregistered role in a health and care setting.
- Had an NMC registrant as their line manager.
- Had the same line manager for at least 6 months (supporting information from up to two NMC-registered line managers covering 12 months or full-time equivalent is accepted).

In this case, the staff member's line manager will be asked to provide information through a link to the NMC website to confirm direct experience of that staff member's English language competence in the missing domain. The line manager should be an Agenda for Change (AfC) NHS Band 6 (or non-NHS equivalent) or above (NHS, 2022i).

This information also needs to be countersigned by an NMC registrant who is at the NHS Band 8a (or non-NHS equivalent) level or above to confirm that the process has been fair and consistent.

Visit the NMC website (NMC, 2023f) for further information on accepted English language tests and the provision of English language evidence (NMC, 2023g).

2.5.6 IELTS ACADEMIC EXAMINATION CERTIFICATE

An IELTS academic examination certificate that confirms that the individual achieved a score of at least 7 for reading, listening and speaking, and of at least 6.5 for writing, is accepted. Both the paper- and computer-based IELTS Academic test, which are completed at a test centre, are accepted.

A range of IELTS preparation resources are available to help staff pass their IELTS exam (IELTS, 2023).

Combining IELTS test scores: individuals can achieve the required mark across two IELTS test sittings if:

- They sit the tests within 12 months of each other.
- They complete all four sections at the same time.
- They achieve a score of at least 7 for reading, listening and speaking, and of at least 6.5 for writing, in at least one of the two test sittings.
- No scores in either of the two test sittings are below 6.5 for listening, reading or speaking, or below 6 for writing.

2.5.7 OET ACADEMIC EXAMINATION CERTIFICATE

An OET examination certificate (OET, 2023a) that confirms that individuals achieved at least a B grade (score of 350 or above) for reading, listening and speaking, and at least a C+ grade (score of 300 or above) for writing, is accepted. Paper, OET on Computer, and the OET Home are all accepted.

Combining OET test scores: individuals can achieve the required mark across two OET test sittings if:

- They sit the tests within 12 months of each other.
- They are tested on all four sections at the same time.
- They achieve at least a grade B (score of 350–440) for reading, listening and speaking, and at least grade C+ (score of 300–340) for writing in at least one of the two test sittings.
- No scores in either of the two test sittings are below grade C+ (score of 300–340) for listening, reading or speaking, or below grade C (score of 250–290) for writing.

Refer to the NMC website (NMC, 2023f) for guidance regarding combining OET and IELTS test scores and review the NMC Test Combining Calculator for more information (NMC, 2023h).

2.5.8 SUBMITTING THE OET CERTIFICATE

If individuals are submitting an OET certificate as part of their application, they will need to give permission for their results to be verified through their 'my OET account'.

Further information on how individuals can grant institutional access to their results is available on the OET website (OET, 2023b).

2.5.9 PREPARING TO TAKE AN ENGLISH LANGUAGE TEST

It is recognised that taking an English language test can cause anxiety. There are various materials that individuals can access and use to prepare for the test, including the test format (OET, 2023c) and sample test questions (OET, 2023d).

Available OET (2023e) preparation materials include study guides, an introduction to nursing medicine and AHP course, general study and learning tips, training videos, and sample listening, speaking, writing and reading tests (NMC, 2023f).

2.5.10 OBJECTIVE STRUCTURED CLINICAL EXAMINATION

The OSCE is the second part of the official practical exam used by the NMC (2023b) to test the competence of nurses and midwives, including clinical and communication skills. Preparation materials for nursing, midwifery, and nursing associates (NMC, 2023i) taking the OSCE are available prior to sitting the exam to support successful completion of both parts thereof before progressing the application for initial registration or readmission to the NMC (2023b) register.

There are five approved OSCE test providers: Oxford Brookes University, the University of Northampton, Ulster University, Northumbria University, and Leeds Teaching Hospitals NHS Trust (NMC, 2023b).

Additional information regarding the OSCE's structure, including assessment, planning, implementation, evaluation and the skills tested; the 10 stations included in the OSCE; the content of the Test of Competence; fees and booking; and the elements associated with taking the OSCE can be found on the NMC (2023b) website under OSCE Test of Competence section, including for nurses and midwives.

The NMC test of competence measures candidates against the current UK preregistration standards for nursing and midwifery. It covers what is done before and on the day of the OSCE and it also provides guidance on the actions to take following receipt of the test results, including appeals and retesting in the event of failure to pass the OSCE (NMC, 2023j).

Further resources and support to ensure success when preparing for the IELTS exam, OET and OSCE are available on the RCN (2023a) website.

This includes information on preparing internationally recruited healthcare staff (IRCS) for successful completion of the IR process, where exam preparation, sitting and progression are key success criteria. Other hints and tips on passing your exam include creating and using a study log and planner.

IR staff contribute significantly to filling the staffing gaps in the healthcare system, which in turn contributes to the delivery of high-quality and safe care across the health and care system.

Support to ensure successful recruitment and retention includes pastoral care and resources for effective onboarding for IR staff covering the following topics:
- Top tips for onboarding new international employees (European Commission, 2023).
- New employees coming to work from abroad (GOV.UK, 2023n).
- The nursing workforce—IR (NHS England, 2023e).

- The Pastoral Care Guide for International Recruitment in Social Care (National Care Forum (NCF), 2023).
- Building understanding of IR through lived experience (Health Education England (HEE), 2023a).

2.5.11 SUPPORT AND RESOURCES IF INDIVIDUALS FAIL THEIR OSCE OR ENGLISH IELTS TEST

It can be disappointing and frustrating to fail to get the desired score on the IELTS exam. There are various resources to support staff to retake and achieve the best result in their IELTS exam, OET and OSCE, including for overseas qualified nurses who want to register with the NMC (RCN, 2023a). Resources and support are also provided by various associations and professional bodies (Box 2.2) and a dedicated IR team and leader in recruiting organisations.

2.5.12 NMC REVALIDATION

NMC revalidation must be undertaken every 3 years by all nurses and midwives in the UK, and by nursing associates in England, to maintain their registration with the NMC. Revalidation includes continued professional development (CPD) and reflection on practice in alignment with the NMC code (NMC, 2021b) (Box 2.3). There are lots of resources (including guidance and information, forms and templates, training materials and films) which can be used to help staff with their NMC revalidation (NMC, 2023k). NMC revalidation promotes effective practice and strengthens public confidence in health and care service delivery from nursing and midwifery professionals (NMC, 2021b). However, revalidation does not include assessment of staff's fitness to practice; instead, revalidation contributes to a culture of sharing, reflection and improvement, benefiting the nurse, midwife or nursing associate and the individuals who are cared for. Staff can access case studies (NMC, 2023l) and stories on the NMC website from other staff regarding how they found undertaking the NMC revalidation process. The NMC revalidation requirements (NMC, 2023m) exist so staff can demonstrate that they are keeping their skills and knowledge up to date and maintaining safe and effective practice. They include the submission of practice hours; hours of CPD and participatory learning; five pieces of practice-related feedback; five written reflective accounts; reflective discussion; a health and character declaration; and a professional indemnity arrangement and confirmation.

BOX 2.2   **IELTS Exam and OSCE: Personal Testimony**

I found the NMC and RCN resources to be very helpful, and they have been a great source of support and guidance to help me achieve my dream of working as a nurse in the UK after passing my IELTS exam and OSCE. I am really grateful to all colleagues who have contributed to providing these resources to assist me in my journey. I strongly recommend the NMC and RCN resources for the IELTS exam and OSCE for all nurses, midwives and other staff who wish to work in the UK.

An IR registered nurse

BOX 2.3	**NMC Revalidation**

NMC revalidation (2023l) is an important part of the NMC code (NMC, 2023c) and standards, ensuring nurses and midwives remain up to date and fit for practice throughout their careers. It strengthens professionalism through ongoing reflection on the NMC code (NMC, 2023o), with feedback provided by colleagues and services users, and it encourages best practice and guards against isolation.

Important parts of the NMC code (NMC, 2023c) and standards focus on areas including:

Compassionate care: kindness, respect and compassion.

Team work: working cooperatively.

Record keeping: six clear standards to support all record keeping.

Delegation and accountability: delegate responsibilities, be accountable.

Raising concerns: this aligns the NMC code with the raising concerns guidance (NMC, 2023c):

Cooperation with investigations and audits: includes investigations and audits of individuals or organisations and acting as a witness at hearings.

The Code also covers:

Duty of candour

Social media

Fundamentals of care

Medicines management and prescribing

Conscientious objection

End of life care

(NMC, 2023c)

Further information on the NMC revalidation process can be found on the NMC website (NMC, 2021b), including application submission, creating an online NMC account, and support with revalidation such as extensions.

There is also a guidance sheet with information regarding how the NMC supports and helps staff revalidate (NMC, 2023n), including how to apply for this support. Finally, there are various additional resources to help nursing and midwifery professionals (NMC, 2021b) get the best from the NMC revalidation process, including resources and templates (NMC, 2023k) that can be downloaded.

2.5.13 ENABLING PROFESSIONALISM

Enabling professionalism, as defined by the NMC code (NMC, 2023o), and supporting professional standards of practice and behaviour for nurses and midwives encompasses:

- Accountability to practice effectively: problem solving and challenging practice; reflective and evidenced based
- Leadership to promote professionalism and trust: be autonomous, delegate and coordinate, be honest, innovative and demonstrate systems thinking
- Advocate for and prioritise people: be emotionally competent, resilient, impartial and compassionate
- Competence to help people: demonstrate technical competence, critical thinking and inquisitiveness

(NMC, 2023o)

2.6 Health and Care Professions Council

The HCPC is a regulator of health and care professions in the UK, with the role of protecting the public and ensuring that, by law, people in this professional group are registered to work in the UK. The HCPC works with other UK health regulators to share best practice in areas including HR, education and equality (HCPC, 2023).

2.7 The General Medical Council

The General Medical Council (GMC) regulates healthcare in the UK (GMC, 2023). The GMC website includes information on checking a doctor's registration status; information for doctors such as becoming a doctor in the UK, professional standards and revalidation; and information for patients such as who the GMC are and what they do, what patients should expect from their doctor and how to raise a concern about their doctor (GMC, 2023).

2.8 Trade Unions

Formally recognised trade unions that support nursing, midwifery and other healthcare staff are detailed in the following sections.

2.8.1 ROYAL COLLEGE OF NURSING

The RCN is the largest nursing union in the UK and it aims to represent, educate and protect nurses through committee meetings, online training, forums, conferences, networks and the RCN congress (Box 2.4). Further information, including on how to join the RCN, can be found on the RCN (2023b) website.

2.8.2 THE RCN EXECUTIVE NURSE NETWORK

The RCN Executive Nurse Network offers opportunities to extend professional networking and get involved in the work of the RCN and other healthcare- and staff-related matters. This network enables staff to share existing working practices, learn from each other and develop new ways of working (RCN, 2023c).

2.8.3 ROYAL COLLEGE OF MIDWIVES

The RCM is the only professional organisation and trade union dedicated to serving midwifery, with the mission of promoting the voice of midwives. The union is dedicated

BOX 2.4	Trade Union: Personal Testimony

I was introduced to the RCN very early, when I first started working in the UK health and care system. This helped me to build confidence, and I went on to become an accredited RCN representative and RCN board member where I support others to thrive in the workplace.

Deputy director

to serving the whole midwifery team. Further information, including on how to join the RCM, can be found on the RCM website (RCM, 2023).

2.8.4 FURTHER INFORMATION ON OTHER TRADE UNIONS

- The British Medical Association (BMA) (2023) is the trade union and professional body for doctors and medical students in the UK.
- UNISON (2023) is among the largest trade unions in the UK, representing staff who provide public services in the public and private sectors.
- Unite The Union (2023) is dedicated to serving the best interests of its members, protecting workers' rights and promoting equality and diversity in the workplace.
- Managers in Partnership (MIP) (2023) is the specialist union for health and social care managers.
- The Public and Commercial Services (PCS) Union (2023) provides staff with security at work.
- The British Dental Association (BDA) Trade Union (2023) is the voice of dentists and dental students in the UK, supporting members through education, advice, *British Dental Journal* (BDJ) publications and campaigning.

This group of trade unions work together to form a partnership forum of trade unions and support staff across all professional groups, although different unions represent different staff groups. They represent staff across the different professions and pay bands in NHS England, although not all staff are members of trade unions.

2.8.5 FACULTY OF PUBLIC HEALTH

The Faculty of Public Health (FPH) is the professional home for public health in the UK and abroad, with a growing and engaged membership forming part of its community. The FPH supports over 5000 members across all career stages, enabling them to drive the profession forward and achieve our vision of improving public health (FPH, 2023) including through professional development, education, policy, advocacy and special interest groups.

2.9 Summary: Preparing Internationally Recruited Staff for Successful Completion of the International Recruitment Process

This chapter covered how to enter the UK healthcare system from abroad, NMC registration, competencies, exams such as the IELTS exam and OSCE, NMC revalidation and other elements that are required for compliance with the NMC code of practice. Professional organisations, healthcare registration bodies (NMC, HCPC and GMC) and trade unions (RCN, RCM and BMA) ensure standards are maintained to provide the best care possible.

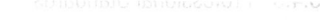

CHAPTER 3

Basic Guide to the National Health Service Structures

3.1 Introduction

This chapter includes an introduction to the National Health Service (NHS), a basic guide to the NHS structures and healthcare organisations in the United Kingdom (UK) and insights into the organisation and regulation of healthcare. It also includes information on healthcare and service delivery, nursing and other healthcare processes and models of nursing.

3.2 An Introduction to the NHS

The NHS is a complex system that can be difficult to understand, particularly in terms of determining who is responsible for what (NHS England (NHSE), 2023b). It includes an extensive number of different organisations with different roles, responsibilities and specialities. These organisations deliver various services that support patients, carers and other service users. In recent years the NHS structures and way of working have experienced ongoing change, although some of this change may not be noticeable as it may not affect access to local doctor or hospital services. However, the changes affect health service decision makers and budget holders (NHSE, 2023b). Further information regarding the NHS structure in England, including who does what, can be found on the NHS website (NHSE, 2023f). The King's Fund (2021) has produced a structure diagram providing information about the NHS.

3.2.1 A BASIC GUIDE TO THE NHS STRUCTURES

The King's Fund (2021) provides information on a basic guide to the structures, including the government, treasury, Department of Health and Social Care, NHS England, the CQC, integrated care system (ICS), providers of services, other regulators and commissioners of care.

3.3 Healthcare Organisations in the UK

Organisational insights into health and care institutions in the UK, including their roles and duties, can be found by visiting the websites of the following organisations.

In 2023, Public Health England (PHE), Health Education England (HEE) and NHS Digital merged to form a single organisation, NHS England (NHSE, 2023f).

3.4 Organisation and Regulation of Healthcare

The organisation and regulation of healthcare in the UK involves many regulatory and professional bodies, as well as policy, strategy and legislative bodies. Information on organisations that regulate healthcare in the UK, including professional and regulatory bodies, can be accessed as outlined below.

3.4.1 THE HEALTH AND CARE ACT 2022

The Health and Care Act 2022, as newly updated legislation, is explained by the King's Fund, which provides information to help staff make sense of the Health and Care Act. The King's Fund also provides information on other key factors and challenges related to health and care in the UK (King's Fund, 2023c).

3.4.2 CARE REGULATIONS AND STANDARDS

Carers UK provides information on care regulations and care standards nationwide, including help and advice, getting involved, news and campaigns, policy and research, information for professionals and how the Care Quality Commission (CQC) regulates and monitors care standards (Carers UK, 2023, and Care Quality Commission (CQC), (2023)).

3.4.3 THE HEALTH FOUNDATION

The Health Foundation believes good health and healthcare are important in ensuring the population thrives and it supports assessment of the impact of regulation on NHS organisations (Health Foundation, 2023). The Health Foundation explores the strengths and weaknesses of the approaches to regulation in the NHS and compares the approaches taken in healthcare with those of other high-risk industries. The Health Foundation examines the relationship between regulators and the services they regulated in the NHS and assesses the impact of regulation services on the regulated services in safety-critical industries (Health Foundation, 2023).

3.4.4 NHS ENGLAND

NHSE provides oversight and regulation of the NHS through a mix of external control, self-regulation and varying forms of agency, using new regulatory techniques and instruments including risk-based profiling, national quality standards and outcome indicators to measure improvements in patient safety, organisational activity and performance and patient outcomes (NHSE, 2023f). Effective regulation is one of the foundations of high-quality, safe patient care, and significant emphasis is placed on the measurement of quality and safety via inspections by the CQC (NHSE, 2023f).

3.4.5 MEDICINES AND HEALTHCARE PRODUCTS REGULATORY AGENCY

The Medicines and Healthcare Products Regulatory Agency (MHRA) regulates medicines, medical devices and blood components for transfusion in the UK, providing information on:

- The MHRA itself
- All MHRA services
- Alerts, recalls and safety: medicines and medical devices
- Drug safety updates
- The Yellow Card Scheme (reporting a problem with a medicine or medical device)
- Marketing authorisations and licensing guidance
- Medicines
- Medical devices (regulation and safety)
- Latest guidelines for patients
- Coronavirus disease 2019 (COVID-19) (GOV.UK, 2023o)

3.4.6 HUMAN FERTILISATION AND EMBRYOLOGY AUTHORITY

The Human Fertilisation and Embryology Authority (HFEA) oversees the use of gametes and embryos in fertility treatment and research (HFEA, 2023), providing information about in vitro fertilisation (IVF) clinics and other fertility treatments from the UK government fertility regulator.

3.4.7 CARE QUALITY COMMISSION

The CQC regulates all health and social care services in England and oversees a register of health and care organisations and professionals requiring regulation according to parliamentary legislation (CQC, 2023).

3.4.8 HEALTH AND SAFETY EXECUTIVE

The Health and Safety Executive (HSE) is the national independent regulator of health and safety in the workplace, including in private and publicly owned health and social care settings in Great Britain. The HSE works in partnership with coregulators in local authorities to inspect, investigate and, where necessary, take enforcement action (HSE, 2023).

3.4.9 PROFESSIONAL STANDARDS AUTHORITY

The Professional Standards Authority (PSA) protects the public by overseeing the regulation and registration of healthcare professionals, i.e. by improving the regulation and registration of people who work in health and social care. The PSA sets standards for organisations holding voluntary registers of people working in unregulated health and care occupations and accredits those organisations (PSA, 2023).

3.5 Models of Healthcare Service in the UK

Models of healthcare service in the UK can be summarised as follows: providing care, commissioning care, improving public health (PH), empowering people and local communities, supporting the health and care system, providing education and training and safeguarding parents' interest. Fig. 3.1 (Department of Health, 2013) provides a guide to the Healthcare System in England, including a guide for NHS Accountability of healthcare for England.

3.5.1 HOW DOES THE NHS WORK?

It is important to understand the way the NHS works (King's Fund, 2023f) to be able to navigate its processes and functions. An understanding of the key organisations that make up the NHS and how they collaborate with partners in the health and care system to deliver joined-up care can be obtained via some key resources that help make sense of the reformed health and care system. These include:

- Integrated care systems (ICSs) and how they work under the Health and Care Act are explained in the videos, diagrams and figures by The King's Fund (2023g).
- The Health and Care Act: six key questions (explainer) (King's Fund, 2023h).

3.5.2 HEALTHCARE IN THE UK: A GUIDE TO THE NHS

A guide to healthcare in the NHS in the UK (NHS, 2023o) is detailed in the following sections. This explains how the healthcare system in the UK works, including how to access doctors, dentists, emergency services and more, this is useful information for new individuals entering the UK (Buswell, 2023). Individuals who are permanently living in the UK will be entitled to free healthcare through the NHS (2023o). However, there is also the option to take out private health insurance in the UK, which can offer quicker access to specialists, better facilities and shorter waiting times (Buswell, 2023). An introduction to the UK, understanding how the government works and the languages used in the UK, and knowing about people and society, the cost of living, housing, food and transport are all important to settle in the country. The following sections provide a guide to healthcare in the UK (Buswell, 2023) to help new staff settle in their new environment.

3.5.3 THE UK HEALTHCARE SYSTEM

An overview of healthcare in the UK is provided here. The NHS (2023o) is a free, publicly funded healthcare system funded by taxpayers rather than health insurance. There is also a private healthcare sector in which services can be paid for based on personal choice.

Each country in the UK has its own NHS body, but the information provided here focuses on NHSE (2023f). More information about health services in other UK countries can be found in Section 3.0 of the websites for NHS Scotland (2023), NHS Wales (2023) and NHS Northern Ireland (2023). The differences between these four healthcare systems mainly relate to structure and service delivery.

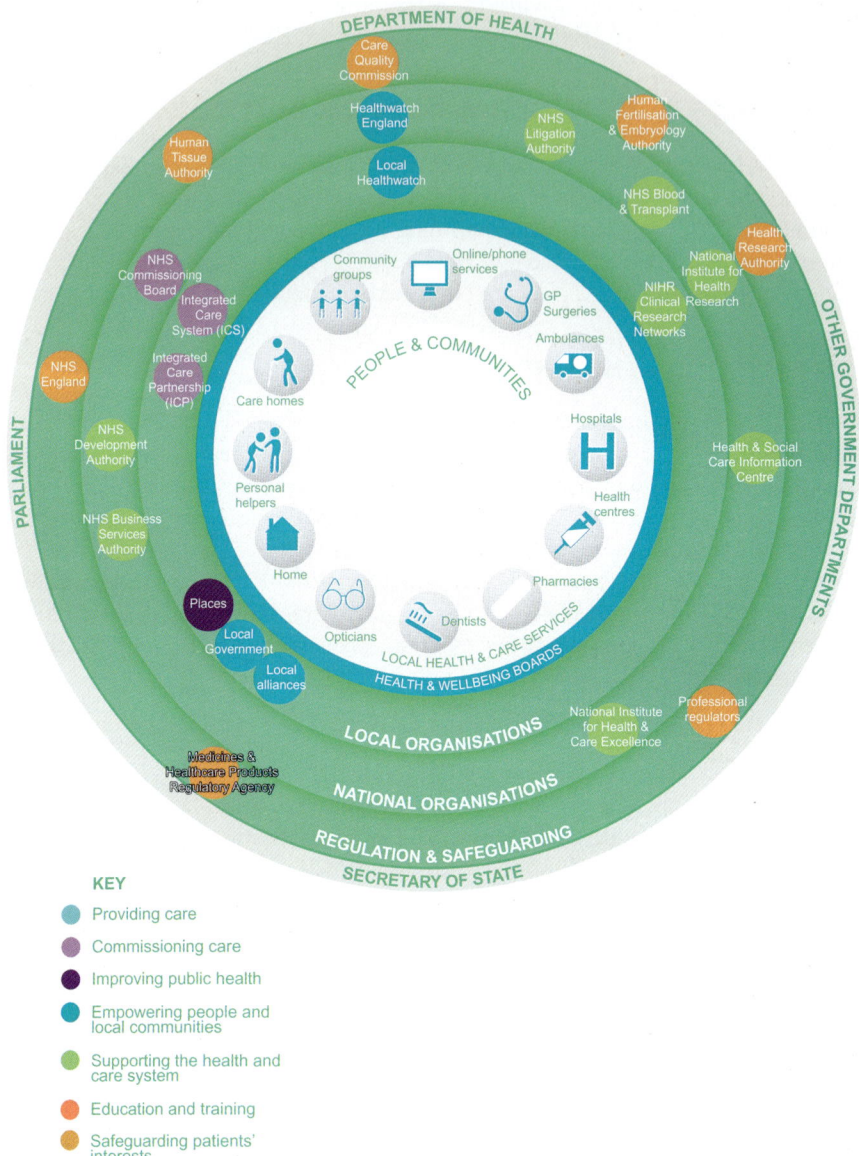

Fig. 3.1 The healthcare system in England from April 2013. (With permission from Department of Health (2013). *The health and care system explained. Department of Health.* https://www.gov.uk/government/publications/the-health-and-care-system-explained/the-health-and-care-system-explained.)

The NHS in England is overseen by the Department of Health and Social Care (GOV.UK, 2023t). NHSE is responsible for commissioning primary care service providers such as doctors, dentists and pharmacists, in addition to key specialised services.

3.5.4 INTEGRATED CARE SYSTEMS

ICSs were established in July 2022. These geographically based partnerships bring together providers and commissioners of NHS services with local authorities and other local partners to plan, coordinate, commission and deliver health and care services (King's Fund, 2023d). ICSs have the responsibility for commissioning secondary care services in local areas, including planned hospital care, rehabilitative care, urgent and emergency care, most community health services, and mental health (MH) and learning disability services. ICSs aim to improve the lives of people who live and work in their area (NHSE, 2023d).

3.5.5 ACCESS TO HEALTHCARE IN THE UK

The NHS is a residence-based rather than an insurance-based system, meaning that all UK residents including newly arriving international individuals can access services for free. Third-country nationals may be required to pay a surcharge but can access NHS services on the same basis as others. Some countries have a reciprocal healthcare agreement with the UK and some individuals may qualify for an exemption (NHS, 2023p).

3.5.6 HEALTHCARE COSTS IN THE UK

NHS healthcare is funded mainly by taxation and most services are delivered free at the point of care to residents. However, some services such as dental treatment (NHS, 2023q) and prescriptions (NHS, 2023r) are chargeable, and the prices change yearly. Some residents, including low earners, those aged over 60 years and children, are exempt from payment or benefit from reduced NHS charges.

3.5.7 REGISTERING FOR HEALTHCARE ON ENTRY TO THE UK

Residents register for healthcare in the UK by registering with a general practitioner (GP) within the local area. GPs accept patients who are from the local population they cover, providing they are not at full capacity. The General Medical Services (GMS) GMS1 form (NHS, 2023s) is completed to register with a GP. The 'GMS1: user guide for GP practices' (NHS, 2023b) document is available to help GP practices explain the form to patients. The form can be printed, filled in and returned to the chosen GP to register. Proof of identify is needed to register, requiring a valid form of identification (ID) such as a passport as well as proof of address such as a UK utility bill (e.g. council tax letter). Once registered, a medical card will be issued, which can be used to record appointments (NHS, 2023b).

3.5.8 DOCTORS AND SPECIALISTS IN THE UK

Local GPs are the first point of contact for routine medical queries, but not for emergencies, providing assessments and advice for general illnesses and complaints, prescriptions for medications and referrals to a specialist if necessary. GP surgeries operate by appointment booking, and some may also offer a 'walk-in' service for a few hours in the morning or evening. Some surgeries now offer an online booking service and GPs mainly open between Monday and Friday. For emergencies and out-of-hours care, individuals should attend the accident and emergency (A&E) department or an urgent care centre, or alternatively call an out-of-hours number or use the 111 service (NHS, 2023t) for urgent but nonemergency advice.

3.5.9 PRIVATE HEALTHCARE IN THE UK

A smaller proportion of UK residents (approximately 10.5% of the population) choose to pay for private health insurance compared with other European countries. Private health insurance has various benefits including in cases of an urgent illness or injury, as private patients can access specialists' services more quickly, avoid long waits and access additional environmental facilities such as private en-suite rooms (rather than sharing wards with other patients). There are several payment arrangements for private healthcare, including on an individual or family basis, depending on the level of cover required to suit the patients' lifestyle, age and preexisting medical conditions. However, private healthcare can come with significant cost.

3.5.10 WOMEN'S HEALTHCARE IN THE UK

A range of women's healthcare services is provided by the NHS and wider healthcare services. Some of these services, which can be accessed through GPs or well woman clinics (NHS, 2023u), include access to gynaecology services, access to free sexual health services, free contraception, maternity care services, IVF treatment for women under 40 years of age who meet certain criteria and screening programmes for cervical and breast cancer, among many other services including abortion services. Abortion is legal in most parts of the UK if it is carried out within the first 24 weeks of pregnancy. Further information on childbirth and maternity, including on care choices and personalised care in maternity services, is available on the NHS (2023v) website.

3.5.11 CHILDREN'S HEALTHCARE IN THE UK

The NHS works with the local authority and numerous specialist agencies to deliver children's services aimed at improving children's health. Paediatricians and paediatric services can be accessed through the NHS (2023w) website. Children should also be registered with the family's GP to access their children's healthcare services as needed. More information on children's health (NHS, 2022n) and children and young people (CYP) (NHS, 2022o) is available at the NHS website (2023w).

Community healthcare services for families and children are available through local children's centres (GOV.UK, 2023p), including Sure Start centres; these provide help and advice on child and family health, parenting, money, training and employment. Early learning and daycare are also provided for preschool children at some centres.

Nurses and other children's healthcare professionals in the NHS and wider healthcare service offer care and advice, including on nutrition, healthy weight and breastfeeding. Programmes regarding healthy eating, physical activity and mental well-being are delivered through schools, such as 'Mytime Active' (Mytime Active, 2023) programmes.

A free vaccination programme is available for children in the UK, including vaccines against diphtheria, tetanus, whooping cough, polio, hepatitis B and *Haemophilus influenzae* type B; the measles, mumps and rubella (MMR) vaccine; children's flu vaccine; and, more recently, the COVID-19 vaccine for certain age groups (NHS, 2023x).

3.5.12 DENTISTS IN THE UK

Dental care is a paid service available through both the NHS and private healthcare, but it is free for those aged under 18 years (or under 19 years if in full-time education), pregnant women and those who have given birth in the last 12 months. The amount paid for dental care depends on the band of care required and the type of dental treatment, such as examinations, scale and polish (first band); fillings, root canal work and removal of teeth (second band); and crowns, dentures, bridges and lab work (third band). There is also an NHS Emergency Dentist (NHS, 2023y) covering treatments such as pain relief or temporary fillings in England (2023f). The prices for NHS dental care are different across the four UK nations and full details are available in the NHS Scotland (2023), NHS Wales (2023) and NHS Northern Ireland (2023) websites.

3.5.13 HOSPITALS IN THE UK

Hospitals provide secondary care services in the UK and a GP referral is needed for all treatments except emergency treatment, where individuals should attend the A&E department. In the UK, there are both NHS hospitals run by NHS Trusts (government funded) and independent hospitals run by private companies or charities, for which a charge is usually made. Most NHS general hospitals offer A&E, maternity, surgery, elderly care and outpatient services. Additionally, specialist hospitals such as eye hospitals and orthopaedic hospitals are available to the public. The NHS provider directory (NHSE, 2023k) gives an overview of each NHS trust and foundation trust, with information provided on regulatory action, corporate publications and contact details.

3.5.14 HEALTH CENTRES, HEALTH CLINICS AND URGENT TREATMENT CENTRES IN THE UK

There are numerous NHS walk-in centres and urgent treatment centres (UTCs) (NHS, 2023z) providing healthcare in the UK all year round, including outside office hours. Walk-in health centres can deal with a range of minor injuries and illnesses, with some centres offering access to doctors and nurses providing a limited list of services such as treating infections/rashes, fractures, minor cuts (via stitching and dressing), burns and bruises and vomiting and diarrhoea. They also provide GP, dental, pharmacy, urgent care, MH, hospital, sight test, sexual health and pregnancy services, among other NHS services (NHSE, 2023l).

3.5.15 PHARMACIES IN THE UK

Local pharmacies in the UK can be found in town centres, next to GP practices, in large retail stores such as Boots and in supermarkets such as Tesco, among other local areas. Certain types of medicine require a GP prescription, which can then be filled at the pharmacy. The payment of a standard charge per prescription item is required in England unless there is an exemption (NHSE, 2023m).

3.5.16 MENTAL HEALTHCARE IN THE UK

There is a significant commitment to delivering high-level MH (NHSE, 2023n) services in the UK, which can be accessed free of charge via the NHS to support adults and children who experience mental illness. Individuals can be referred by a GP and people can also refer themselves to a mental healthcare service; these include psychological therapy, counselling services, drug and alcohol services, children's MH services and eating disorder services (NHSE, 2023n).

3.5.17 ALTERNATIVE THERAPIES AND OTHER FORMS OF HEALTHCARE IN THE UK

There are limited alternative therapies provided through the NHS, but they are accessible across the UK, including osteopathy, chiropractic treatment, acupuncture, reiki and herbal medicine. Therapists should be registered with regulatory bodies such as the Federation of Holistic Therapists (FHT) (2023).

3.5.18 HEALTHCARE CHARITIES

Many charities also deliver healthcare in the UK, with some being commissioned and others being part-funded by the NHS (Charity Choice, 2023).

3.5.19 WHAT TO DO IN AN EMERGENCY

Emergency services are free of charge in the UK and can be accessed by calling 999 (NHS, 2023bb) and having an ambulance sent where required. Alternatively, where possible and appropriate, the A&E department at the nearest hospital, which is open 24 hours per day, can be visited. Where required, individuals may be admitted to an NHS hospital and placed on a ward where other people with similar illnesses are treated, such as a surgical or medical ward.

3.6 Nursing and Other Healthcare Processes

3.6.1 THE NURSING PROCESS

There are many components of the nursing process, including assessment, diagnosis, planning, implementation and evaluation (Hector, 2009). This five-step process is used by nurses to provide proper, standardised care to patients (Indeed, 2022b), forming the foundational principles which healthcare staff should follow throughout their careers in hospitals, nursing homes or other clinical settings. The purposes of the nursing process include assessment of the client's health status and healthcare problems or needs, establishing plans and implementing nursing interventions to meet the identified needs,

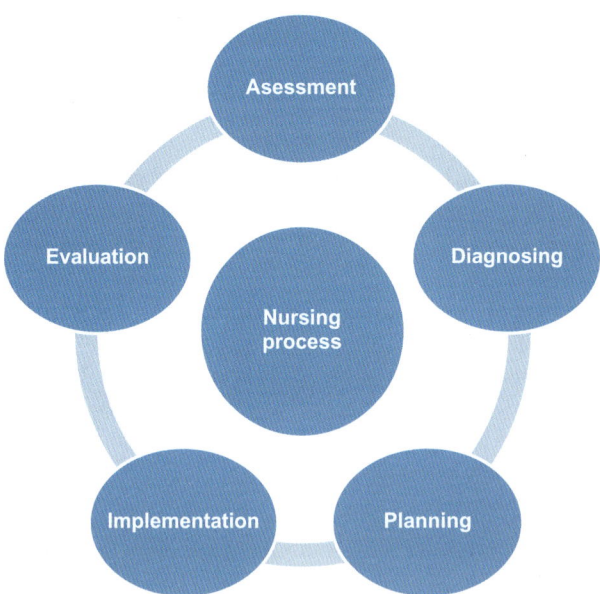

Fig. 3.2   The nursing process. (Reproduced with permission from Stellenbosch University. From Hector, DS. (2009). *A retrospective analysis of nursing documentation in the intensive care units of an academic hospital in the Western Cape.*)

applying the best available caregiving evidence, and promote human functions and responses to health and illness (Parandeh et al., 2016).

The nursing process (Fig. 3.2) is also designed to protect nurses against legal problems related to nursing care, provided the standards of the process are followed correctly, and to help nurses practice in a systematically and organised way. A database covering the client's health status, health concerns, response to illness and ability to manage health-care needs should also be established (Wayne, 2023). The nursing process promotes a unique, patient-centred, interpersonal approach. It emphasises collaborative working among interprofessional teams, promoting open communication, mutual respect and shared decision-making to achieve quality patient care. It is a dynamic, cyclical process in which each phase interacts with and is influenced by the other phases. It also enables nurses to engage in critical thinking, which is a vital nursing skill for identifying patient problems and implementing interventions to ensure effective care outcomes (Wayne, 2023).

3.6.2 OTHER HEALTHCARE PROCESSES

Healthcare processes relating to allied health professionals (AHPs), midwifery, perinatal care, healthcare assistants (HCAs) and other healthcare staff are detailed later.

3.6.3 WORKING IN MULTIPROFESSIONAL TEAMS IN THE HEALTH AND CARE SETTING

Multiprofessional teamworking and multiagency teams are important to the future of healthcare and general practice, especially with the national and regional integration of ICSs and primary care networks (PCNs) (as described in the section on PCNs). These groups of practices in England work together to focus on local patient care, with primary care nurse clinical directors providing system leadership in areas including acute care, MH, learning disabilities and autism (LDA) and community care. New roles and models of care are being introduced, creating multidisciplinary environments. Ensuring these teams function effectively is a complex task (King's Fund, 2023b). The clinical director in a PCN is responsible for providing leadership to improve quality in the delivery of services (Royal College of Nursing, 2023k). Further information about team working is found in Section 5.3 on professional leadership in healthcare.

3.6.4 DAILY AND LONGER-TERM CHALLENGES IN HEALTHCARE

There are major challenges facing the healthcare system (Siwicki, 2020), particularly given the impact of the pandemic, which can be addressed by expanding the workforce, joining up virtual and in-person care and embedding the use of new digital health tools. The updated NHS Long Term Plan (LTP) (NHSE, 2022a) and NHS Operating Plan (NHSE, 2022e) include contents to help the NHS recover and progress through the postpandemic period over the next 10 years. This follows on from the previous NHS Five Year Forward View (NHSE, 2023aa), with goals including making sure everyone gets the best start in life, delivering world-class care for major health problems and supporting all to age well.

3.7 Models of Nursing Care Delivery in the UK

There are many different models of nursing care delivery in the UK and priorities for their development are detailed in the following sections. The four main types of nursing in the UK are MH, LDA, adult and children's nursing, which are further classified into specialities as detailed in the following sections. There are also nursing associate (NA) roles (NHSE, 2023bb).

3.7.1 LEARNING DISABILITIES AND AUTISM, MENTAL HEALTH AND SPECIAL EDUCATIONAL NEEDS OR DISABILITY NURSES

Priorities for MH, LDA and special educational needs or disability (SEND) nurses include career development, supervision and physical health training. The Learning Disability in the Long-Term Plan (NHSE, 2024) is designed to support people with learning disabilities. This includes improving the learning disability standards of NHS trusts (NHSE, 2024) in relation to all services, including specialist services; providing advice to staff and managers; being advocates for service users and families; and compliance with the British Institute of Human Rights (BIHR), the UK Health Security Agency (UKHSA) (previously PHE), NHSE and CQC quality teams in assessing treatment. The learning disability standards cover human rights, the inclusion of all people, staff knowledge and hospital and community services pertinent to learning disability. Metrics and questions for managers and staff are used to monitor learning disability improvement standards in NHS trusts (NHSE, 2024). The standards also provide guidance on preserving the quality of life of people with learning disability, including by using tool kits and working with aspects of the wider system in alignment with the CQC Key Lines of Enquiry (KLOE). This also aligns with the contracting, commission and benchmarking of services to ensure exemplary practice based on the learning disability improvement standards for NHS trusts (NHSE, 2024).

3.7.2 CARE HOME NURSES

Training, learning and understanding language and health and care values is especially important for staff working in care homes, including nurses from abroad, to help familiarise them with systems and processes.

3.7.3 INDEPENDENT SECTOR AND SOCIAL ENTERPRISE

Care delivery in the independent sector and social enterprise should be aligned with NHS standards, practices, values, shared learning and the voice of nursing.

3.7.4 PRIMARY CARE NETWORKS, COMMUNITY NURSING, DISTRICT NURSING, GENERAL PRACTICE NURSING AND SCHOOL NURSING

These are supported by the general practice nursing (GPN) 10-point plan (NHS) and the community nursing and LTP support 'ageing well' and personalised care (NHS).

3.7.4.1 Primary Care Networks

PCNs are key to the future of general practice, community services and social services. PCNS focus on prevention and self-care and involve extended community teams focusing on diabetes, frailty, dermatology, respiratory care, musculoskeletal (MSK) physiotherapy, pain management, paediatrics, bladder and bowel services, neurology, tissue viability and skin care and prison health services. Members of the practice teams include clinical pharmacists, MH therapists, community nurses, social prescribers and physiotherapists. Moreover, an anticipatory and urgent care team, discharge planning, infection prevention and control (IPC) and safeguarding help the wider primary care team including in terms of community pharmacy, dentistry, ophthalmology, podiatry, speech and language therapy (SALT), CYP, APHs and the wider voluntary sector (GPN 10-point plan programme (NHSE, 2019a, 2019b)).

3.7.4.2 Primary Care

The NHS Leadership Academy works collaboratively with a range of primary care stakeholders, nationally and within regions, including primary care training hubs, PCNs, practice managers and other systems leaders within ICSs. The NHS Leadership Academy offers world-leading practical, targeted, locally available and accessible leadership development for everyone working in primary care (NHS Leadership Academy, 2023m).

An ambitious plan is to transform primary care within a generation, offering patients with diverse needs a wider choice of personalised, digital-first health services than ever before with support from the NHS LTP. This encompasses general practice, district nursing (DN), dentistry pharmacists talking to patients undergoing eye examinations, eye health, nurses, PCNs and doctors in surgery rooms (NHSE, 2023x).

3.7.4.3 Community Services

The National Community Nursing Plan 2021–2026 engagement document sets out how community nursing can be enhanced to deliver high-quality care to the population, including through integrated and reablement care delivery. Community teams deliver preventative community programmes to help with issues such as frailty (Box 3.1), working with PCNs and multidisciplinary teams (MDTs) to improve the healthcare outcomes of the population (NHS, 2022a).

The LTP integrated care commitments include assessing the risk of poor health outcomes in the local population, working with community services to support people and supporting care home residents including by providing enhanced healthcare in care homes (EHCH) (NHSE, 2022a).

3.7.5 ENHANCED HEALTHCARE IN CARE HOMES

This model helps to reduce variation in the access to healthcare and ensure that all care home residents receive holistic and integrated care (Box 3.2). This involves the delivery of enhanced primary and specialist support through regular reviews of residents by MDTs, aligning with rehabilitation services including out-of-hours support and end-of-life care.

3.7.6 URGENT COMMUNITY RESPONSE

Urgent community response (UCR) increases the capacity and responsiveness of community services, allowing the early identification of people with urgent needs and the

---

BOX 3.1   Community Services: Case Study

Cambridgeshire Community Services NHS Trust used a model to identify over 800 people with high healthcare needs relating to the frailty, who were then supported by MDTs thereby reducing acute hospital usage among the population by 15%.
Community Nursing Plan (NHS, 2022a) and the Long-Term Plan (NHS England, 2022a)

BOX 3.2   Enhanced Healthcare: Case Study

The Wakefield EHCH programme achieved a reduction in ambulance calls from care homes due to falls by 27% and a reduction in hospital stays (in bed days) of 28%.
Community Nursing Plan (NHS, 2022a) and the Long-Term Plan (NHS England 2022a)

BOX 3.3   **Integrated Care: Case Study**

For people over the age of 65 years, the Dorset integrated care system, involving health and social care partners, reduced the number of unplanned hospital admissions for trauma and orthopaedic surgery by about 17% over a 2-year period.
Community Nursing Plan (NHS, 2022a) and the Long-Term Plan (NHS England, 2022a)

BOX 3.4   **Comprehensive Community Programme: Case Study**

The author of this book was a regional director of nursing who led a comprehensive community programme. This involved leadership of the community team, designing the right structure, recruiting the team, supporting programme delivery across accelerator sites and supporting cross regional and system-wide programme delivery.
Director of Nursing

---

provision of timely care (in line with the community health services' 2-hour standard UCR time) through recovery and rehabilitation services (Box 3.3; NHS England, 2022n).

3.7.7 NURSING DIRECTORS LEADING COMMUNITY PROGRAMMES

Effective leadership of community teams by nursing leaders (Box 3.4), commissioners and directors is key to changing perceptions of the community services detailed in the NHS LTP, moving from task-oriented care to person-centred and holistic care (NHS, 2022f).

3.7.8 GENERAL PRACTICE NURSING

The GPN 10-point plan (NHSE, 2019a) is key in primary nursing care delivery. It includes: (1) GPN leadership development, educator networks, conferences and nurses voice networks; (2) student ambassadors and hubs for placements; (3) an induction template and preceptorship–Queen's Nursing Institute (QNI); (4) return to practice; (5) integration of other PH programmes and a single information hub for GPN/healthcare support workers (HCSWs), GPN digital ambassadors and clinical protocols; (6) a GPN education programme; (7) advanced nurse practitioner (ANP)/advanced clinical practitioner (ACP) competencies for GPN, including capital nurses; (8) a GPN apprenticeship scheme and conferences for NAs, new GPNs and HCAs; (9) a GPN bank, digital supervision, a supervision model and collaboration with NHS jobs; and (10) national GPN workforce engagement, a workforce online tool kit for the online workforce and workforce demographics and planning. This ensures that there are ongoing efforts to grow the GPN workforce, with a focus on the competencies underpinning this nursing role that are required to deliver on population health through integrated care (NHSE, 2019a, 2019b).

3.7.8.1 General Practice Nursing Induction Template

This GPN induction template (NHSE, 2018) promotes a consistent and comprehensive system, ensuring that all newly qualified GPNs who are new to primary care and general practice are provided with the right induction support. It covers key areas including an introduction to, and the aims and objectives of, GPN; a glossary of terms; information on GPN; orientation; information about employers; and education and resources (NHSE, 2018).

3.7.8.2 General Practice Nurses

General practice nurses work as part of an MDT within GP surgeries and assess, screen and treat patients across the lifespan, as detailed in Fig. 3.3. This includes a patient-focused approach, management, collaboration, education, knowledge, skills and leadership.

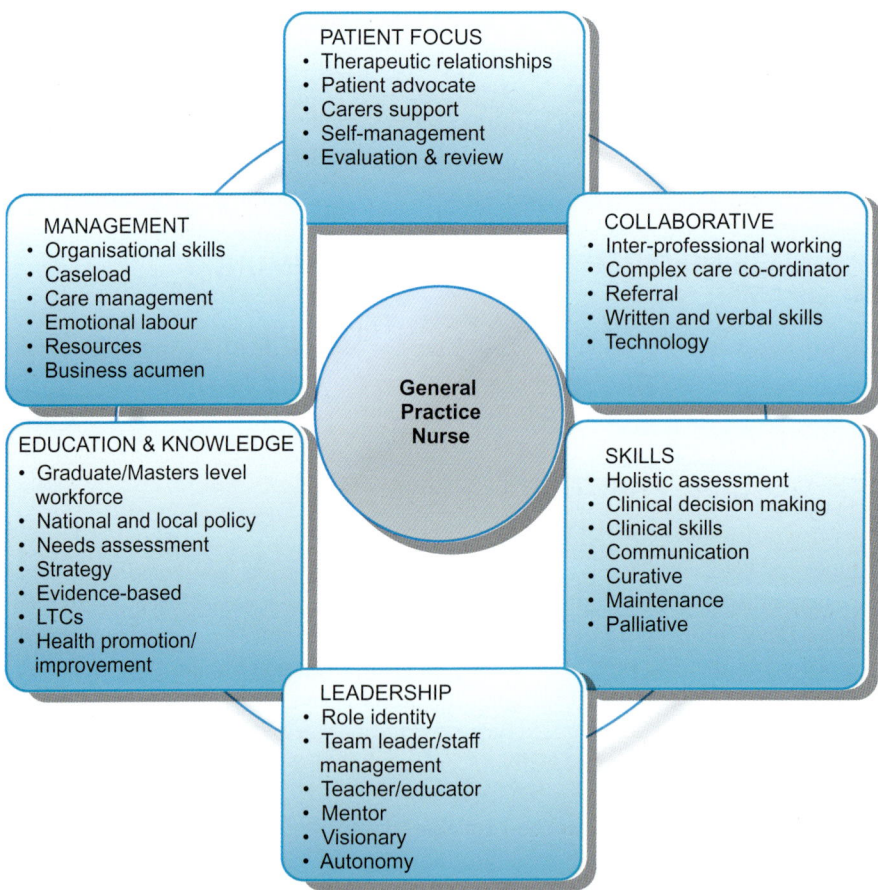

Fig. 3.3 General practice nurses. (With permission from NHS England (2018). *The Queen's Nursing Institute: General practice nursing induction template.* https://www.qni.org.uk/wp-content/uploads/2019/05/General-Practice-Nursing-Induction-Template.pdf. Accessed 3 September 2023.)

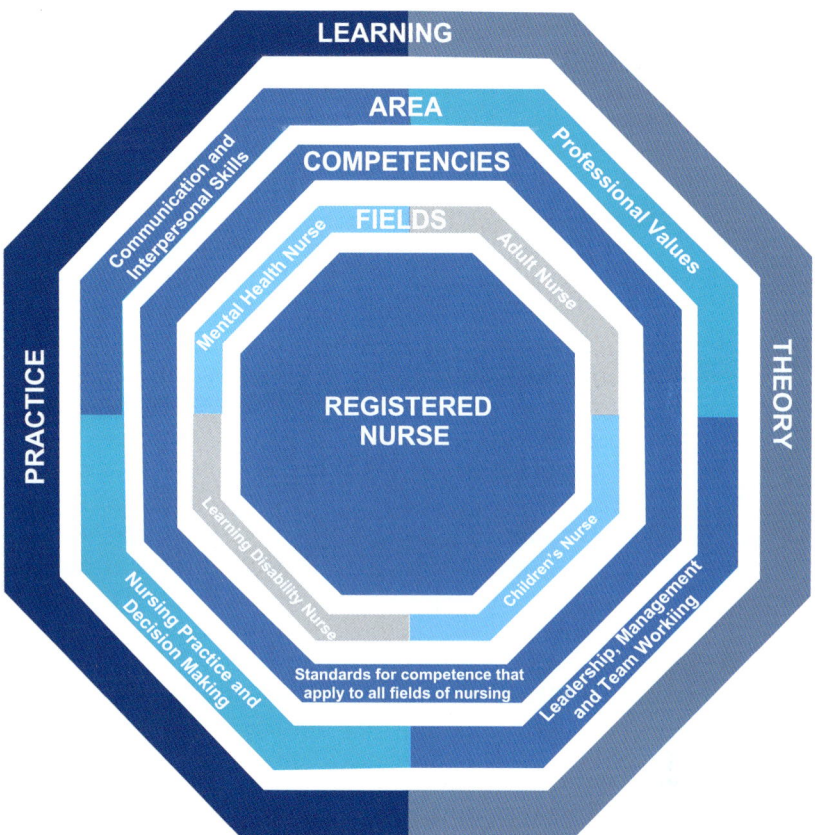

Fig. 3.4 Competencies for general practice nursing. (Diagram developed by Aaron Bent, in NHS England (2019a). *General practice – Developing confidence, capability, and capacity: A 10-point action plan for General practice nursing, milestone report.* https://www.england.nhs. uk/wp-content/uploads/2018/01/general-practice-nursing-ten-point-plan-v17.pdf. Accessed 3 August 2023.)

Competencies for GPN are detailed in Fig. 3.4. The GPN induction template (NHSE) also includes a clinical competencies checklist; a GPN checklist; strengths, weaknesses, opportunities and threats (SWOT) analysis; and information on general support, preceptorship, clinical supervision, methods of building resilience, assessment, record keeping, management of incidents, child protection, duty of candour, safeguarding adults and children, consent and the Mental Capacity Act (MCA). GPN also requires skills related to a person- and relationship-centred approach to care, skills assessment, health screening, medicine management, vaccination and immunisation, travel health, ear care, sexual health, contraception and cervical screening, wound management, long-term conditions, frailty, diabetes, respiratory care, coronary vascular diseases, health protection (supported by a local health protection forum with respect to flu vaccination, emergency preparedness, resilience and response (EPRR), IPC, infectious diseases, screening and environment hazards), smoking cessation, falls, loneliness and isolation, aspects of

MH and dementia, learning disability and end-of-life care. The general practice nurse works with the wider system and integrated care to perform these duties and there is an example induction checklist template for general practice to help staff settle into their roles. Information is provided on resources for GPN, including an example induction checklist template for MDT staff to use in general practice (NHSE, 2023o) to use.

3.7.9 PERSONALISED CARE

Supporting self-management and personalised care (NHSE, 2019) is led by the personalised care group. Personalised care is where people are having choice and control over decisions that affects their health and well-being within a system that harnesses the expertise, capacity and potential of people, families and communities in delivering better outcomes and reducing health inequalities (NHS England, 2023c). This comprehensive model for personalised care takes a whole-population approach, supporting people with long-term physical and MH conditions and empowering people with complex needs to ensure that they have more choices and legal rights. The model also incorporates specific personalised care commitments and goals in the LTP, including personalised care budgets, social prescribing, community-based support, self-care management, quick elective care, staff training on personalised care conversations, the use of shared decision making and planning support tools and ensuring that the least effective interventions are not routinely performed. The model also includes health coaching and training to help people set goals and take actions to improve their health or lifestyles, with support from subject matter experts (SMEs), a supported self-management (SSM) guide, health coaching quality standards, webinars and incentives/levers in PCN.

3.7.10 BETTER CARE FUND

The Better Care Fund (BCF) is used by local systems to support integrated working across the health, social care, housing and voluntary and community sectors in a way that supports person-centred care, sustainability and better outcomes for people and carers (Local Government Association, 2023).

3.7.11 INTEGRATED CARE

Integrated care involves building strong and effective ICSs within the NHSE, in accordance with the NHS LTP and planning and contracting guidance; the COVID-19 pandemic response, learning and recovery; the devolution of functions and resources; provider collaboratives; place-based partnerships; local government; clinical and professional aspects of care, primary care, specialists and wider clinical leadership. It also covers governance, accountability and regulation, including via use of the national oversight framework; individual organisations; the financial framework; and digital and data health transformation and services. Moreover, strategical, clinical and specialised commissioning of services is achieved through national service specifications, multi-ICSs, national engagement and clinical networks. Commissioning of services is achieved using the allocated funding and legislative protocols relating to tendering, competition, procurement, tariffs, NHS and foundation trusts, capital investments and joint and collaborative commissioning, with improvement of the health outcomes of citizens as the central focus of care in accordance with the triple aim of better population health, better quality care and better finance.

3.7.12 MIDWIVES AND PAEDIATRIC STAFF

Support pertaining to culture, supervision and resilience is provided to midwives and paediatric staff as part of national delivery plans for maternity and paediatric services, as described in this book.

3.7.13 ACUTE HEALTHCARE ORGANISATIONS: NURSES AND AHPs

Mentoring and coaching, in addition to an extensive range of services, are available to support nurses and AHPs in acute healthcare organisations.

3.7.14 INTERNATIONALLY RECRUITED STAFF

There are five high-impact actions that can be used to develop and retain the internationally recruited (IR) workforce, including career conversations, coaching and mentoring, preceptorship and on-boarding, induction and the provision of funds for IR provided by the government. There are also dedicated resources to support staff from Black, Asian and minority ethnic (BAME) and global majority backgrounds, including in relation to identity, equity and progression, as detailed in the chapters of this book.

3.7.15 CONTINUING HEALTHCARE (CHC) WORKFORCE

Assessment skills and dedicated training are provided for this group of staff.

3.7.16 SAFEGUARDING STAFF

Safeguarding staff includes supporting them in relation to trauma-informed care delivery.

3.7.17 STUDENT NURSING ROLES

Regarding student nursing roles, a pool of local students can be set up for pre-registered staff placements, while also meeting the needs of the students.

3.7.18 NURSING ASSOCIATE ROLES

NAs are supported in the process of registration, including for nursing degree apprenticeships. The NA is a new and autonomous role regulated by the Nursing and Midwifery Council (NMC) that is designed to address the skills gap between the HCA and RN roles. NAs provide support to patients and service users while working within set parameters in line with the NMC (2023c) code, supported by dedicated training and placements covering areas including health and well-being, deteriorating patients,

BOX 3.5	Standards of Proficiency

The NMC (2023p) standards of proficiency set out the knowledge and skills that an NA needs to meet, including in relation to education, supervision, assessment, pre-registration and return to practice.

(NMC, 2023p)

pharmacology, team work and leadership, complex care and other key areas. The NA's roles are supported by the Practice Placement Assessment Document (PLAD) and dedicated learning supervisors (NMC, 2023p).

The models and types of nursing are supported and regulated by the NMC (2023c), as per Section 2.4, according to the code of professional standards that nurses, midwives and NAs must uphold to be registered to practise (Box 3.5).

3.8 Summary: Basic Guide to the NHS Structures

This chapter provided a basic guide to the NHS structures, covered the organisation and regulation of healthcare and provided insight into healthcare organisations in the UK. It also included information on healthcare and service delivery, nursing and other healthcare processes and models of nursing.

Cultural Competency

4.1 Introduction

This chapter outlines the cultural competency that is required for supporting internationally recruited (IR) staff and ensuring a smooth transition through the healthcare system. This includes insights for all nurses about achieving successful and positive interactions with diverse international groups; addressing all forms of diversity-related issues, given that there are differing national perceptions; and communication challenges and solutions, including in the domain of professional communication, such as assertive communication. The chapter also covers record keeping in health and care strategies. relating to nursing and midwifery. These communication approaches include elements specifically from the perspective of IR staff and the content will also be useful for all nationally qualified nurses (NQNs).

4.2 Cultural Competency to Support Internationally Recruited Staff

The cultural competency required for all staff to support IR staff and ensure a smooth transition through the healthcare system is discussed here.

Cultural differences and challenges impact on the success of the transition of IR staff into their new healthcare settings (Sherman & Eggenberger, 2008). This is because nursing in other countries is significantly different, especially in the areas of nurse autonomy, accountability for patient assessment and technology. In India and China, physicians direct care and are present on patient care units. In the United Kingdom (UK), healthcare professionals including nurses independently assess some elements of patient care, and assertiveness and leadership are increasingly encouraged at all levels in healthcare organisations. Areas that require focus for both IR staff and their line managers include the following.

Managers should ensure training programmes are in place to help international nurses undertake practices that they may not have done in their home countries, including:

- Using stethoscopes in their practice to listen to lung, heart or bowel sounds.
- In addition to generic drugs, administering brand-name drugs used in the UK, which are often unfamiliar or newer drugs.
- Using newer technologies or computerised charting.
- Adapting to the new UK care delivery systems.

Managers should also:

- Support UK staff to understand the languages and cultures of IR staff as they transition into the UK healthcare system.
- Put processes in place to increase patient awareness and understanding of IR staff and the immense benefits they bring to the health service. Clinicians and other leaders should contribute to supporting IR staff to adjust to the UK healthcare setting, including in relation to communication, accent and language.

4.2.1 CULTURAL COMPETENCY FOR INTERNATIONALLY RECRUITED STAFF

Supporting the transition of IR nurses into clinical settings is key. Building an environment that respects and values the diversity and individuality of all staff is an important step in helping IR nurses succeed in their new environment. Increasing numbers of health and care organisations are recruiting international nurses and other healthcare staff as part of their work force strategy, which will contribute to addressing the growing shortage of healthcare staff. Therefore it is important for organisations to invest significant resources in IR staff to help them transition into practice environments, as they are outside their countries of origin and in an unfamiliar environment. This includes educational and other support to fulfil the needs of international nurses and staff, from both their perspective and that of managers and other UK staff with experience in supervising IR nurses, to ensure staff development (Sherman & Eggenberger, 2008). Cultural competency is important for transitioning IR nurses into clinical settings (Tables 4.1 and 4.2).

TABLE 4.1 ■ Managers' and Leaders' Questions to Support IR Staff

Managers and leaders should use the following questions designed to support internationally recruited (IR) staff

1. How many staff has your institution or unit recruited internationally during the past 2 years and from where?

2. Based on the information received from existing staff, supervisors, preceptors and the international staff themselves, what challenges face international staff in transitioning to the local clinical setting?

3. What are the agreed responsibilities for mentoring international staff toward a successful transition to the clinical setting?

4. What resources and best practices are currently invested in to help international nurses and other staff transition to the local clinical environment?

5. What are the needs of mentors and preceptors assigned to international nurses?

6. What local transitional programmes are in place to support international nurses and other staff considering the competencies, skills, content areas and leadership skills that are needed for international staff and nurses to develop?

7. Are there any additional transitional challenges for international nurses according to their country of origin (specifically Asia, India, China, South Africa or the Caribbean)?

8. How have patients in the local environment responded to international nurses and staff who have been recruited?

9. Are there any relevant religious or cultural beliefs of IR nurses and other staff, and what elements have been put in place to enable adjustment to the patient care setting?

10. From a manager's perspective, what are the learning needs of nursing and other leaders who recruited international staff and nurses to join their team?

Reprinted with permission from SLACK Incorporated. Sherman, R. O., & Eggenberger, T. (2008). Transitioning internationally recruited nurses into clinical settings. *The Journal of Continuing Education in Nursing, 39*(12), 535–544. https://doi.org/10.3928/00220124-20081201-04.

This section focusses on international recruitment and selection of staff, including ensuring supportive processes are put in place, as international employment is important to assist healthcare organisations in delivering effective services globally (Scullion and Collings, 2006).

These include:

- Examining expatriate failure and making adjustments; this is an important area due to the high cost of failure in international assignments in both economic and human respects, highlighting the importance of effective international recruitment and selection.

- Addressing the core competencies of the global manager, contributing to increasing knowledge in this area.

- Examining three broad alternative approaches to resourcing strategies.

- Evaluating the different approaches to attracting and sourcing international managers, including some key methods that international companies use for sourcing; attracting and selecting international managers; and adapting the techniques based on the country being recruited from (Scullion and Collings, 2006).

TABLE 4.2 ■ Questions to Support the Transition of IR Staff to the UK

IR staff should ask the following questions designed to support their transition to the UK

1. What have been your biggest challenges as you have transitioned into the work environment here in the UK?

2. Has the work setting been what you anticipated based on the information you received when recruited? If not, what surprised you or what did you not expect about your transition to the work setting?

3. What are the differences between what is expected of you as healthcare staff in your country and here in the UK?

4. Who have you spoken to about the concerns you have about your transition to the work environment?

5. Was your orientation what you needed, and what could have been done differently or more effectively to help you transition into your clinical setting?

6. What are the differences in your practice situations with patients in the UK compared with your home country?

7. Were there questions related to your practice setting that you were too embarrassed to ask and did you discuss this with anyone?

8. Was there anything in the clinical setting that you were asked to do that conflicts with your religious or cultural beliefs? How did you deal with the situation? Did you feel supported?

9. Are there any clinical skills or forms of healthcare or nursing knowledge that would have been helpful to learn or review when you first entered this country?

10. What advice would you give to a nurse from your country who is considering coming to the UK to live and work?

11. What additional skills, knowledge and content do you think needs to be added to the local transition programme for IR nurses and other staff?

12. What do you think healthcare leaders in the UK need to know to help them successfully transition into the healthcare setting?

Reprinted with permission from SLACK Incorporated Sherman, R. O., & Eggenberger, T. (2008). Transitioning internationally recruited nurses into clinical settings. *The Journal of Continuing Education in Nursing, 39*(12), 535–544. https://doi:10.3928/00220124-20081201-04.

4.2.2 CULTURAL AWARENESS AND OVERSEAS STAFF

Cultural awareness (Morris & Morris, 2021) is critical to success when working across borders and cultures, contributing to the achievement of organisational objectives as well as leadership development, which ultimately improves the performance of individual employees as well as their ability to adjust to a new culture and settle quickly. IR staff are exposed to significant emotional and work-related issues that have the potential to disrupt their duties. Lack of cultural awareness can cause miscommunication, embarrassment and offence within the host culture, which may lead to workplace disputes, financial loss and reputational damage. Employers should support their IR staff to help them deal with the pressures of working and living in a new country. As well as the management of job duties, IR staff should be assisted in developing intercultural competence; navigating these issues is necessary to achieve personal and job-related success. Elements necessary to ensure the success of IR staff include critical intercultural competencies and cultural awareness training.

4.2.3 CRITICAL INTERCULTURAL COMPETENCIES FOR STAFF

Intercultural competence ensures staff are equipped to respect cultural differences, and to embrace them, improving self-awareness and the ability to adjust how they act and react within the new culture. This helps staff to fulfil their duties in all interactions on a daily basis by increasing resilience and coping strategies, to avoid issues and misunderstandings and allow them to perform their roles. Intercultural competence addresses issues regarding behaviour, language and decision-making, promoting staff success in their duties. Cultural competences are also important for building relationships, rapport and loyalty in the new working environment, and to improve understanding and communication between employees and employers, as well as management, to allow for a more positive professional and life experience. This can include welcoming new ways of doing things and showing an interest in how things are done within the new environment. It also involves reading body language and other forms of nonverbal communication to understand others effectively. This contributes to the building of resilience and reduces the likelihood of culture shock and feelings of isolation. The acceptance and tolerance of differences by both the employee and the employer will contribute to a more positive and rewarding experience, personally and professionally.

4.2.4 CULTURAL AWARENESS TRAINING

Personal and professional competences should include cultural awareness training, for both employees and the employer, to support the adjustment and adaption of all to the new working environment. This should also be included in the support and development programme undertaken prior to commencement of the new international role, aimed at developing cultural skills to align with the technical capabilities required for the challenges of the role. Cultural awareness training can be delivered using different methods including bespoke, on-site training provided on a face-to-face basis; ongoing coaching; or e-learning, webinars or other online platforms that provide practical guidance. Support should be provided for families travelling with IR staff to support their integration into the new culture, including supporting them with the logistics of relocating such as finding a home and school and orienting to their new working environment.

Cultural awareness is important, enabling organisations to benefit from positive working environments and stronger workforce performance and relations through enhanced understanding, connection and appreciation of those from different cultural backgrounds and ethnicities, ensuring cultural diversity when recruiting staff.

Some examples of steps individuals can take to promote cultural awareness in the workplace include training on global citizenship and communication skills and encouraging staff to express interest in each other's cultural backgrounds and identities.

This holistic approach to supporting IR staff with preparation and integration will improve overall success and performance for the employee and employer.

This book provides support and signposts regarding key aspects of global mobility, including assisting employers and employers in developing provisions to manage the logistical demands of relocating, thereby supporting the wellbeing of IR staff.

Further education and training is available to meet the challenge of cultural competence in the workplace. Some staff believe that cultural competence training should be 'regular' and 'mandatory', including cross-cultural educational initiatives for all professionals and not only for IR staff (Shepherd et al., 2019).

4.2.5 CULTURAL COMPETENCE IN HEALTHCARE

This includes referring to the Code of Practice for International Recruitment, which applies to the appointment of all international health and social care personnel, both clinical and nonclinical, to work in the UK (National Health Service (NHS) Employers, 2023c).

4.2.6 FURTHER INFORMATION ON CULTURAL COMPETENCE IN HEALTHCARE

Resources provided by Nair and Adetayo (2019) and Handtke et al. (2019) should be explored; these relate to:
- Challenges of cultural competence in healthcare.
- Barriers to cultural competence in healthcare.
- Engaging with the international civil service.
- Examples of cultural competence in the workplace.
- Barriers to cultural competence in nursing.
- Cross-cultural competence.

Cultural competence in the NHS (NHS England, 2022 m), an e-learning tool designed to support staff to gain knowledge and understanding of issues regarding culture and health, including how they may influence healthcare outcomes.

4.2.7 DEVELOPING CULTURAL COMPETENCE FOR LEADERS

Cultural competence for mid-level to senior leaders is transformational, helping leaders to openly engage with diversity-related matters and visibly demonstrate inclusive leadership across organisations (NHS Professionals, 2023b). This includes elements such as willingness to engage, visible commitment, humility, setting the cultural tone, awareness of bias, curiosity about others, creating an inclusive environment, cultural intelligence and effective collaboration (NHS Professionals, 2023b).

4.3 Addressing All Diversity-Related Issues, Including Differing National Perceptions

4.3.1 ACHIEVING SUCCESSFUL AND POSITIVE INTERACTIONS WITH DIVERSE INTERNATIONAL GROUPS

An important first step for any healthcare organisation to be successful at scale is embracing cultural diversity at all levels in the organisation. There are many benefits of cultural diversity in the healthcare setting, although areas such as working across borders, cultures, communication, language and accent may need further dialogue and support for success. There are various organisations, groups, policies and guidelines in place in the UK that are designed to address all forms of diversity-related issues, including differing national perceptions.

4.3.2 THE NHS'S MISSION TO ADDRESS DISPARITIES

The enduring mission of the NHS is high-quality care for all. This means tackling the relative disparities in access to services, patient experience and outcomes. This is outlined in the resources of the NHS England Equality and Health Inequalities Hub (NHS England, 2023 g). These resources, which provide insights for all nurses and other healthcare staff regarding achieving successful and positive interactions with diverse international groups in the healthcare setting, are detailed in the following sections. The resources are aimed at preparing and developing all international staff and students, who constitute a diverse group, to thrive in this fast-paced and changing healthcare environment and to be leaders in healthcare. Some of the key benefits and challenges that an international and diverse group may face in the healthcare setting are detailed next.

4.3.2.1 Benefits

- Diverse cultural perspectives can inspire creativity and drive innovation.
- Diverse healthcare knowledge and insight makes organisations more effective.
- Cultural sensitivity, insight and local knowledge means higher-quality and safer patient care.
- Drawing from a culturally diverse talent pool allows organisations to attract and retain the best talent.
- A diverse skills base allows an organisation to offer a broader and more adaptable range of products and services.
- Diverse teams are more productive and perform better.
- Diversity provides greater opportunity for personal and professional growth.

4.3.2.2 Challenges

- Staff from some cultures may be less likely to let their voices be heard.
- Integration across multicultural teams can be difficult in the face of prejudice or negative cultural stereotypes.
- Professional communication can be misinterpreted or difficult to understand across languages and cultures.
- Navigating visa requirements and employment laws, and the cost of accommodating workplace requirements, can be difficult.
- Different understandings of professional etiquette.
- Conflicting working styles across teams.

This book aims to address these challenges, as outlined in the following sections. This includes information to support diverse international staff like Black, Asian and minority ethnic (BAME) and Black and minority ethnic (BME) background, as well as other international and diverse staff. There may be debates regarding the use of various terminologies to describe individuals from an international and diverse group, including Global

Majority, BAME and BME, which are used interchangeably in this book. However, it is important to focus on the support that these staff need to thrive and succeed in their new working environment.

The 'We Are the NHS: People Plan for 2020/2021' (NHS England, 2021) described actions through which we can all support and retain our workforces. This includes ensuring a sense of belonging in the NHS, particularly as staff from diverse groups have been more significantly affected by the COVID-19 pandemic and challenged by the response to and recovery from this period. These pressures, more than ever before, have driven our leaders to work towards more compassionate and inclusive leadership and to put more processes in place to support international and diverse staff to thrive in the workplace. As highlighted in Section 5.3.2 on leadership in the healthcare setting and Section 5.3.5 on the development of leadership skills, clinical and distributed leadership is more critical than ever in driving the agenda to make culture an important element of the NHS and other healthcare settings. This includes universal understanding, being kind and inclusive based on the principles of social justice, equity and conscience in the UK, and collectively supporting staff from international and diverse groups. This supports the NHS in achieving excellence in healthcare through identifying and using the best talent, thereby reducing health inequalities and improving population health through service changes. Following recent national and international events such as the COVID-19 pandemic and the Black Lives Matter campaign, it is more urgent for leaders to act and create an organisational culture where everyone feels they belong, particularly to improve the experience of people from BAME backgrounds. In the UK, healthcare organisations welcome all, with a culture of belonging and trust promoting understanding, providing encouragement and celebrating diversity in all its forms. This comes with the aim of eradicating discrimination, violence and bullying via role modelling, where both staff and patients from international and diverse groups are treated equitably and as individuals. Further information to support the achievement of these principles and agenda is detailed later.

4.3.3 A TIME OF NATIONAL AWAKENING

The COVID-19 pandemic intensified social and health inequalities, having a disproportionate impact on our BAME colleagues, families and friends, as well as on older people, men, those with obesity and those with a disability or long-term condition. The NHS is the largest employer of BAME staff in the UK and BAME colleagues lost their lives in greater numbers than any other group. Leaders who manage BAME staff are responsible for ensuring risk assessments are done to identify at-risk staff, implementing processes to ensure physical and psychological safety, and contributing to eliminating systemic inequalities in the NHS to improve the working lives of NHS and other healthcare staff recruited from the diverse communities we serve.

There is strong evidence (NHS England, 2021) that when the NHS and wider healthcare workforce is representative of the community that it serves, patient care and experience is more personalised and improves. Therefore patients and staff from diverse backgrounds should be treated equitably. The NHS Workforce Race Equality Standard (WRES) (NHS England, 2023 h) contributed to progress in some areas, such as increasing the number of BAME senior management staff. NHS England and the NHS Confederation established the NHS Race and Health Observatory (NHS England, 2023i), an expert research centre on health inequalities bringing together UK and international experts to provide analysis and policy recommendations to improve health outcomes for NHS staff, patients and communities. This is vital for accruing evidence to drive progress in the commitment to equality, diversity and inclusion (EDI), leveraging integrity, intelligence, empathy, openness and a learning culture. This NHS leadership observatory provides an evidence base, highlighting areas of best practice globally, commissioning research and translating learning into practical advice and support for NHS leaders.

4.3.4 COVID-19 IN THE UK

The COVID-19 pandemic has been a difficult time for everyone, with many staff from abroad finding themselves separated from family and friends in their home countries. Important information regarding COVID-19 infection rates, local measures, restrictions and vaccinations, and general coronavirus-related health information can be found by visiting the NHS COVID-19 website (NHS, 2023aa) and reading guides on the COVID-19 pandemic in the UK (Buswell, 2023). There are COVID-19 guidance and support (GOV. UK, 2023r) resources in the UK covering testing, vaccinations, what to do if someone has COVID-19, how to reduce the spread of COVID-19 and advice on travelling abroad. COVID-19 guidance and resources are also available on the use of personal protective equipment for non-aerosol-generating procedures (GOV.UK, 2023 s).

4.3.5 INFECTION PREVENTION AND CONTROL

Infection prevention and control (IPC) is everyone's responsibility, including compliance with standard infection control precautions (SICPs) and transmission-based precautions (TBPs) to ensure prevention of infection development and transmission (NHS England, 2023j). There are additional IPC resources in Section 7.2.8 on IPC competencies, Box 7.3 on IPC competency testimonials.

4.3.6 INFECTION PREVENTION SOCIETY

Joining and volunteering for the Infection Prevention Society (IPS) are good means of professional development, providing the possibility of involvement in the work of the IPS aimed at informing, shaping and leading the IPC agenda locally, nationally and internationally (IPS, 2023).

4.3.7 EXPECTATIONS OF STAFF FROM INTERNATIONAL AND DIVERSE GROUPS REGARDING THEIR EMPLOYER'S ACTIONS IN VARIOUS AREAS

4.3.7.1 Leadership With Diversity

All NHS trusts, foundation trusts and Integrated Care Systems (ICSs) (which have replaced clinical commissioning groups (CCGs)) must publish progress reports according to the model employer's (NHS England, 2023p) goals of increasing BME representation at senior levels across the NHS, where the senior workforce (Band 8d and above) is representative of the overall BAME workforce. This includes ensuring that senior leadership (very senior managers (VSM) and board members) represents the diversity of the NHS, spanning all protected characteristics and involving international and diverse groups of staff.

Leadership with diversity is also supported by the *Chairs and non-executive* directors (NEDs) *in the NHS* report on the need for diverse leadership (NHS Confederation, 2019), which recommended that future chairs and NEDs on NHS boards be diverse and independent where, for their development and support, the focus should be on governance and EDI (NHS Confederation, 2019).

4.3.7.2 Recruitment and Promotion Practices

Employers, in partnership with staff representatives, should improve recruitment and promotion practices to ensure that their staffing reflects the diversity of their community, and regional and national labour markets. This should include ensuring accountability for outcomes, agreeing diversity targets and addressing bias in systems and processes. These efforts must be supported by training and leadership focusing on why this is a priority for our people and, by extension, patients. Divergence from these new processes should be the exception and agreed between the recruiting manager and board-level lead on EDI (in NHS trusts, this is usually the chief executive). This includes ensuring that staff from international and diverse groups are part of interview panels to represent BAME backgrounds and ensure equity in the processes.

4.3.7.3 General Recruitment and Selection Process

Fair and effective assessment, selection and recruitment processes are key to choosing the best talent, as detailed in the following seven steps:

Understand the job: Selection is about matching the right person to the right job, which requires understanding of what the job entails, including the basic requirements, main duties and accountabilities, as detailed in the job description.

Be open-minded about the qualities needed for the role: The skills, knowledge, expertise and qualifications required in the relevant field, combined with the attributes, behaviour and personal characteristics needed for the role as per the personal specification, are vital. There should be consideration of setting requirements for the role at the right level while not deterring high-potential candidates who might lack exposure to the role. There should be a balanced approach to identifying candidates with the qualities, experience, skills, qualifications and personal attributes needed for the role. There should also be consideration of the job environment, team skills, characteristics of the locality and the customer profile.

Search widely for the required candidate: A strong and diverse pool of candidates is an important part of the recruitment process, encompassing internal, external and international applicants to meet the needs of the diverse mix of patients and service users of the health and care system. This should include reaching into different social and community networks and advertising widely using web-based adverts, newspapers, newsletters and magazines.

Record evidence of candidates meeting the recruitment criteria: After candidates apply for the role, there should be a shortlisting process to select those to take forward to interview based on the requirements in the job description and the person specification for the role. This process should be documented for future reference in an open, consistent and systematic manner using simple metrics and a scoring system based on the essential and desirable criteria in the job description and person specification.

Understand stereotypes impacting on the recruitment process: Assess for and guard against the use of stereotypes in the recruitment process, avoiding the unconscious bias of being drawn only to people like ourselves. The value that difference brings to a team should be welcomed, and being open-minded to change during the recruitment process supports this.

Have more than a gut feeling about the recruitment process: Gut feeling should be tested out via the job-related questions asked in the interview, for example regarding the candidate's ability to build relationships at work, based on concrete evidence acquired during the recruitment process. This should be related to the candidate's ability to perform the job effectively.

Be clear about the recruitment decisions being made: Good practice should be maintained to ensure that there is clear written evidence of the decision and outcome of the interview process. This complies with legal requirements and ensures clarity in the feedback provided to candidates, ensuring that unsuccessful candidates can address areas that need strengthening. The successful candidate should be informed as soon as possible following completion of the interview.

4.3.7.4 Health and Wellbeing Conversations

Line managers should discuss EDI as part of the health and wellbeing (HWB) conversations described in the NHS People Plan (NHS England, 2021) to empower people to reflect on their lived experience, support them to be more informed on issues and play their part in contributing to further progress (Box 4.1). Internal and external HWB support are outlined in the following sections.

4.3.7.4.1 Internal HWB Organisational Support

The wellbeing team offers a wide range of support networks and training for employers including relaxation days, salary sacrifice schemes and mental health (MH) training.

Confidential care services include counselling, practical advice and emotional support with work or personal issues.

BOX 4.1   Health and Wellbeing Success Story

My duties include ensuring access to resources and support aimed at investing in people.

I do this by facilitating a reciprocal mentoring programme at my trust, and I was part of the first cohort that really benefited from this.

My reciprocal mentoring benefits junior band 4, 5 and 6 staff members from a BAME background by pairing them up with a senior band 8a or above manager/specialist to form a mentoring relationship; the senior staff member helps to make a difference by acting as a role model.

This in turn helps boost confidence, allowing junior staff to showcase skills and knowledge in executive meetings where they may not have had this opportunity otherwise.

Service manager at a hospital

The occupational health service offers a range of staff services including health supervision and screening, health promotion, safety legislation, a sharps injury service, immunisation and blood tests, protection at work, record keeping and fast-track referrals.

Chaplaincy provides spiritual and pastoral care; support in coping with illness, bereavement, caring for others and workplace problems; and someone to talk to.

Freedom to speak up (FTSU) is emphasised to ensure everyone feels comfortable in speaking up and raising concerns within the workplace, including regarding malpractice, discrimination or other types of wrongdoing. This contributes to an open and honest culture in the workplace.

FTSU uses staff experiences, learning from the handling of whistleblowing and best practice to provide a basis for policy, guidance and resources. These experiences help leadership teams to improve operational arrangements based on the FTSU concept. This supports the safety of patients, where staff can report concerns to FTSU guardians in the organisation, networks, executive leads and the national guardian's office, supported by changes in legislation and national policies. This supports staff who raise concerns about unsafe working conditions, unethical behaviours, inadequate staff induction or training, bullying and harassment, and EDI. The vision for raising concerns is to ensure that staff feel confident and safe in speaking up and that concerns raised are investigated and learnings shared to make a difference (NHS England, 2023q).

4.3.7.4.2 External HWB Support and Resources

Mind provides a confidential MH information service, helping people to make choices about treatment, personal rights and sources of support (Mind, 2023).

Single point of access (SPA) helps to provide the right out-of-hours care for people in crisis all year round. When individuals feel unsafe, at risk or unable to cope without professional advice, trained MH advisors and clinicians will work with them so that they can manage their difficulties without having to access other services.

NHS One You (Every Mind Matters) represents a step towards better health and more sustainable services, helping staff manage and maintain good MH and enabling relaxation to achieve more and enjoy life (UK Health Security Agency (UKHSA), 2023a).

Samaritans provides confidential, nonjudgemental emotional support for people who are experiencing feelings of distress, despair and desperation (Samaritans, 2023).

Citizen's Advice provides independent advice, including immigration advice, to those facing problems, giving them knowledge and confidence to find a way forward (Citizens Advice, 2023).

Free access is provided to HWB apps and hubs, allowing for rapid referrals and quick access to expertise.

4.3.7.5 Tackling the Disciplinary Gap

Leaders across the NHS and wider healthcare service must implement processes to reduce the number of staff with a diverse ethnicity background who enter formal disciplinary proceedings. The actions to do this are outlined in the 'A fair experience for all' (NHS England, 2020) document, supporting organisations in taking practical steps to achieve this goal including establishing robust decision-tree checklists for managers, post-action audits on disciplinary decisions and pre-formal action checks (Box 4.2).

| BOX 4.2 | **Dealing With Disciplinary Matters** |

The RCN provides help and advice for staff who are involved in disciplinary matters. *'If you are being involved in a disciplinary process, read the following information provided and contact he RCN without delay, by phone or online, through the RCN website, the discipline section' (RCN, 2023e). Advice is also provided on writing a statement, acting as a witness and immigration.*

(RCN, 2023e)

4.3.7.6 Governance to Support International and Diverse Staff

All NHS organisations should review their governance arrangements to ensure that BAME and other international and diverse staff networks can contribute to and inform healthcare decision-making processes. These staff networks (NHS England, 2023r) provide a supportive and welcoming space for staff; they have extensive expertise on EDI matters and support executive boards and teams. Staff networks should look beyond the boundaries of their organisation to work with colleagues nationally, across systems, and at 'place' level including supporting staff who work in hospitals, primary care, the community, domiciliary care, nursing homes, MH services, care homes, NHS 111, NHS 999, the independent sector and voluntary services. These services meet the changing needs of the ageing population, treating chronic conditions, episodes of illness and long-term conditions, and developing new treatments to meet the increasing demand on services.

4.3.7.7 Information and Education

There are resources, guides and tools (NHS England, 2021) to help leaders and individuals engage in productive conversations about race, and to support each other to make tangible progress on EDI for all staff. This includes NHS EDI training for all staff, which will contribute to more impactful and focused actions based on E-Learning for Health resources — Equality, diversity and inclusion (NHS England, 2023 s).

4.3.7.8 Accountability for Equality, Diversity and Inclusion

Competency frameworks for all NHS Trusts, commissioning and ICS board-level positions outline the accountability of executive staff for equality and diversity in the workplace. These frameworks reinforce that it is the explicit responsibility of the chief executive to lead on EDI, and of all senior leaders to hold each other to account regarding the progress they are making. The accountability of line managers is included in the competency frameworks for board positions in NHS organisations, which cover the requirements for the recruitment, appraisal and development of individuals in these crucial leadership roles.

These include the HR Framework for Developing Integrated Care Boards (NHS, 2022b) and the career framework competency-based job descriptions (NHS, 2022c).

4.3.7.9 Regulation and Oversight

The Care Quality Commission (CQC) assessments of trusts place increased emphasis on whether organisations have made measurable progress on EDI and whether they can demonstrate the positive impact of this progress on staff and patients (CQC, 2023).

4.3.7.10 Building Confidence to Speak Up

A joint training programme for FTSU guardians and WRES experts is available to support staff with leading roles in this area to support the workforce, named Freedom to Speak Up (NHS England, 2023t).

4.3.7.11 Ensuring Staff Have a Voice

It is important to ensure all staff feel safe and confident when expressing their views; if something concerns us, we should feel able to speak up about it. This may involve sharing different and better ways of doing something, thereby shaping roles, the workplace, the NHS and our communities, improving the health and care of the nation. Staff take time to really listen to each other, hearing what they have to say, as they progress through challenges and changing times and make the most of new opportunities as they arise. These strategies will prevent staff from feeling unable to speak up or that they have been ignored. Support needs to be provided to BAME staff to enable them to speak up, including sharing their lived experience. When staff speak, leaders must listen and then take action.

Following the experience of COVID-19, which resulted in a great need to engage with and listen to staff, the NHS People Pulse for all NHS and provider organisations was implemented (NHS England, 2021) to understand the experiences of NHS staff during the COVID-19 pandemic and the recovery period. To build on this, leaders should use the NHS Staff Survey to solicit views from staff, reflect on the current context and take actions to implement strategies aimed at improvement of the healthcare setting, including actions to boost staff morale.

Networks and digital spaces are also helpful ways of conveying staff experiences, ensuring staff are empowered to speak up and, based on what is heard, taking key actions to create a culture where patients and staff feel safe. These key strategies help staff to feel valued and confident that their insights are being used to shape learning and improvement.

The NHS (NHS England, 2021) works with the National Guardian's office to support leaders and managers to foster a culture of listening and speaking up. Board members of NHS and foundation trusts already have specific executive board responsibilities to embed the 'just culture' and FTSU concepts.

4.3.7.12 Just Culture

A just culture guide supports consistent, constructive and fair evaluation of the actions of staff involved in patient safety incidents. All employers are also encouraged to ensure staff complete just culture training and accredited learning packages to help create a fair, open and learning-oriented organisation where staff feel they can speak up. NHS England (2021) also aims to take demonstrable action to promote leadership behaviours among employees, supported by NHS England (2023 u).

4.3.7.13 Patient Safety Incident Response Framework

The Patient Safety Incident Response Framework (PSIRF) processes and procedures help ensure serious incidents are identified correctly, investigated thoroughly and, most importantly, learned from to prevent similar incidents happening again, as part of the patient safety strategy (NHS England, 2023 v).

4.3.7.14 Compassionate and Inclusive Leadership

Inclusive cultures are driven by inclusive leaders, requiring powerful leadership at all levels, across all roles and in all teams in the NHS, irrespective of titles and seniority, building on the distributed leadership described earlier. All NHS leaders and other leaders, especially those in formal management positions, are expected to act with kindness, prioritise collaboration and foster creativity in the people they work with so that teams and staff can flourish.

4.3.7.15 Leadership Development

This includes line managers and leaders training to enhance their proficiency in the new approach to NHS leadership, to in turn help leaders to continue to build a more compassionate and inclusive culture in their teams, supporting the operating environment. Means to achieve this include expert-led seminars on health inequalities and racial injustice and action learning sets for senior leaders across health and social care.

4.3.7.16 Clinical Leadership

Leadership and management development in various organisations has been expanded to encompass the number of yearly placements available for talented clinical leaders within systems and organisations, focusing on improvement projects across clinical healthcare pathways.

4.3.7.17 Shared Governance

Strengthening leadership in the clinical environment is vital in creating leaders, from ward to board, providing excellence in healthcare. This involves shared governance (Box 4.3),

---

BOX 4.3   Shared Governance

EXAMPLES OF SHARED GOVERNANCE WORK TARGETED FOR IMPROVEMENT INCLUDE

Phlebotomy: decrease waiting times for patients having blood taken.

Medicine management: using drug trolleys to increase care times and safety while reducing interruptions and variation in practice.

Managing and **streamlining** ward stock: ensuring cost savings and ordering reduction.

Ear, nose and throat (ENT) and **cardiology** pathway: using X-ray diagnosis to reduce the need for additional consultation and appointments, ensuring cost savings and saving clinical time.

Orthopaedic theatres: use of standardising dressings to improve effectiveness and reduce cost.

Pre-operative assessment (POA): using telephone assessments to reduce clinic appointments, improving effectiveness and reducing cost.

SHARED GOVERNANCE CARE OUTCOMES INCLUDE

Reduction of pressure ulcers, falls, catheter-associated urinary tract infections (CAUTIs), methicillin-resistant *Staphylococcus aureus* (MRSA) infections and *Clostridioides difficile* infections (CDI).

SHARED GOVERNANCE PATIENT OUTCOMES INCLUDE

Improvements in patient engagement, patient-centred care, patient education, courtesy and respect, safety, pain and active listening.

Trust shared governance lead

which has key cornerstones including accountability, ownership, partnership and equity (NHSE, 2022b) that support the following:

- Workforce recruitment and retention.
- Increased staff autonomy and enhanced skills to make and recognise changes.
- Giving staff expertise in providing the best care to patients.
- Encouraging frontline staff to take ownership.
- Empowering staff to work effectively in their organisation.

The principles of shared governance are associated with the following benefits:

- Giving a greater voice to staff in clinical decision-making.
- Supporting professional practice.
- Use of evidenced-based practice for service improvement.
- Making positive changes in patient and staff satisfaction, safety and experience.

Shared governance contributes to the recognition and development of talent, with benefits for clinical ward leadership and culture, career pathways and the valuing and support of staff using the shared governance cycle of define, attract, develop, manage and evaluate.

Shared governance promotes excellence, education research and development opportunities in:

- Elective care: specialist, advanced, clinical/academic and international learning.
- Leadership training in shared governance systems, patient safety, senior leadership in acute care, all routes into healthcare and research studies.
- Core skills: acute care skills, preceptorship, critical care, children's care, surgery, health care of older people (HCOP), community, specialist training (such as endoscopy) and wider workforce training.
- Shared governance: collective leadership is about everyone taking responsibility not just for their own job or role but also for the success of their team and organisations (NHS England, 2022b).

4.3.7.18 Talent Management

Talent management refers to leadership development as well as the approach used to source, develop, manage, engage and deploy individuals with high potential to progress faster and further in their career, enhancing their potential to help organisations achieve common business goals in the short and long term. These individuals demonstrate the highest potential to make a difference by improving an organisation's performance through immediate and long-term contributions. Therefore strong and effective talent management is important to high-performing organisations, identifying, growing and developing people such that they can become the responsible managers and leaders of tomorrow. This ensures that everyone feels supported in terms of developing their career in their chosen direction, achieved through having honest conversations about their prospects and helping them to fulfil their aspirations while also meeting the needs of the team, the organisation and the system (NHS Leadership Academy, 2023a). Talent management processes should ensure there is a greater prioritisation and consistency of diversity in talent in executive director, senior manager, chair and board roles. This requires clearer guidance on the recruitment process and metrics to track progress.

TABLE 4.3 ■ **Talent Management, Development and Success**

Are you a leader wanting to develop your career?

Do you want to progress to the next level?

Do you want to achieve your full potential?

Do you want to be a top leader?

Do you want to work in the health and care system?

Do you want to have your talent recognised and developed?

Do you want to be part of a talent management scheme that works for you?

From NHS Leadership Academy. (2023a). *Talent management hub*. https://www.leadershipacademy.nhs.uk/talent-management-hub/. Accessed 6 October 2023. NHS Leadership Academy. (2023b). *Talent management toolkit*. https://www.leadershipacademy.nhs.uk/talent-management-hub/talent-management-toolkit-home-page/. Accessed 6 October 2023.

Talent management is beneficial for staff who answer 'yes' to the questions in Table 4.3. These staff can access the talent management resources referred to throughout this book, including those in the further information section. These resources support staff to develop and maximise their potential. There are various processes that can support this, such as communities of practice (CoPs) where people with a shared vision collectively come together to embed leadership and develop talent (NHS Leadership Academy, 2023a, 2023b).

4.3.7.19 Digital Line Management Training

Free online training material for all NHS line managers is available for those who seek to progress and a management apprenticeship pathway is also available.

4.3.7.20 Online Leadership Resources

NHS leadership programmes, which can be accessed from the relevant digital platforms, emphasise the principle of inclusion and provide practical resources on team effectiveness, crisis management, retention and talent management.

4.3.7.21 Response to the Kark Review

Ensuring high standards of leadership in the NHS is crucial; well-led organisations and better-led teams with strong teamwork translate into greater staff wellbeing and superior clinical care. This includes implementing the government's response to Tom Kark QC's review of the Fit and Proper Persons Test, ensuring board leaders are fulfilling their duties including driving EDI (NHS England, 2021).

4.4 Communication Challenges and Solutions

Professional communication, particularly assertiveness, includes key elements to ensure effective communication such as empathy, active listening, clarity, use of nonverbal communication, being personable, respect and an appropriate medium of communication

(Evolution, 2021). Effective communication helps to resolve and prevent numerous workplace disputes and contributes to resolving and improving many other issues, such as employees' wellbeing and feeling valued, which can increase staff retention in organisations. The key elements of effective communication to ensure messages are being delivered clearly and effectively every time are detailed next.

Empathy is a skill that all leaders should have, enabling delivery of a message (after considering how it affects those who are receiving it) in the best and most effective way to the target group of individuals. This is especially useful in conversations where there is disagreement with what another individual is saying, by helping people see things from another's perspective, understand where they are coming from, and identify areas of mutual agreement.

Listening is an important element to consider when communicating with others, creating an environment where individuals feel comfortable and able to speak up and voice their concerns, in turn enabling the creation and use of collective solutions.

Clarity prior to message delivery, achieved by pausing to consider what is being said, is vital. Clear and concise messages help individuals get their point across in a manner that is easy for others to understand, without causing confusion.

Nonverbal communication is vital as over 90% of our communication is nonverbal. Therefore it is important to get the body language 'right' to compliment the intended message (Evolution, 2021). It is important to maintain an open, relaxed stance and maintain eye contact without prolonged staring when communicating.

Being personable, including when communicating in a professional environment, is beneficial, particularly with junior staff; people want to be treated like people. Therefore it is helpful to take time to ask questions about others when communicating.

Respect is undoubtedly vital for all conversations in the workplace and it is important to ensure that colleagues are respectful in every conversation; this can be achieved by using the other person's name and staying focused on the conversation, listening actively to responses.

The medium of communication is important and, depending on the type of message being conveyed, communication can be via email, phone call or face-to-face meeting. However, an email can be easily misconstrued and a face-to-face meeting can cause unintended anxiety; phone calls can be effective, especially for urgent and sensitive matters. It is important to take the time to choose the best medium to ensure the most effective communication, which benefits all individuals involved, while taking into consideration the seven key elements of effective communication (Evolution, 2021).

4.5 Documentation and Record Keeping in Nursing

Documentation and record keeping in nursing are important to ensure continuity of care and for communication among the multidisciplinary teams who care for patients. Various types of record keeping are used in the UK, including electronic patient records (EPRs). Healthcare organisations are moving towards this type of digitalised service to ensure innovative and seamless care delivery, improving patient experience, quality of care and job satisfaction and also saving time and money by reducing duplication in documentation. Good record keeping and documentation are important for legal reasons, providing evidence of care delivery and future services. The patient's record must provide an accurate, current, objective and comprehensive yet concise account of the patient's stay in hospital (National Institutes of Health, 2023). Patient records therefore act as a vital communication tool that help ensure safety (Royal College of Nursing Institute (RCNi), 2022). Records of all evidence and decisions must be kept, including from all nursing and midwifery professionals involved in the patient's care (Nursing and Midwifery Council (NMC), 2021c). As per best practice in nursing and midwifery documentation (NMC, 2021c), patient record keeping/care plans should include the following sections/elements: a drug chart; information about the patient; patient risk assessments for IPC, falls, pressure ulcers, continence, manual handling, nutrition and hydration; a nursing assessment proforma; intentional rounding; ward rounds; and vital signs/observation. There should also be care plans for breathing, pain, manual handling, eating and drinking, sleeping, self-care, care of the dying person, diabetes and bladder and bowel functions.

The Whitepaper on Patient Safety Communication (Occupational English Test (OET), 2021) reinforces the importance of communication to patient safety. It covers areas including the impact of communicative ability on healthcare; patient satisfaction and quality of care; patient engagement and compliance; and patient safety. It is particularly important in supporting staff with limited language proficiency (OET, 2021).

Guidance is also provided by the National Institutes of Health (2023), RCNi (2022) guidance on record keeping and documentation in nursing and NMC (2021c) standards on keeping records of all evidence and decisions.

Additional details on record keeping and documentation competencies are presented in Section 7.4. A glossary of linguistic phrases, terms and colloquialisms can be found in Section 8.5. The Royal College of Nursing (RCN) (2023f) guide to common English expressions is another resource that staff can refer to for familiarisation with everyday terminology.

4.6 Summary: Cultural Competency

This chapter covered the cultural competencies required for supporting IR staff, ensuring a smooth transition through the healthcare system. This involves insights, support, development and resources for all staff aimed at achieving successful and positive interactions with diverse international groups, as well as addressing all diversity-related issues and differing national perceptions. This chapter also covered communication challenges and solutions, including elements of professional communication such as assertiveness, as well as documentation and record keeping in nursing.

CHAPTER 5

Strategies for Coping With and Flourishing in Your Healthcare Staff Role

5.1 Introduction

This chapter describes professional elements of leadership, including details on the available career and study pathways in the UK healthcare system; career conversations regarding professional leadership in healthcare, including career options; and working in multiprofessional teams in health and care settings, including daily and longer-term challenges in healthcare.

Tailored development and career pathways aligned to foster inclusion and diversity are important parts of the framework for staff development in healthcare. These efforts support staff in managing everyday complexities and challenges in the working environment, by providing resources for staff including resilience training, workforce balance and role modelling. Support for staff may include quality improvement (QI) initiatives, as well as ensuring staff have a clear understanding of clinical standards and how they can use their personalities and have the right tools for the job. Goals include ensuring commitment to patient-centred care and more direct clinical care, through leading change, adding value and helping staff grow and achieve their best. These efforts enable staff to be respectful, open, collaborative, consistent and compassionate, thereby ensuring better outcomes, experiences and use of resources in healthcare delivery (NHS England, 2016) by leading change and adding value.

5.2 Career and Study Pathways in the UK Healthcare System

Diverse and exciting career and study pathways are available in the UK healthcare system. According to a recent survey, nursing has been the most trusted profession by the public for 21 consecutive years (Nurse.org, 2022).

5.2.1 CAREER PATHWAYS FOR NURSES, MIDWIVES, NURSING ASSOCIATES AND ALLIED HEALTH PROFESSIONALS

The diverse career pathways available in the UK for nurses, midwives, nursing associates and allied health professionals (AHPs) (Fig. 5.1) offer many opportunities for staff to develop, specialise and progress in their professions. These opportunities include progressing from newly qualified registered nurse, midwife, nursing associate and AHP roles, with support through preceptorship and effective induction in specialities such as medicine, surgery, paediatrics or clinical specialities, in hospital, community and GP settings. Staff can further progress to leadership positions, such as ward managers and related roles; advanced and specialist practitioner roles; research and clinical academic roles; clinical educator or academic lecturer roles; or corporate roles, including infection prevention and control (IPC), prevention of pressure ulcers, safeguarding, patient safety and experience. Skills and expertise from these roles can prepare staff to advance to more senior roles, such as matron or lead specialist nurse; head of nursing; associate director of nursing; deputy director of quality and governance/education; or deputy director of nursing, midwifery and AHPs. Staff can subsequently advance to the level of director of nursing, midwifery and AHPs, or of chief nursing officer, and then to the top of the career ladder, as chief executive officer (CEO). Career development for staff can be accessed through various routes, including the staff's own organisation.

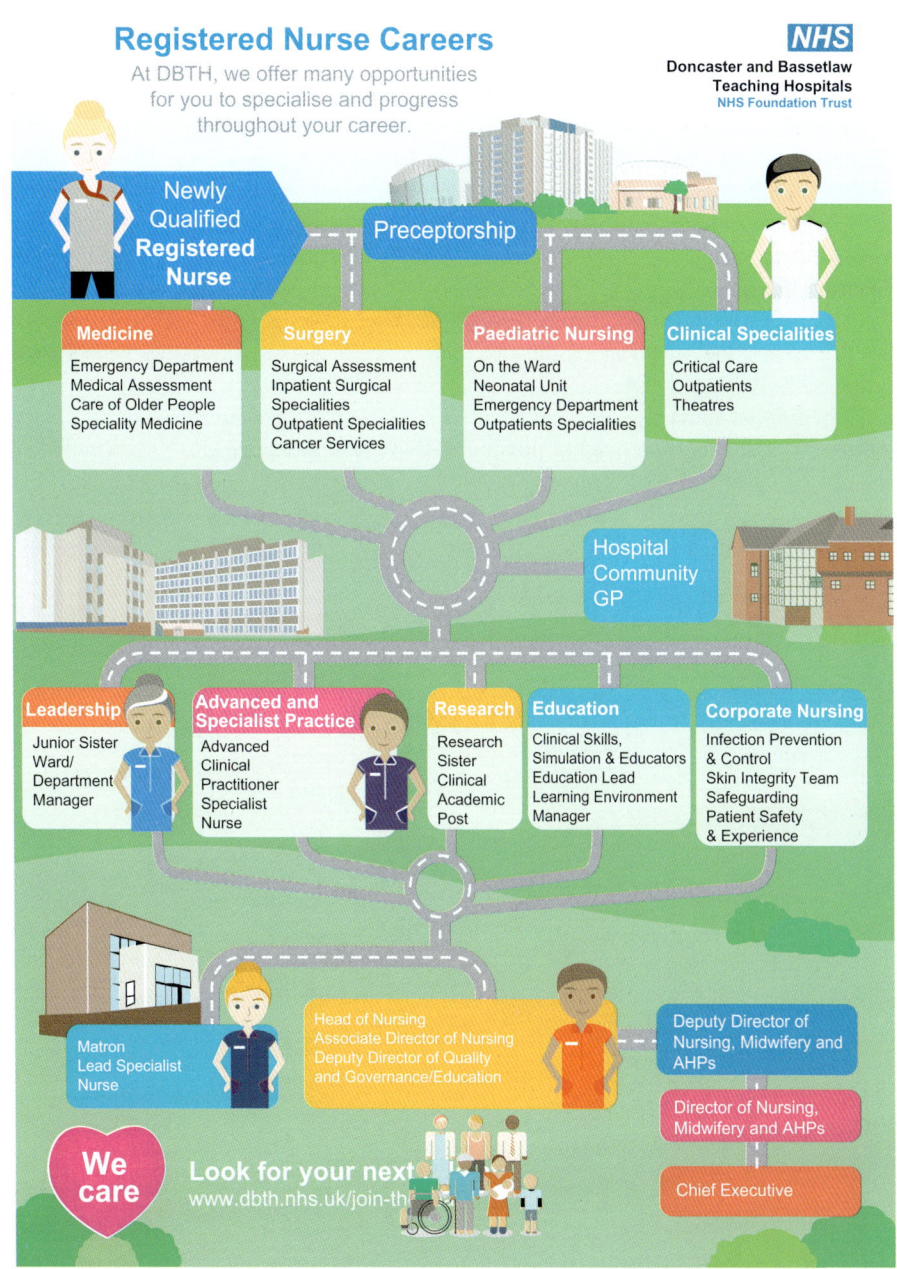

Fig. 5.1 Sample registered nurse career pathway in the UK. (With permission from Doncaster and Bassetlaw Teaching Hospitals NHS Foundation Trust. (2021). Registered Nurse Careers. https://www.dbth.nhs.uk/news/dbth-jobs-week-newly-qualified-adult-nurse/. Accessed 27 March 2021.)

5.2.2 CHIEF NURSE/DIRECTOR OF NURSING/DIRECTOR OF MIDWIFERY CAREER PATHWAY/DEVELOPMENT

The preparation of senior health and care clinical leaders for executive director roles (Fig. 5.2) delivering organisational and integrated systems leadership expertise includes the use of QI, inclusive and compassionate leadership, and talent management. Talent management processes (NHS London Leadership Academy, 2023) are required by the NHS People Plan 2020/21 (NHS England, 2021) and should be used to ensure diversity among talented staff in executive director roles, by matching the diversity within the health service at the senior level to that at the junior level. The career pathway and development for chief nurse/director of nursing (DON)/director of midwifery (DOM) roles include a targeted talent management approach providing access to programmes for aspiring directors. This includes undertaking the executive director pathway, to support the career pathways of health and care staff undertaking director roles in healthcare organisations, the integrated care system (ICS), and regional and national roles (NHS, 2021).

A traditional route to DON and DOM is ward manager/team leader/coordinator, followed by matron, then head of nursing/midwifery and deputy DON/deputy DOM.

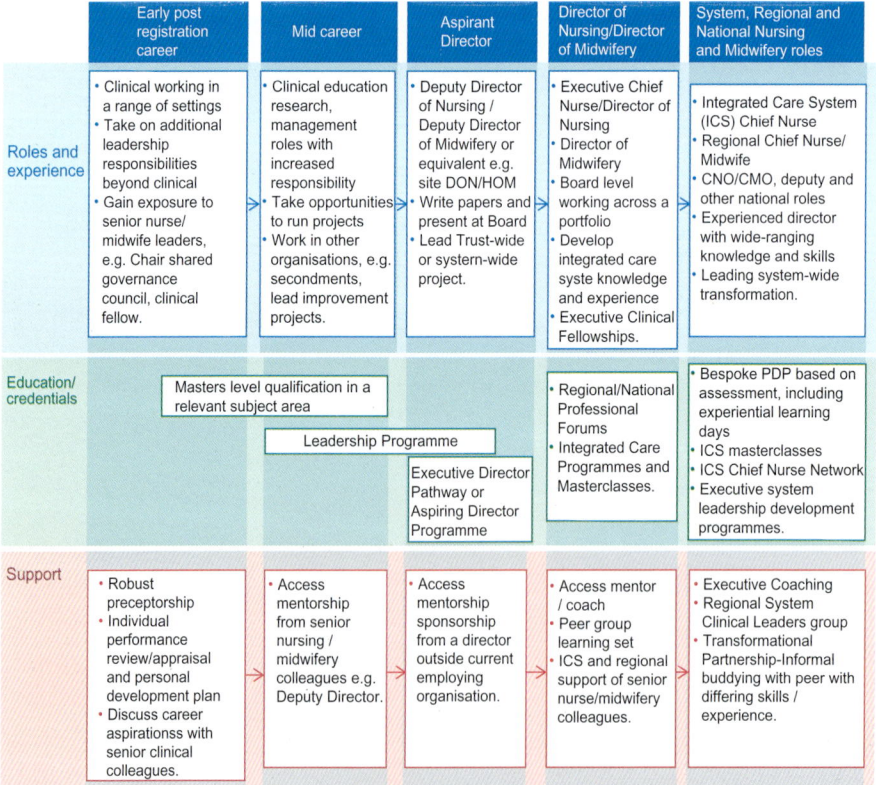

Fig. 5.2   Chief nurse/director of nursing (DON) and director of midwifery (DOM) career pathway. *PDP*, Personal development plan. (With permission from NHS. (2021). *Chief nurse, director of nursing, director of midwifery career pathway summary key finding*. London: NHS England.)

However, ensuring both breadth and depth of experience is considered crucial; therefore, at earlier stages in their careers, aspirant directors are encouraged to plan and gain experience in other roles and settings, e.g. operational, research and educational roles, across sectors. There has been a move to less of a focus on 'years chalked up' to more of a focus on the outcomes and skills/experience that aspirant chief nurses/DONs/DOMs have delivered and acquired (NHS, 2021).

Talent management to support effective nursing and midwifery leadership in an ICS is necessary to prepare ICS chief nurses with advanced systems leadership expertise across their wide-ranging portfolios. Candidates must demonstrate an ability to work in a senior team approach and develop their clinical voices while using critical business language at both the provider and system levels (NHS, 2021).

A more transparent career pathway creates senior leaders and directors who are curious, courageous, compassionate, collaborative and transformative, and support shared decision-making. The accountability framework for chief nurses and DONs/DOMs includes inclusive talent management for nursing, midwifery and AHPs in their organisations, including career coaching, mentorship, allyship/sponsorship and explicit career pathways; these aspects are modelled by executive directors (NHS, 2021).

The early career pathway for progression into DON/DOM roles should include a foundation of clinical work, robust preceptorship and induction, in a range of clinical settings, with individual performance reviews, appraisals and personal development plans (PDPs) developed through career-based discussions. Exposure to senior clinical leaders is encouraged, e.g. through internal clinical fellowships and chairing of shared governance forums.

The organisation's appraisals and PDP tool (Table 5.1) and policy provide internal information on career development, including the appraisals process, inclusive opportunities, people and human resource processes, objective setting, performance assessment, pay progression, monitoring and compliance, study leave arrangement and funding for personal development.

Guidelines are available for accessing nursing, midwifery, nursing associates, carers and other professionals, including AHPs' education and training, and funding for clinical professional groups in bands 5–9 and unregistered clinical workers. These guidelines include information on receiving and using the allocated national training funding, and on line managers discharging their responsibilities of ensuring equitable opportunities for use and access.

5.2.3 INTERNAL ORGANISATIONAL TRAINING AND DEVELOPMENT COURSES (TABLE 5.2)

Training and development courses and information in e-learning and face-to-face formats may include the following:

5.2.3.1 Clinical Audit e-Learning Courses and Quality Improvement (QI) Training

Examples of clinical audit e-learning courses and QI training:

The Institute for Healthcare Improvement (IHI) (2023b): Quality Improvement and Management Programme such as the IHI Quality Leaders Professional Development Programme applies global best practices to quality management across systems.

TABLE 5.1 ■ **Appraisal and Personal Development Plan Tool**

Section 1: Background Information

Appraisee's name:	Job title:
Directorate:	Ward/department:
Date of last appraisal:	Date of this appraisal:
Appraiser's name:	Job title:

Section 2: Mandatory Core Skills Training Compliance

Mandatory Core Skills	Date Last Completed	Date Due or Date Booked	Mandatory Core Skills	Date Last Completed	Date Due or Date Booked
Conflict resolution			Mental capacity		
Emergency resilience			Moving and handling		
Equality and diversity			Preventing radicalisation		
Fire safety			Resuscitation		
Health and safety			Safeguarding adults		
Infection prevention and control			Safeguarding children		
Information governance					

Section 3: Managerial Responsibility for Appraisal and Training Compliance

What percentage of your staff has a current appraisal?

Excluding information governance; this area of responsibility and compliance   Yes/no
  is required as part of the mandatory core skills above.

Section 4: Review of Achievements and Objectives, and Demonstration of Our Values

Our values

The organisation's values are, e.g.:

- Delivery of high-quality care with compassion to every patient
- Demonstrating respect and dignity for patients, their carers and our colleagues
- Striving to excel in everything we do
- Sustaining the highest professional standards, and showing honesty, openness and integrity in all our actions
- Working together to achieve the best outcomes for our patients

Summarise your achievements, including current work objectives and your personal development plan, and how you demonstrate the organisation's values.

Appraiser's summary of your achievements, including your current work objectives and your personal development plan (potentially including discussions of health and well-being)

TABLE 5.1 ■ Appraisal and Personal Development Plan Tool—cont'd

Section 5: Review of Performance Against Our Values

Trust Values	Discussion Summary	Select Agreed-Upon Position
Care with compassion		Exceeds expectations Meets expectations Partially meets expectations
Respect and dignity		Exceeds expectations Meets expectations Partially meets expectations
Striving to excel		Exceeds expectations Meets expectations Partially meets expectations
Professional standards		Exceeds expectations Meets expectations Partially meets expectations
Working together		Exceeds expectations Meets expectations Partially meets expectations

Section 6: Agreed-Upon Objectives and Personal Development Plan (SMART = Specific, Measurable, Agreed, Resourced and Timely)

What Are My Agreed-Upon Personal/ Development Objectives?	What Activities Do I Need to Undertake to Achieve These Objectives?	What Support/ Resources Do I Need to Help Achieve These Objectives?	Target Date for Completion	Date Achieved
Objective 1				
Objective 2				
Objective 3				
Objective 4				
Objective 5				
Personal objectives				
Clinical and professional training to undertake over next 12 months:	Agreed-upon career plan internally within the trust:			

What development do you require over the next 12 months: personal objectives planned for senior management development:

Clinical and professional training undertaken over the past 12 months:

Signed by individual: ....….......................…....... Date: ....….

Signed by appraiser: ....….....................…. Date: ....

Note for appraisers: Where an internal system exits for PDP, complete and submit (a) the appraisal online form and, where applicable, (b) the pay progression manager's confirmation form, to align with the Agenda for Change (AfC) staff pay awards/increments process.

TABLE 5.2 ■ Internal Organisational Training and Development Courses

Statutory and mandatory training

This training includes but is not limited to the following:

Section 1: Statutory and Mandatory Training

Safeguarding children and adults

Prevent awareness: It is linked to safeguarding to protect the vulnerable individuals from exploitation (HM Government, 2024).

Mental Capacity Act (2005) and deprivation of liberty training

Fire and evacuation training for all staff

Fire warden training

Venous thromboembolism, including ensuring completion of venous thromboembolism assessments

Clinical systems and information technology training

Conflict resolution training for frontline staff

Equality, diversity and inclusion training

Information governance training

Mandatory training days for paediatric nurses and staff working with children

Training in manual handling and other safe handling practices

Resuscitation and basic life support training for adult, paediatric and neonatal patients, including intermediate life support and advanced life support

Emergency planning

Section 2: Statutory and Mandatory Training

Health and safety training

Control of Substances Hazardous to Health (COSHH) training

First aid at work

General risk assessment training

Risk management training

Incident management training, such as Datix

Food hygiene training

Section 3: Statutory and Mandatory Training

Infection prevention and control (IPC) training

This training is for clinical staff with hands-on care/patient contact and nonclinical staff with no hands-on care/patient contact, including allied health professionals and domestic staff. Additional IPC training at universities may include postgraduate certificate modules on microorganisms, disease and the epidemiology and surveillance of HCAI, and decontamination; postgraduate diploma modules on advanced IPC, research methods and techniques, qualitative enquiry, host defence and protection, healthcare outbreak management, informatics in health and social care, and patient safety; and MSc training with a dissertation.

Section 4: Statutory and Mandatory Training

Clinical skills training including:

Palliative end of life care (PEoLC).

Dementia awareness.

Blood transfusion.

Blood handling.

Blood glucose monitoring.

Note taking and record keeping.

Drug administration.

Medicines management.

Section 5: Statutory and Mandatory Training

Personal development patient first programme

TABLE 5.2 ■ **Internal Organisational Training and Development Courses—cont'd**

This programme focusses on assertiveness, communication, customer care and continual improvement in the quality of care delivered to patients; it provides opportunities to consider services from the patient's viewpoint and to improve both patients' and visitors' experiences.

Section 6: Statutory and Mandatory Training

Health and well-being training, including

Stress awareness and management programme to support individuals experiencing substantial stress, by recognising and managing causes of stress

Resilience training to help staff address high work pressure, through exercises, discussion and teaching of positive psychology to boost personal resilience and staff counselling; prevent stress and ill health; enable staff to flourish; and support both personal and organisational resilience

Section 7: Statutory and Mandatory Training

Development for clinical staff

This training is for clinical staff delivering hands-on care to patients, to provide the knowledge and understanding necessary to identify patient risk factors, implement interventions to modify risks and optimise care delivery in the following areas. This training is beneficial for occupational therapists and physiotherapists but is not mandatory.

Section 8: Statutory and Mandatory Training

Fall prevention training

This training covers National Institute for Health and Care Excellence (NICE) guidelines, internal policies, risk assessment tools, equipment/interventions, fall management protocol, and incident reporting and management.

Section 9: Statutory and Mandatory Training

Clinical audit, effectiveness and QI training

This training is useful for all staff, to increase the quality and effectiveness of clinical audit projects aligned at the national and local levels; improve patient care and experience; and increase service productivity. These resources support staff to complete the required clinical audits appropriately, at the correct frequencies and intervals.

Healthcare Quality Improvement Partnership (HQIP) (2023): HQIP tools include clinical auditing; the Plan, Do, Study, Act (PDSA) model for improvement; LEAN/Six Sigma performance benchmarking; process mapping and statistical process control. The HQIP provides staff with optimal skills to deliver QI projects and programmes.

Quality, service improvement and redesign (QSIR) by the Act Academy (2023) and AQUA (2023): The purpose of the QSIR programme is to provide a platform for healthcare organisations and systems to build improvement capability at scale, in line with the aims set in the NHS Long-Term Plan (NHS England, 2022a). QSIR (AQUA, 2023) covers leading improvement, project management, measurement of improvement, sustainability of improvement, engaging and understanding others, creativity in improvement, process mapping, and demand and capacity.

QI support resources and training are also provided by the following organisations:

The Royal College of Paediatrics and Child Health (RCPCH) (2023): The RCPCH provides QI resources in child health and shares QI projects and posters in medicine, safety, patient-centred care and systems of care.

The Royal College of Physicians Quality Improvement (RCPQI) (2023): The RCPQI uses QI work within the RCP, including developing new infrastructure and approaches to support and promote continual improvement in the healthcare system.

The RCNi QI (2023): This QI framework supports nurses undertaking efficiency programmes and QI projects by enhancing their understanding of QI processes.

The Royal College of General Practitioners (RCGP) QI programme (2023): This programme is aimed at continued improvement in the quality of healthcare through focusing on the needs of service users. It uses an evidence-based approach, which helps primary care staff free up time to deliver initiatives and embed new approaches more effectively and efficiently into practice.

Royal College of Psychiatrists (RCP) QI (2023): This QI framework is aimed at improving the quality of care delivered to patients through best practices in the routine delivery of care, including improving service delivery for patients receiving mental health treatment.

The National Mental Health Act Quality Improvement programme (Public Service Consultants (PSC), 2023): The PSC puts principles of the Mental Health Act reforms into practice, to meet the needs of patients with mental health conditions.

QI processes helps staff best utilise their systems, organisations, talents and expertise to deliver better outcomes for patients (Table 5.3).

5.2.4 PALLIATIVE AND END-OF-LIFE CARE STUDY DAYS

Study days are usually provided by the palliative care team internally, to enable effective communication with patients, family members and other professionals; ensure effective advanced care planning and development of personalised palliative and end-of-life care (PEoLC) plans; and provide end-of-life symptom management for individuals.

5.2.5 MANAGEMENT DEVELOPMENT AND BESPOKE PROGRAMME

The **APPRECIATE** management programme covers communication, customer care, assertiveness, attitude, behaviour and a framework for addressing difficult situations, as detailed later in Table 5.4 on internal organisational leadership programmes.

5.2.5.1 Performance and Development Review

This review includes the use of tools such as Actus, which aids in setting specific, measurable, achievable, relevant and time-bound (SMART) objectives, in delivering mid-career and end of year career reviews, planning, and recording development and career aspiration goals and one-to-one meetings.

5.2.5.2 Recruitment and Selection Training

This training for managers covers the essential requirements of the recruitment and selection process, including those relating to fair and transparent recruitment, employment check standards and safer recruitment.

TABLE 5.3 ▪ **Sample QSIR Change Concepts Tool**

QSIR Change Concepts Tool: Guides to Improvement Concepts

Area of Focus	Area of Focus	Date Completed/ Progress/ Comments
Eliminating waste includes:	**Improving workflow includes:**	
Eliminating processes and systems that are not used or required to increase efficiency.	Synchronise and use automation in processes.	
Eliminate multiple entries related to activities such as documentation and use of electronic systems to reduce duplication and save time.	Schedule workflows into multiple processes to save time.	
Reducing or eliminating excess activities beyond what is required or suitable for duties being undertaken.	Minimise handing over activities to others to retain understanding of the background of the work at being undertaken and to save time.	
Reduce the controls on the system and processes to increase innovation.	Move steps in the process close together to reduce waiting time and maintaining momentum in activities.	
Recycle or reuse resources as suitable or required.	Find and remove bottlenecks, whic h are points in a process where the flow of work becomes delayed or breaks down completely.	
Use opportunities and situations as they occur to innovate and implement solutions in systems and processes.	Smooth workflow, which refers to the efficiency and effective flow of tasks and information within an organisation by optimising processes, eliminating bottlenecks and ensuring that work moves seamlessly through systems and processes.	
Reduce classifications and stratification in systems and process to enable flexibility in daily activities.		
Remove unnecessary intermediaries to processes to be completed quicker and smoother.	Perform tasks in parallel, where possible to reduce repetition and duplications in activities.	
Match demand and need to the service capacity to prevent backlogs in systems, processes and activities.	Ensure people in the same system are working together as a unit.	
Use sampling where required to test out new projects and programmes, so that process corrections can be made before full implementation.	Use multiple processing units based on the types of activities to reduce the overall length of time processes take to be completed.	
Change targets or objectives based on the progress made during process implementation.	Adjust work activities to meet and align with peak demand to reduce work pressure.	

(Continued)

TABLE 5.3 ■ Sample QSIR Change Concepts Tool—cont'd

QSIR Change Concepts Tool: Guides to Improvement Concepts

Area of Focus	Area of Focus	Date Completed/ Progress/ Comments
Change the work environment by: Giving people access to information regarding activities, systems and processes. Use the recommended standards and measures to reduce complexity and ensure that outcomes can be compared to each other. Ensure basic practices and principles are in place to lay the foundation for more innovative work. Reduce de-motivating aspects of pay systems by ensuring pay and wards systems are fully implemented. Conduct training on new and ongoing processes and activities Implement cross-training where multiple processes are aligned. Invest more resources in improvement and learning from audits and investigations. Focus on more patient care process and purpose to improve quality of care and services. Share risks across broaders systems and processes to increase to number of mitigation to reduce the risk. Emphasise natural and logical consequences as a result of the various processes used. Develop alliances/cooperative relationships with key individuals within and outside the organisation.	**Enhance the product and customer relationship by:** Listening to patients and service users and integrating their feedback in service delivery. Support patients and service users in service use through adequate provision of information and resources. Focus on patient safety, quality and health outcomes in designing improvements and innovations. Use a coordinator to manage and align process flows. Agree on expectations at the start of activities and process redesign. Gain 'free' of cost external input into product implementations and customer relationship by engaging individuals company and product representatives. Ensure regular inspections are embedded within processes so that findings can be addressed to improve outcomes. Work with suppliers in the implementation of their products and services to increase efficiency.	
Managing variation: Standardise improvements by creating formal processes which are implemented and embedded within the organisation. Develop operational definitions and criteria for people to use to ensure standardisation. Improve predictions in processes and services by setting forecost and objectives and putting processes in place to address them.	**Manage time by:** Reducing setup or startup time, through planning and organisation. Extend specialists' time to sure increased investment into more complex and technical areas. Reduce wait times through address key issues which affects waits. Reduce wait times	

TABLE 5.3 ▦ Sample QSIR Change Concepts Tool—cont'd

QSIR Change Concepts Tool: Guides to Improvement Concepts

Area of Focus	Area of Focus	Date Completed/ Progress/ Comments
Develop contingency plans, which can be implemented when there are breakdown in the processes or if there are periods of emergencies. Sort products into grades where required to ensure ease in selection and use. Review and explore variations so that processes can be implemented to ensure standardisation in service, systems and processes.		
Optimise inventory by: Matching inventory to predicted demand with supply. Use pulls systems and automation to manage stock rotation and use. Reduce choice of features to reduce decision and maximise use of the right products for the right purpose. Reduce multiple brands of the same items to ensure ease in selection and use.	**Design systems to avoid mistakes, by using:** Reminders and automation. Differentiations, by specifying the difference between products and services used. Constraints, limitation or restriction on products or services which should not be used in certain instances. Affordances, which is the features of products and services that prompts or promotes a specific use or interaction.	
Focus on the patient and the service and user by: Mass customisation of products and services. Offer products and services any time and place to ensure maximum access. Influence or take advantage of seasonal trends, to increase uptake. Reduce the number of components in products and services used by patients to ensure ease of use. Address defects or problems with systems and processes to improve patients and service users experience. Differentiate services and resources by using quality dimensions to ensure ease of use.	**Staff support and engagement by:** Supporting staff health and well-being by ensuring access to resources which balances home-life with work-life. Provide staff with resources they need to undertake the duties they are allocated. Provide administrative and Project management office (PMO) support to maximise service outcomes.	

(Continued)

TABLE 5.3 ■ Sample QSIR Change Concepts Tool—cont'd

QSIR Change Concepts Tool: Guides to Improvement Concepts

Area of Focus	Area of Focus	Date Completed/ Progress/ Comments
Change the order of process steps to improve access, where the current process is not working. Manage uncertainty in tasks to improve experience, use and access.		
Staff name:..Date completed:......................................		

Modified from Act Academy. (2023). QSIR practitioner programme: Change concepts. In G. L. Lanely, R. Moen, K. M. Nolan, et al. (Eds.). (2009). *The improvement guide* (2nd ed., pp. 357–408). San Francisco: Jossey-Bass Publishers.

TABLE 5.4 ■ Internal Organisational Leadership Programmes

Development programmes include
Becoming an outstanding manager.
Band 2–5 development programmes.
Band 6–7 staff progression course.
Trust board development.
Divisional director and assistant managing director leadership programme.
Divisional triumvirate programmes.
Clinical leads and clinical directors' programme.
Senior leader programme.
Senior service line management development programme.
Management development programme.
Leadership and partnership working short course.
Short course in using patient feedback and insight to transform services.
Short course in professional development.

Apprenticeship training includes
Nursing, midwifery, radiography, AHP, business administration; medical administration; human resources support; finance and budgeting; perioperative support; pharmacy; customer service; healthcare support; engineering; digital and technology solutions; data analysis; estates/infrastructure; and healthcare science or engineering.

Internal learning and development directory
The internal learning and development directory lists further career pathways, new starter support and opportunities regarding apprenticeships; foundation degrees in health; flexible nursing and nursing associate courses; improving patients' and carers' experience; budget and finance management; human resources and workforce information; report and business case writing; conducting investigations and disciplinary reviews; managing change; and leadership and management skills.

TABLE 5.4 ■ Internal Organisational Leadership Programmes—cont'd

APPRECIATE Tool

Good People Management Guide: raise managers' awareness of the importance of practising the basics of good people management.

Aims: agree upon **aims**, **purpose**, **priorities** and **SMART objectives** with staff, covering the fundamentals of management and effective leadership.

Performance management: review performance for successful people management, including learning and development based on shared understanding; strategic, integrated involvement; development; managing behaviours; and using tools such as appraisals to support performance management.

Personal and professional development: ensure development and growth, including coaching, mentoring, action learning sets (group learning to resolve issues), masterclasses, technical training, psychometrics and personality review with tools such as MBTI (Myers-Briggs Foundation, 2023), secondments and learning opportunities on the job.

Recognition: recognise good work and celebrate success, including noticing staff actions and praising their work; promoting a culture of recognising a job well done; and using rewards and recognition schemes (e.g. annual trust awards; monthly chief executives' excellence awards; monthly executive nursing awards; long service awards; successful achievement awards; leadership awards; behind the scenes awards; customer service awards; quality, safety and cost improvement awards; patients' choice awards; the chairman's cup; and service improvement awards).

Empowerment: empower staff to make decisions and take actions by ensuring that team members have opportunities to act autonomously; avoiding micromanaging or overmonitoring; being clear regarding responsibilities and delegated duties; encouraging staff to find their own solutions; adopting a no-blame culture; and managing challenging situations well.

Communication: ensure effective communication and negotiation, have regular one-on-one meetings with staff, be sensitive to staff concerns, actively support staff health and well-being, hold regular meetings, elicit feedback from senior team briefings, conduct effective appraisals and conversations with staff, and recognise and manage stress.

Involvement: be involved in decision-making affecting staff work, seek input when making decisions on how to achieve goals in the department, ask staff about situations affecting their teams and services, manage teams through change and encourage staff to find their own solutions.

Accountability in team **management** and **development**: take accountability for the delivery of objectives and outcomes, and model accountability for one's own behaviour; recognise staff who take ownership of their work and outcomes; hold staff accountable to their role objectives; and seek continuing improvement the team, service and self.

Teamwork: ensure effective team development activities, so that team members have a clear sense of purpose; hold regular meetings; ensure clear understanding of roles; use the available teamwork tools and development opportunities; value team members' strengths and respect their weaknesses; share knowledge and experiences; and use a range of skills in the team to effectively perform tasks (foundations for effective teams also include real team interdependencies, membership and development).

Environment and equipment: ensure health and safety in the job by promoting a positive culture and eliminating harassment and bullying.

Modified from NHS Leadership Academy. (2023d). *Programmes to help you grow as a leader*. https://www.leadershipacademy.nhs.uk/programmes/. Accessed 31 October 2023.

5.2.5.3 Human Resources Policy and Procedure Workshops

These workshops are for new managers seeking to refresh their management knowledge and skills, to improve their confidence in managing, and to enhance team performance.

5.2.5.4 Training on Managing Grievances, Bullying and Harassment in the Workplace

This is aimed at increasing managers' awareness and ability to address grievances, bullying and harassment in work settings. Topics include ways of enabling informal resolution before formal disciplinary action, understanding the roles of staff representatives, investigating complaints and resolving disputes.

5.2.5.5 Training on Managing Capabilities and Conduct

This training provides skills and knowledge to manage capabilities and conduct, including monitoring and reviews to address performance issues. The disciplinary process should be used appropriately, including ensuring that appropriate investigation is conducted before disciplinary action is considered.

5.2.5.6 Sickness Absence and Attendance Management

This training includes use of systems, such as first care absence management systems, to manage long- and short-term sickness and absences, including using the resources provided by the occupational health department, undertaking return to work interviews as needed and considering the Disability Discrimination Act regarding how disability affects sickness management.

5.2.5.7 Managing Workplace Investigations

When required, investigations should be held to establish the facts of individual cases and grounds for formal hearings, as necessary, to enable fair investigation, ensure equality and avoid discrimination.

5.2.5.8 Bespoke Development for Managers and Teams

The Aston Team Performance Inventory (ATPI) (Aston Organisational Development, 2023) measures effective teamwork, thus leading to the delivery of high-quality patient care, improving innovation, decreasing mortality and avoiding errors. The Myers-Briggs Type Indicator (MBTI) (The Myers-Briggs Company, 2023) is a self-reported questionnaire for assessing personality type and increasing self-awareness, thereby enabling teams to work with individuals' personality types.

5.2.5.9 Coaching

Coaching is an effective way of way of helping individuals develop new attitudes and behaviours; build confidence; enhance their leadership skills, potential and growth; and develop skills for practice, such as assertiveness, prioritisation, interpersonal awareness and communication. Coaching is often available internally to organisations and can help achieve individual and organisational goals by identifying clear aims that are measured against expected outcomes. Leadership coaching by external providers is detailed in

Section 7.9 on coaching for leadership, through partnership with the NHS Leadership Academy and other providers.

5.2.5.10 Healthcare Leadership Framework

These efforts are facilitated by a 360-degree framework, a tool used to identify leadership strengths and areas for development through feedback from peers, direct reports and managers, as also detailed in the NHS Leadership Academy (2023d) resources. The process is supported by leadership training, as also detailed in Section 5.2.6 on mid-career leadership programmes and Section 7.5 on ward and department manager leadership development programmes.

5.2.5.11 Apprenticeships Schemes

Apprenticeship schemes are available in various forms and settings for adults and young adults, to create career pathways for key professional groups, and develop a motivated and skilled workforce. Apprenticeships allow staff to learn on the job, build knowledge and skills, and gain qualifications and apprenticeship framework completion while earning a salary.

Apprenticeship training includes academic leadership and management through the apprenticeship levy, at levels 3, 4 and 5. The NHS Leadership Academy works with apprenticeship providers to offer access to leadership development programmes as part of apprenticeships (NHS Leadership Academy, 2023c). Apprenticeship is also detailed in Table 5.4 on internal organisational leadership programmes; Section 5.2.12.5 on new career pathways for nursing support workers; and Section 5.2.12.13 on training routes to NHS careers.

5.2.5.12 Bespoke Learning Activities and Planning for Retirement

These activities are for staff thinking about retirement, to consider options for lifestyle changes, post-retirement opportunities such as interim work and consultancy, development of new skills, financial options and updated pension information.

5.2.5.13 Healthcare Assistant Training and Development Programme

The Qualifications and Credit Framework (QCF) and National Vocational Qualification are often provided as part of internal organisational healthcare assistant (HCA) training and development programmes.

5.2.5.14 Other Training Provisions by Organisations

The learning and development team provides general information and resources to facilitate continuing professional development (CPD), which contributes to competent practice. This training is provided at post-registration and vocational levels, thereby supporting staff in identifying and fulfilling their potential, and ensuring safe quality care for patients in ever-changing work environments. **These additional educational programmes include the following**:
- Intravenous therapy and central line care
- HCA training for new starters with certificate on completion

- Preceptorship programme for newly qualified staff nurses
- Deteriorating patient study day
- Cannulation
- Venipuncture
- Twelve-lead electrocardiography

Workshops are also provided, including:
- Work-based learning with a practice educator
- NMC revalidation guidance and support
- Competency packages
- Evidence-based learning packages
- Packages for new staff wanting to use skills in intravenous therapy, cannulation and venipuncture gained elsewhere
- Mentorship updates

Specialist study days are also available on:
- Blood glucose monitoring
- Catheter care
- Dementia
- Tissue viability (TV) and pressure ulcer prevention study days

These training programmes are often co-ordinated by organisations' training and development teams. They may be available online via intranet under the training and development section, where staff can search for and book selected training to remain updated, extent their knowledge and skills, and undertake personal development. Team development opportunities may also be provided through methods such as The Aston Tool (Aston Organisational Development, 2023), which assist with support and development of managers to embed best practice. Principles such as APPRECIATE (as detailed in Table 5.4) in internal organisational leadership programmes can be used to ensure good people management. These programmes provide useful resources to help individuals and managers meet training and development needs.

5.2.5.15 Postgraduate Training Centre Resources

These resources include providing venues for educational events for all health professionals, including staff presentations, tutoring, grand rounds, Schwartz rounds, SWARM (patient safety processes), study days, courses, teaching and videoconferencing.

5.2.5.16 Library Information Service

This service includes details regarding health information skills training and provides information on database searching for evidence-based practice and research purposes, to help staff remain up to date. Further details can be found in the internal library information service.

Training and development resources on the following are included:
- NHS careers at (NHS, 2022j)
- Working for Department of Health and Social Care (DHSC) (2023b)
- NHS 'experience' opportunities (Health Education England (HEE), 2023f)
- Work experience and work-related learning activity (HEE, 2023f)
- Healthcare careers (National Careers Service, 2023)
- UK universities' websites

5.2.6 MID-CAREER LEADERSHIP PROGRAMMES

These programmes are designed to help all staff in the NHS discover their full leadership potential and achieve the highest standards in health and care. The mid-career pathway to director roles should incorporate roles and settings outside previous career experience, to incorporate 'stretch experience' beyond that in the normal working environment in addition to increasing seniority/responsibility. Examples include undertaking leadership projects, operational roles or secondments. A trusted, experienced mentor who can effectively provide career coaching should be identified. Some national programmes that can aid in mid-career pathway progression are detailed in Table 5.5.

TABLE 5.5 ▦ **National Programmes for Mid-Career Pathway Progression**

Edward Jenner Programme

This programme supports staff preparing for their first leadership or management role and builds foundation-level leadership skills for staff. A self-guided suite of short courses is available online with interactive discussions (NHS Leadership Academy, 2023d).

Mary Seacole Programme

This programme is also for staff in their first leadership role. The Mary Seacole programme develops knowledge and skills in leadership and management, through 100 hours of online learning plus three behavioural workshops (NHS Leadership Academy, 2023d).

Rosalind Franklin Programme

This programme is for mid-level leaders aspiring to lead large and complex programmes, departments, services or systems. The training includes 120 hours of online learning, 4 days of workshops and small group work (NHS Leadership Academy, 2023d).

Elizabeth Garrett Anderson Programme

This programme for middle to senior leaders helps staff challenge the status quo, drive lasting change and prepare for senior roles. The training includes a 24-month programme leading to an MSc in healthcare leadership (NHS Leadership Academy, 2023d).

Foundations in System Leadership; Collaborating in Health and Care

This programme is for people working in health and care who want to improve the ways in which they collaborate across organisational and professional boundaries, to design and deliver better health outcomes (NHS Leadership Academy, 2023d).

Core Managers: Developing Inclusive Workplaces Programme

This programme is for managers or supervisors in health and care seeking to develop inclusive leadership skills. It includes a suite of self-guided online short courses (NHS Leadership Academy, 2023d).

Sustainability Leadership for Greener Health and Care Programme

This programme is for staff seeking to develop their leadership skills and knowledge, to build a more environmentally friendly and sustainable health system. This 16-week programme includes a choice of online learning or face-to-face learning (NHS Leadership Academy, 2023d).

Hope (Hospitals of Europe) European Exchange Programme

This exchange programme offers NHS staff leadership positions and with managerial responsibilities in healthcare a unique opportunity to swap roles with an EU member state for 4 weeks (NHS Leadership Academy, 2023d), to understand the challenges in healthcare systems outside the UK.

(Continued)

TABLE 5.5 ▦ National Programmes for Mid-Career Pathway Progression—cont'd

Development Support for Clinical Leaders

Development support for clinical leaders includes schemes, forums and resources to ensure that clinicians at every level have career development pathways to develop the skills they need (NHS Leadership Academy, 2023f, 2023d).

NHS Graduate Management Scheme

The NHS Graduate Management Scheme contributes to leading teams and driving change at the heart of the NHS. It enables staff to develop the skills to innovate, undertake project management, inspire others and support the vision for the future (NHS Graduate Management Training Scheme (GMTS), 2023). The GMTS applications open yearly and staff can register and apply to join the programme.

Coaching and Mentoring

Coaching and mentoring (as detailed in Section 5.2.5.9 on coaching, Table 7.12 on coaching for leadership and Section 5.3.7 on mentoring) are helpful tools supporting health and care leadership development. Staff can review or sign up with the Coaching and Mentoring Register and explore offerings from the NHS Leadership Academy (2023e).Section 5.3.7

From NHS Leadership Academy. (2023d). *Programmes to help you grow as a leader*. https:// www.leadershipacademy.nhs.uk/programmes/. Accessed 31 October 2023.

5.2.7 INTERNAL ORGANISATIONAL MANAGEMENT PROGRAMMES

Table 5.4 includes internal organisational management programmes for good people management, which correlates with high-quality patient care.

The **aspirant-director career pathway** should usually include a deputy or equivalent role within the chief nurse/DON and DOM infrastructure. The DON/DOM infrastructure in organisations should be designed with sufficient roles according to portfolio complexity, so that the pipeline to directorship includes individuals who have led system-wide or trust-wide improvement efforts.

Aspirant directors'benefit from seeking mentors/sponsors outside their current organisations and should be encouraged to invest time and energy in networking. The chief nurse/DON and DOM career pathway (Fig. 5.2) (NHS, 2021) involves knowledge, experience and skills development; accessing support; and heightened leadership thinking. Achievement of a master's degree (MSc) and a leadership programme, such as the Nye Bevan programme (NHS Leadership Academy, 2023d) from the NHS Leadership Academy, is required for aspirant DONs/DOMs, in preparation for the increasingly complex and ambiguous leadership responsibilities inherent at the director level.

Talent management for director-level appointments should assess aspirant directors' potential to advance in the executive director pathway (NHS Leadership Academy, 2023g) or similar aspirant-director programmes including the Florence Nightingale Foundation (2023a) Leadership Programmes and the Aspiring Mental Health Nurse Directors Programme (NHS Confederation, 2023).

5.2.8 DIRECTOR LEADERSHIP PROGRAMMES

The director leadership programmes (Table 5.6) are for senior executive level leaders and directors seeking further development and support. These programmes support individuals who are undertaking stretch assignments involving thinking differently; being challenged in new areas of leadership; and developing, adapting, enhancing and broadening their leadership style (Box 5.1).

5.2.9 EXECUTIVE DIRECTOR OF BOARD LEVEL LEARNING AND DEVELOPMENT OPPORTUNITIES

Executive director development programmes are detailed in Table 5.7. The contents include board director support offers, and programmes and networks from other

---

TABLE 5.6 ■ **Director Leadership Programmes**

Nye Bevan Programme

Accelerates movement towards executive roles spanning organisational boundaries and supports senior leaders to move beyond leadership within their areas of expertise (NHS Leadership Academy, 2023d)

Aspiring and current executive directors

Aimed at the development of aspiring and current executive directors, to enable them to reach their full potential

Aspiring chief executive officer programme

Aimed at senior leaders aspiring to lead at the CEO level in an NHS accountable role focused on both service provision and system development, within the next 12–24 months (NHS Leadership Academy, 2023h)

Senior executive programme

Helps staff challenge their thinking and reignite their ambition through a flagship executive development programme designed for senior leaders with an average of 15–20 years' management experience (London Business School, 2023).

Executive director pathway

A talent scheme for individuals demonstrating high potential and interest in becoming an executive director on an NHS Provider Trust Board within the next 12–24 months (NHS Leadership Academy, 2023g).

BOX 5.1   Executive Director Pathway (EDP): Personal Testimony

The EDP programme has been transformational. I was new in my first Director of Nursing role and needed both the challenge and the support the programme offered. The programme is innovative, enabling me to develop as a leader, through reflecting on my leadership, personal resilience, with the values of supportive feedback and excellent facilitation.

The EDP also offers a combination of shared learning and leadership experience, coaching and mentoring, developing my leadership and growing in my role.

Director of Nursing

TABLE 5.7 ■ **Executive Directory of Board Level Learning and Development Opportunities**

These offers, if provided for NHS staff and wider healthcare organisations, may cover **chief executive development network**

Designed to support chief executives with their development and ensure that they achieve the best possible performance in these challenging roles, for themselves and for patient care (NHS Leadership Academy, 2023i).

Collaborate Well Podcast for all board directors and chairs

Resources for examining and sharing learning in integrated care system (ICS) development. Series of podcasts and webinars in topics including clinical leadership, complex needs and inequalities.

Healthcare financial management for board members.
Assortment of resources and learning, including bite-sized sessions.
Support for roles working in NHS finance at the board level.
Provided by the Healthcare Financial Management Association.

Disabled NHS Directors Network for all board roles including chairs
Designed for executives and nonexecutives; provides mentoring and coaching support to strengthen collective impact and voice of the network of leaders with disabilities.
Toolkit commissioned for recruitment and retention of nonexecutive directors with disabilities for boards.

Explore and rethink the new CEO lens
Resources to support the first 100 days in the role, in three modules:
Transitioning into the role.
Systems leadership.
Leading an effective executive team.

First time chief executive/CEO programme
Peer support and development for first time CEOs.
Bi-monthly meetings with national leaders from across the system.

Chief executives/new CEO development network
Three 2-day development days per annum.
Access to online resources.
Meetings with a dedicated transition coach twice yearly, including an initial welcome into the network and subsequently aiding in progression of a personal learning agenda and shaping network events.

Peer-to-peer support for new CEOs
Support for new and experienced CEOs.
Confidential and practical support, and peer-to-peer relationship.

Transition coaching for new CEOs
Access and support to a dedicated transition coach, to provide a welcome to the network, help progress personal learning agenda and shape network events.
Provided by the NHS Leadership Academy.

Collaborate Well Podcast for CEOs
Resources examining and sharing learning regarding ICS development.
Series of podcasts and webinars in topics including clinical leadership, complex needs and inequalities.
Provided by the NHS Leadership Academy.

TABLE 5.7 ■ **Executive Directory of Board Level Learning and Development Opportunities—cont'd**

Mentoring offer for all NHS chairs and CEOs
Mentoring from experienced former NHS chairs and CEOs provided to current NHS chairs and CEOs.
Provided by the NHS Leadership Academy.

Network run by NHS Providers, chairs, CEOs and nonexecutive directors (NEDs) of NHS trusts and foundation trusts.
National networking events for NHS board members, who meet several times per year, including one network run by NHS Providers for members.
Includes events specifically designed to help members obtain necessary information, guidance and inspiration.

Onboarding for new chairs, as part of the NHS Providers board development
Onboarding event; 6-month induction programme.
Chair mentoring support network.
Provided by NHS Providers.

Chair Development Network, for **chairs**
The **Chair Development Network** (**CHADN**) is designed to provide personalised, flexible and accessible learning, and offers the following core elements:
Three 2-day network meeting days per annum.
Access to online resources.
Access to coaching and mentoring.**coachingmentoring**
Dedicated transition coach for first-time chairs.
Provided by the NHS Leadership Academy.

Aspirant chair programme, for current NEDs aspiring to a chair role
New programme for current NEDs ready to assume chair roles in the next 12–18 months, aimed at supporting a strong, diverse pipeline of candidates for chairs on NHS Provider boards.
Provided by the NHS Leadership Academy.

Network for all BAME NEDs and NHS chairs
Designed for aspiring/existing **NEDs** with **BAME** backgrounds.
Associate membership open to NEDs with other backgrounds who are interested in learning about and supporting the objectives of the group.
Provided by the Seacole Group | National Network for Black, Asian and Other Ethnic NEDS and Chairs in the NHS.

Programme for first time chief finance officers (CFOs) and directors of finance
Designed to support and provide new leaders in their first year with the knowledge and skills required to become high-performing directors

Healthcare financial management for existing board level leaders
Offers to support financial skills for NEDs.
Provision of an assortment of resources and learning.
Provision of support for roles working in NHS finance at the board level.
Provided by Healthcare Financial Management Association.

Nonexecutive leader networks
Arrangement of networks **for non-executive leaders** across health sectors, including mental health chairs, independent ICS chairs and community chairs.
Provided by NHS Confederation.

(Continued)

TABLE 5.7 ▪ **Executive Directory of Board Level Learning and Development Opportunities—cont'd**

Senior leader onboarding for NEDs
A range of resources for new and existing NEDs, including:
NED competencies and appraisal, values and behaviours support, and further reading.
Induction, development framework, governance and support offer.
Designed as a support resource for newly appointed board members in the first year of the role.
Provided by NHS Leadership Academy.
Resources include new NED and chair competencies and appraisals via NHS senior leadership onboarding and support.

NExT director programme for aspiring NEDs and new NEDs of NHS trusts
A 6–12-month programme providing insights into the roles and responsibilities, bridging knowledge gaps and supporting better performance at future NED interviews.**interview**
Provision of support to individuals from under-represented groups on trust boards with the skills and expertise to navigate the NHS boardroom.
NED essential 1-day induction; face-to-face and virtual options.
Provided by the NHS People and Culture Board Level Development and Careers.
Developed to provide deeper understanding of board roles.

Programmes and networks from other organisations
Offers from organisations aligned with healthcare, or offering executive education and support with connections to the public sector:

Strategic clinical leaders/The King's Fund, for board level clinical leaders
Designed for senior clinical and professional leaders (medical directors, chief nursing officers or similar levels).
Learning includes expert insight/challenge, reflection, critical knowledge and problem solving.

Building collaborative leadership across health and care organisations, for senior leaders working in systems/The King's Fund.
Enables senior leaders to collaborate in the newly integrated health and care landscape.
Provides participants with an opportunity to consider how to best lead ICSs.

Release Your Potential: A Programme for New Leaders, for staff new to **leadership** and senior managers aspiring to board level positions.
For aspiring leaders across health, social care, voluntary, third sector and public health
Provided by The King's Fund.

Clinical directors and lead clinicians, for existing **clinical directors**, lead clinicians and those stepping into roles or considering them.
Addresses the knowledge, skills and behaviours needed to lead both operationally and strategically as a clinical director or lead clinician.
Provided by The King's Fund.

Top Manager Programme for senior people in health and social care, public, private and third sector for existing directors.
Focus on connecting with and creating shared purpose, and developing the political and emotional intelligence necessary for leadership in senior roles in an increasingly demanding environments.
Provided by The King's Fund.

TABLE 5.7 ■ **Executive Directory of Board Level Learning and Development Opportunities—cont'd**

The Circles Programme: Leadership Development and online speaker series for women leaders of all levels.
Designed regardless of role or experience, to respond to the leadership challenges facing women.
Open to diverse under-represented groups.
Provided by The King's Fund.

Health and social care integration webinar for CEOs and chairs.
Series of webinars examining ICS **development**, sharing good practices and learning.
Provided by Social Care Institute for Excellence, through integration with NHS England.

CEO and **deputy CEO programme**, for CEOs and deputies.
Short courses and programmes to develop skills, knowledge and networks for CEOs, deputy CEOs and their equivalents in public service.
Provided by The Civil Service College.

The IGNITE leadership programme for new and existing CEOs
Aims to build stronger relationships with peers to support deeper collaboration across local government and within systems.
Provided by The Local Government Association.

The Future Vision programme for existing board level leaders
Delivered by Leadership Centre and the Birmingham Leadership Institute.
Offers development for senior leaders recognise that their knowledge and leadership are not sufficient to address the challenges faced.
Provided by The Leadership Centre.

Onboarding support
Curated resources for newly appointed executive directors, including articles, videos and podcasts in areas such as setting strategy and delivering long term transformation; further information on senior leader onboarding and support is available on the NHS Leadership Academy (2023j) website.

From NHS England. (2023w). *Directory of board level learning and development opportunities*. https://www.england.nhs.uk/long-read/directory-of-board-level-learning-and-development-opportunities/. Accessed 2 August 2023.

organisations. These resources for health and care leaders and aspiring directors help develop staff and prepare them for board level roles, and includes a directory of support offers for executive and nonexecutive board directors. These offers should be considered against a set of quality assurance criteria. The list is not exhaustive and supplements support offers detailed in other sections of this book. Inclusivity and equality of access should be considered for all programmes, so that all relevant staff are aware of and can access these opportunities.

5.2.10 DIRECTOR OF NURSING AND DIRECTOR OF MIDWIFERY ROLES

Key themes in vertical learning include operating at the board level; structural/health inequalities and inclusive leadership; health and well-being of self, staff and the workforce; professional work; workforce; working across organisations and sectors; director portfolio delivery; and the contributions of nursing/midwifery to quality. New DONs and DOMs benefit from 'wrap around' support including access to a trusted and experienced director level mentor (external to their organisation), peer group/action learning set quarterly meetings during the first year in the post which involves group of people solving workplace problems together, coaching, and ICS and regional collegiate support (NHS, 2021).

The use of a nursing and midwifery directors' alumni network aids in strengthening and amplifying the nursing and midwifery leadership voice at the board and system level. Such networks may be developed in collaboration with appropriate agencies, e.g. the NHS Leadership Academy, and have clear links to the Chief Nursing Officer England and Chief Midwifery Officer England infrastructure, thus providing a potential venue to share opportunities for seniors with challenging projects and posts (NHS, 2021).

Equality, diversity and inclusion should be embedded in the chief nurse/DON and DOM roles. Nursing and midwifery talent management should be informed by the lived experience of staff, and leaders should reflect the diversity of the communities they serve. Nursing and midwifery leaders must have self-awareness and openness to think creatively about their talent spotting and succession planning (NHS, 2021).

ICS chief nurse role holders should have previous director level achievement, have broad experience in healthcare work and have demonstrated collaborative relationships with other agencies for leadership in population health improvement (NHS, 2021).

In developing the DON/chief nurse framework beyond the provider DON/chief nurse career framework, the full diversity of talent for these important system leadership roles is a major success factor that must be ensured. Chief Nursing Officer England offers executive clinical fellowships as part of the career framework bridge for directors who are considering an ICS chief nurse or other similar role in their future career progression (NHS, 2021).

During the first year in the role, ICS chief nurses should have access to a development programme of strategic leadership masterclasses, experiential learning in areas in which they may lack familiarity (e.g. local authority social care provision) for a minimum of 30 days, executive coaching, access to a transformational partnership (buddying with an ICS chief nurse with different experience), peer regional groups and organisation development accessed as a member of an ICS executive team (NHS, 2021).

The chief nurse/DON and midwifery career pathway framework encompasses roles extending beyond large provider level director, including ICS chief nurse, and regional and national strategic roles, e.g. chief nurse/chief midwife. Staff within the career pathway should also consider roles outside nursing and midwifery in which their expertise and transferable skills are also valued, including many senior roles (e.g. chief operating officer, CEO and national workforce leadership) (NHS, 2021). These roles are associated with the health and care nursing and midwifery strategies outlined in Table 5.8.

TABLE 5.8 ■ **Health and Care Nursing and Midwifery Strategies**

Health and care strategies are supported by the nursing and midwifery strategy, and are key items in the chief nurse role and duties, which ensure optimal care delivery, as described below:

Leadership development integration and collaboration.

Professional and workforce development, including health and well-being; equality, diversity and inclusion; recruitment and retention; professional auditing, revalidation and professionalism in line with NMC code; and practice development.

Education, teaching and training strategy for staff.

Quality and safety culture of openness and assurance; delivered with project management, legal services, complaints, incident management, risk management, clinical auditing, human factor team, and continuous improvement and learning.

Safeguarding and harm free care, including safeguarding for children and adults, MCA/DOLS, learning disabilities and autism, tissue viability and falls.

Infection prevention and control.

Research and development, including clinical academic careers.

Patient experience and engagement: patient involvement, staff satisfaction, clinical effectiveness, voluntary service, bereavement, spiritual and pastoral care, and PALs in the delivery of care.

Digital and innovation in delivering excellent, modern health and care.

Raising the profile of the health and care workforce through advancing practice, publications and conference presentations.

5.2.11 TESTIMONIAL FROM A PARTICIPANT WHO COMPLETED A DIRECTOR'S PROGRAMME (BOX 5.2)

5.2.11.1 Executive Director of Performance and Improvement Role

Further examples and descriptions of executive directors, such as DON, chief nurse, DOM, chief AHP, chief executive and chairs, are outlined later. A **typical recruitment pack** for this type of role covers the context of the role appointment, including the following:

Introduction: number of staff in the organisation, population served, speciality and type of services delivered

Background: CQC rating of the trust, performance and achievements, financial position, trust strategies and forward planning, and how recruitment for the role is being performed to support the delivery of these aspects; includes an outline of the organisation's values, safety, quality and culture.

Current context of the role: indication of the level of care being delivered, presented through operational, financial and national performance metrics/dashboards, such as A&E waiting times.

Opportunity: covers operational leadership, financial performance, developing systems and staff for the future.

About the candidate required: requirement for a mix of substantial leadership experience in hospital operational management; a strategic mindset; and the ability to develop, sell and implement innovative systems and processes.

BOX 5.2	Director's Programme Testimonial

I cannot recommend the director programme enough. The combination of impact group, the experience and knowledgeable facilitation and the focussed space away from my work environment have given me excellent insights. I have directly applied it to my role and grown as a result. I have learned a great deal and enjoyed it immensely.

Director of Integrated Care

Job description: responsibility for the overall clinical performance of the trust, development and delivery of trust strategy and plans; and delivery of clinical innovation, operational improvement and transformation.

Person specification: requirements for the role, including degree, ongoing CPD, postgraduate management qualification, such as master of business administration (MBA) or MSc, along with knowledge, experience, skills, personal disposition, behaviour and other criteria.

Trust profile and strategy: information on saving lives, improving lives and the strategic direction of the organisation, including improving health and well-being for the people and population of the organisation; the organisation's vision may include providing safe, clean and personal care to the population served.

Board: includes information on the trust board, including the chair, CEO, executive directors, NEDs and other members, including their biographies and experience.

Further information: provides reference to information on the trust website, NHSE, CQC, how to arrange a visit, and academies and universities associated with the organisation.

Timetable and application process: covers the application process for the job, including the advertisement opening date, closing date, long listing, short listing, preliminary one-on-one interviews with the executive team, assessment centre, psychometric assessment (personality, verbal and numeric reasoning tests), reference taking and pre-panel interview preparation provided by NHS Executive Search.

Final selection process: **interview** plus presentation to the interview panel including the chair, CEO, NED and independent expert.

Equal opportunities monitoring form: form completed by the candidate to provide diversity monitoring for equal opportunities.

Fit and proper person requirement: completed by candidates to confirm that they meet the standard required for the role (modified from the NHS Leadership Academy, 2023d).NHS Leadership Academy, 2023d

These **leadership programmes** help meet the demand for talented and capable leaders in healthcare through specific and demonstrated developmental pathways, thus developing outstanding leaders who positively inspire others to do the best they can to improve health, patient care, treatment, experience and sustainability, through staff and patient engagement.

Organisations benefit from filling of healthcare leadership gaps and the creation of a pool of strong candidates who are ready to take on demanding senior roles.

5.2.12 STUDY PATHWAYS FOR NURSES, MIDWIVES, NURSING ASSOCIATES AND AHPs

Numerous study pathways (Fig. 5.3) are available in the UK for nurses, midwives, nursing associates and AHPs, as detailed in the following sections.

5.2.12.1 Nursing Degree Qualification/Registered Nurse

The standard 3-year BSc (Hons) nursing (adult) (Buckinghamshire New University, 2023) involves individual study of nursing at a university or other higher education setting, to develop the combined theory and practice required to provide safe, compassionate care and become a qualified nurse. Additional qualifications can be undertaken, including an MSc degree in IPC, leadership, management or advanced practice, followed by a doctorate in areas of interest, such as public health.

5.2.12.2 Midwifery Qualification/Registered Midwife

To become a midwife (Royal College of Nursing, 2023g), individuals need a degree in midwifery which takes three years to complete. Staff who are already a registered adult nurse can undertake a shorter course instead, which takes 18 months.

5.2.12.3 Health Visitor Qualification

5.2.12.3.1 Becoming a health visitor: Institute of Health Visiting, Excellence in Practice

To become a health visitor, individuals must be a qualified nurse or midwife, then undertake a 1-year (52 week) full-time or 2-year (104 week) part-time programme to qualify as a registered specialist community public health nurse (health visitor) (Institute of Health Visiting, 2023a).

5.2.12.4 Research Careers Through the National Institutes for Health and Care Research

The National Institutes for Health and Care Research help provide clinical academic training for nurses, midwives, AHPs and other health and care professionals in the UK, including instruction on principles and obligations (National Institutes for Health and Care Research, 2023a). Research careers and positions for which staff may apply are outlined by the Florence Nightingale Foundation Chair in Clinical Nursing Practice Research (The University of Manchester, 2023).

Florence Nightingale Foundation Chair in Clinical Nursing Practice Research: This chair includes duties of leading clinically applied research and developing and implementing strategies, policies, practices and pathways across hospital and community services and settings, to facilitate the delivery of outstanding patient care, partly through accessing and using research grants. The quality-of-care delivery to patients is enhanced through the advancement of clinical research and the development of clinical evidence-based practice, through aligning the priorities of the national nursing and

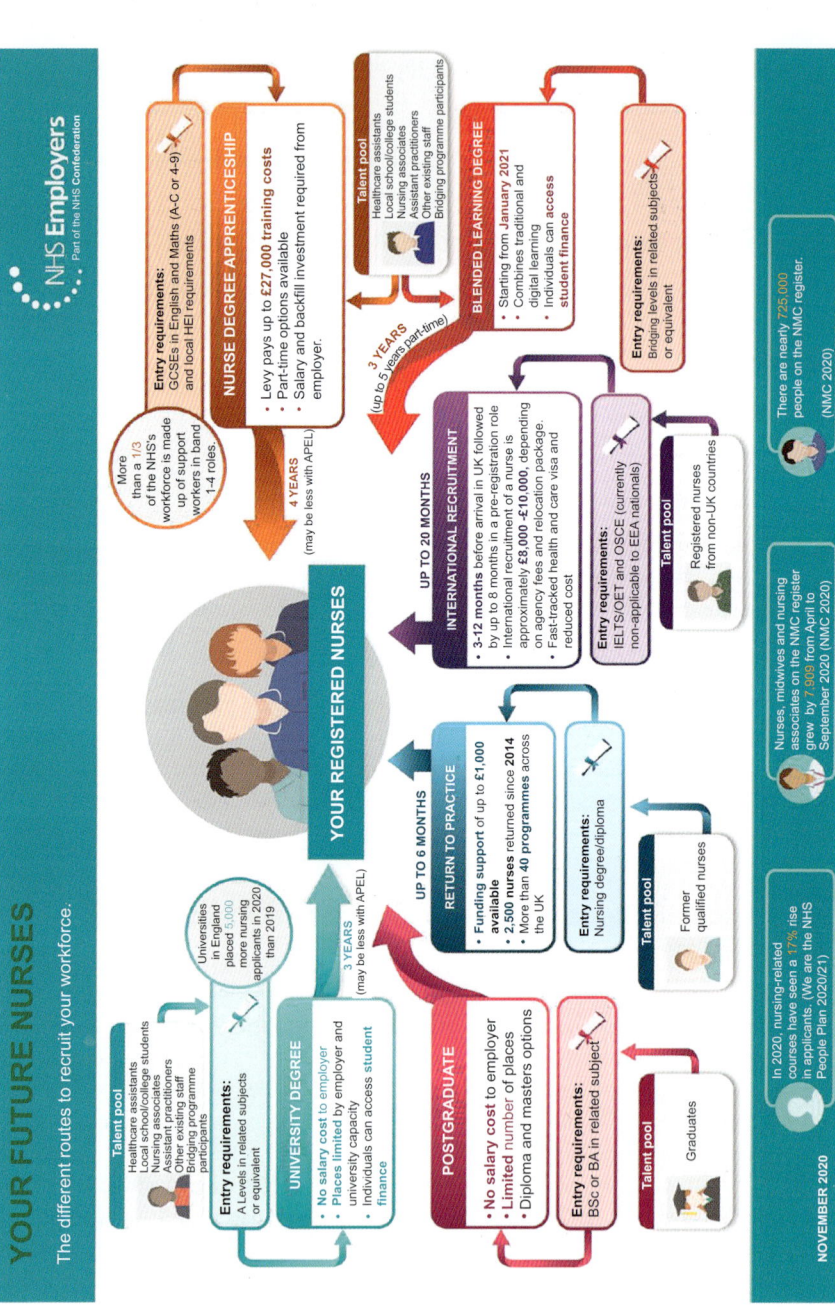

Fig. 5.3 Study pathways for nurses, midwives, nursing associates and AHPs. (With permission from NHS Employers. (2023a). The different routes to recruit your nursing workforce and increase your nursing supply. https://www.nhsemployers.org/articles/your-future-nurses. Accessed 10 July 2024.)

midwifery strategy and the national nursing research strategy. Efforts include building nursing and midwifery research strategies leading to change and improving value, and increasing the provision of clinical academic careers and leadership in research. Other joint clinical research roles include chair in clinical nursing practice research at universities or organisations such as the Florence Nightingale Foundation, where staff can improve clinical practice while undertaking research (The University of Manchester, 2023).

5.2.12.5 New Career Pathways for Nursing Support Workers

New career pathways for nursing support workers, such as nursing apprenticeships, and nursing associate and assistant roles, are open to HCAs or healthcare support workers (Royal College of Nursing, 2023h).

5.2.12.6 Nursing Associate Training and Development Programme

The nursing associate programme requires either functional skills in mathematics and English level 2 or General Certificate of Secondary Education grade 5–9, or C or above, for training nursing associates and TNAs. Nursing associate health careers (NHS, 2022d) include undertaking academic learning 1 day per week and work-based learning during the remainder of the week while being employed in a healthcare setting such as an acute hospital.

Resources for nurse associate support and development include the following:
- Nursing associates (HEE, 2023c), including case studies; employer resources; and workforce planning and deployment of nursing associates.
- Training and development (HEE, 2023d) and career progression for nursing associates, including apprenticeship.
- Standards of proficiency for registered nursing associates (Nursing and Midwifery Council, 2023q), which delineate the knowledge and skills required of nursing associates.
- Become a nursing associate (Royal College of Nursing, 2023i), describing a new role introduced in England to bridge the gap between HCAs and registered nurses.

5.2.12.7 Preceptorships for Newly Qualified Staff

Preceptorships (NHS Employers, 2023d) involve a period of structured transition to guide and support newly qualified staff in the progression from student to autonomous professional, further develop their practice and ensure the best possible start for these health professionals.

5.2.12.8 National Preceptorship Framework for Nursing

The main aim of this framework is to welcome and integrate newly registered practitioners into their new teams and workplaces (NHS England, 2022f). Staff already in the organisation are included in greeting new IR staff and introducing themselves, through methods such as 'Hello, my name is'. Various examples of good practices are available, including the preceptor support testimonial in Box 7.1 and the sample preceptorship programme in Table 7.2. Preceptorship helps professionals translate and embed their knowledge into everyday practice, grow in confidence and achieve the best possible start to their careers. Preceptorship is not designed to replace appraisals, or to substitute for formal inductions and mandatory training.

Preceptorship programmes may cover the following:

- Introduction to preceptorship.
- Clinical skills.
- Nutrition and hydration.
- Admission and discharge planning.
- Acute Life-threatening Events Recognition and Treatment (ALERT), a multi-professional course in the care of acutely ill patients at risk, covering emotional intelligence and resilience; intravenous medication administration; skin care; pain management; cancer and palliative care; cardio-respiratory care, including Airway, Breathing, Circulation, Disability, Exposure (ABCDE); acute care; neurology; leadership; communication; human factors; and potentially IPC (personal protective equipment [PPE], hand hygiene, aseptic technique and sharps), safety, pain with breathlessness, hypotension, disordered consciousness, altered urine output, sepsis and pain (NHS England, 2022f).

5.2.12.9 Skills Development Strategy for Specific Organisations

This strategy includes compassionate care; dementia; emergency care; primary care; and care of children and young people (NHS, 2022e).

5.2.12.10 Return to Practice for Healthcare Professionals

The national return to practice (RtP) programmes for nurses, midwives and health visitors provide information and resources to support healthcare professionals' return to practice in the healthcare setting (NHS Employers, 2023e).

5.2.12.11 Allied Health Professionals

How to become an AHP (NHS, 2022 Fig. 5.3f) is described on the NHS Healthcare careers site. The main route is an undergraduate or postgraduate degree approved by the Health and Care Professions Council (HCPC). Fig. 5.3 shows the study pathways for nurses, midwives, nursing associates and AHPs, and provides further information on the different routes into nursing (NHS Employers, 2023a). Development of AHPs is supported by guidance, publications and resources (NHS England, 2022g) regarding how AHPs can lead change, in addition to the Chief allied health professional's handbook (NHS England, 2022o), which outlines AHP skills for development and multi-professional leadership, and the 'AHPs into Action' strategy. Professional development opportunities and possibilities to support AHP leaders at all levels are also detailed in a guide on developing AHP leaders (NHS England, 2022h).

5.2.12.12 Resources for Midwife Support and Development

Resources for midwives include the following:

Maternity resources (HEE, 2023b) including Advanced Clinical Practice in Midwifery; Maternity Support Workers; Midwifery training places expansion; Neonatal training; Registered Midwifery Degree; Apprenticeship Evaluation Report; and Shortened Midwifery Training for Registered Adult Nurses–Funding Arrangements.

Maternity workforce strategy (NHS England, 2019b), for transforming the maternity workforce

Health career resources (NHS, 2022g) regarding working in the NHS, available roles and career planning.

5.2.12.13 Training Routes Towards NHS Careers

Training routes into the wider NHS (Fig. 5.4), as part of the career pipeline and workforce supply, include employability programmes; work experience; T levels; internships; return to practice; traineeships; and apprenticeships. These routes include the academic leadership and management pipeline through the apprenticeship levy at levels 3, 4 and 5. The NHS Leadership Academy is working with apprenticeship providers to offer access to leadership development programmes as part of apprenticeships, graduate schemes, and university and college programmes (NHS Employers, 2022; NHS Leadership Academy, 2023c).

Training routes into the NHS (Fig. 5.4) are supported by the nursing workforce standards (Royal College of Nursing, 2021), covering responsibility, accountability and clinical leadership; patient safety and health; and safety and well-being.

5.3 Professional Leadership in Healthcare

Effective leaders in the healthcare service ensure the top priority of safe, high-quality, compassionate care by ensuring that the voice of patients is heard at all levels at all times, including patient experience, concerns, needs and feedback (both positive and negative), so that these can be addressed. These efforts are supported by leadership development in healthcare at all levels (King's Fund, 2023a).

Effective leadership is also complex and is a highly valued element of high healthcare education standards, research and clinical practice, and should be part of all leadership training and development programmes (Van Diggele et al., 2020). To meet the needs of healthcare in the 21st century, competent leaders are increasingly important across all health and care professional groups, including allied health, nursing, pharmacy, dentistry and medicine. Modern leadership models include not only leadership by example, but a balance among autonomy, accountability, teamwork and focusing on improving patient outcomes. This balance is achieved by working effectively and collaboratively across disciplines and organisational boundaries, while the titles of professional in senior role are not the only association with the position of leadership. Additional leadership and management courses and programmes outlining the current theories of leadership, skills, competencies and roles within the healthcare setting can be accessed by internationally recruited and other staff.

Leadership includes influencing others, either as individuals or as groups working towards the achievement of a common goal (Van Diggele et al., 2020), while maintaining important values, attitudes and behaviours through a dyadic relationship.

Leadership of professionals within the healthcare systems includes many interrelated professional groups, departments and specialty areas (Al-Sawai, 2013). However, this can be complex at times, owing to the constraints pertaining to various disease areas, multidirectional goals and multidisciplinary staff within large organisations such as healthcare systems. Conflicting priorities and demands among groups may arise, because of their associated subcultures. Effective leadership should capitalise on the diversity

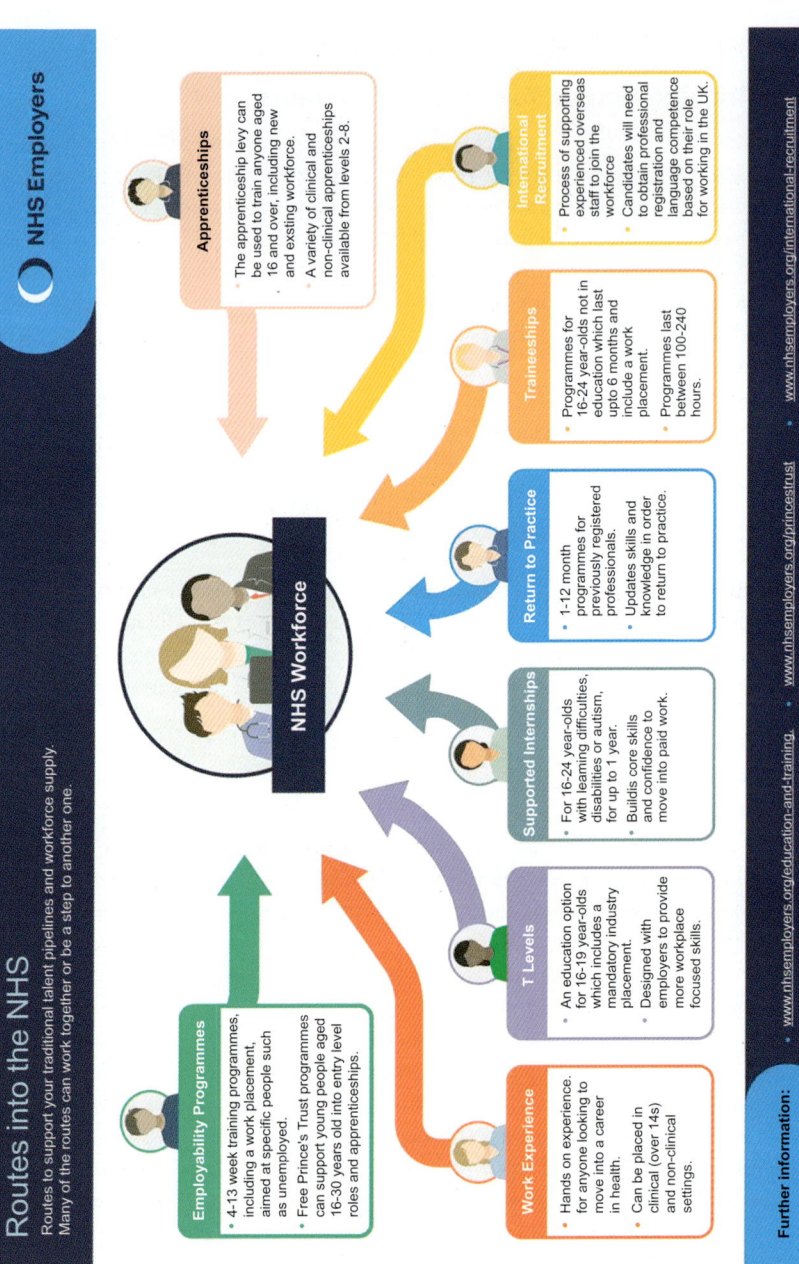

Fig. 5.4 Training routes in the NHS. (With permission from NHS Employers. (2022). The different routes to recruit your nursing workforce and increase your nursing supply. https://www.nhsemployers.org/articles/your-future-nurses. Accessed 10 July 2024.)

within the organisation as a whole and use available resources efficiently when designing management processes, while encouraging personnel to work towards common goals. Various leadership approaches can be used adaptively in the healthcare setting to achieve effective management in this highly complex environment (Al-Sawai, 2013).

5.3.1 MANAGEMENT VERSUS LEADERSHIP

Both management and leadership are important in achieving the goals of an organisation, although they have separate functions (Van Diggele et al., 2020). Management ensures order and consistency (Northouse, 2011) by organising all functions and processes within the organisation, thereby ensuring that the leader's vision and goals are successfully achieved. Leadership delivers change and movement (Northouse, 2011), supported by the effective management processes in place, by creating the vision, setting direction, influencing others and managing change, whereas management's role is to organise resources and ensure the sustainability of the changes affected by leadership (Byrman, 2006; Swanwick & McKimm, 2011).

5.3.2 LEADERSHIP TYPES IN THE HEALTHCARE SETTING

Various types of leadership are used in the healthcare setting.

Transactional and transformational leadership (Van Diggele et al., 2020) are two broad types of leadership. These two models are usually used in combination within organisations to empower staff (transformational) and to hold individuals accountable (transactional) for care and service delivery (Byrman, 2006). Both are necessary for running an effective organisation. However, optimal leaders use primarily transformational leadership, rather than transactional leadership.

Transformational leadership is based on the premise that people work more effectively if they have a sense of mission; therefore, leaders must clearly communicate their visions in a meaningful, exciting and clear manner, to foster unity and collective purpose. Transformational leaders are committed, have vision and can empower and motivate others to perform beyond expectations, through their ability to influence attitudes (Al-Sawai, 2013). Transformational leadership (Van Diggele et al., 2020), in which leaders influence individuals to achieve a common organisational goal, is a contemporary form of leadership based on inspiring individuals and forming teams to achieve goals. Transformational leaders define organisations through articulation of a clear vision and clear values (Van Diggele et al., 2020).

Transactional leadership traditionally focuses on supervision, organisation and group performance. This model is considered an authoritative relationship, on the basis of exchanges between the leader and followers to achieve specific agreed-upon goals, through use of order, structure and formal authority by those in positions of responsibility within organisations (Van Diggele et al., 2020). Transactional leaders achieve organisational goals by using rewards and positive reinforcement; however, leaders should be mindful of the lack of innovation in this style, because individuals are driven by predetermined outcomes and have no incentive and motivation to perform beyond the agreed-upon expectations (Northouse, 2011).

Collaborative leadership uses assertiveness and cooperation by working together with a group of people for the mutual benefit of the organisation; communication of information with staff internal and external to the organisations enables individualised decision-making (Al-Sawai, 2013). These collaborative communication methods improve healthcare management by encouraging dialogue among numerous stakeholders; sharing knowledge and experiences; and decreasing complexity within healthcare organisations. All staff should engage with the leadership process and be actively involved in validating and communicating their needs. This may include identifying modifications in practices that might need to be addressed through changing demands, modifying the various cultures, and facilitating integration and interdependency among multiple stakeholders to meet shared visions and values (Al-Sawai, 2013) and achieve the outcomes of a combined group efforts. Collaborative leaders should model collaborative behaviours to increase staff motivation and nurture interdependency among multiple professionals (Al-Sawai, 2013).

Team leadership through **distributed leadership** is increasingly adopted within healthcare and education settings, and involves multiple professionals sharing and influencing together (Van Diggele et al., 2020). This collaborative role in leadership emphasises the importance of shared leadership and considerate delegation of duties and responsibilities. Under team leadership styles, individuals are interdependent and must coordinate their activities to accomplish shared goals (Burgess et al., 2014). Individual autonomy, accountability, recognition and clarity of roles are important elements contributing to effective team performance, as supported by the organisational culture of involvement and the use of leadership qualities to ensure team success (Pearce et al., 2009).

Team leadership is provided by individuals who meet the specific requirements and abilities of the team at the time. Consequently, rapid responses can be provided to complex issues in organisations, thus enabling good functioning (Van Diggele et al., 2020). For a team to achieve its potential, the operational roles are important in team leadership (Van Diggele et al., 2020). Successful teams function more effectively when they have diversity and can use the strengths that each team member offers (Levi, 2011).

Effective leadership requires good time management and organisational skills, an ability to network professionally, political nous and, most importantly, strong communication skills (Glover et al., 2015). Ready acceptance of feedback and self-awareness are important in the development of leadership skills (Glover et al., 2015). Behaviour, habits and biases can be deliberately corrected by using received feedback. Although no single set of qualities applies to being an effective leader, relevant **leadership competencies** (Table 5.9) for all health professional educators are valued and contribute to the leadership model in different ways (Van Diggele et al., 2020).

5.3.3 LEADERSHIP COMPETENCIES

Key elements regarding leadership competencies and vision are summarised in Table 5.9 and supporting information is provided in Section 4.3.7.15 on leadership development. Leadership competencies are important parts of the leadership strategies of organisations, and include embedding core values of kindness, respect, friendship, helpfulness, caring, excellence, professionalism and understanding (Box 5.3).

TABLE 5.9 ■ Leadership Competencies and Vision

Great Leadership	Engaged, Inspired and Motivated Colleagues	High-Performing Organisations	Excellent Patient Experience
Key Points			
Ongoing support for leaders.	Performing and developing.	Recognised and rewarded for consistently being the best.	Patient-centred care.
Everyone is a leader.	Engagement and involvement.		Organisation of choice.
Good leaders never stop developing.	Enabling and facilitating.	Role modelling excellence.	Increased market share.
Strong leadership community.	Shared purpose.	Great place to work.	Financially stable.
Talent is surfaced so that staff can fulfil their potential.	Staff suggestion scheme.	Fostering innovation.	Engagement in all processes.
	Active listening and communication.	Staff excellence award.	
	Responsiveness.	Recruiting and retaining the best talent.	

BOX 5.3   Conflict Management Tools: Personal Testimony

I used the conflict management tools, modes to frame conversations and resources within and outside my organization. These included a conflict management course completion and conversations with HR colleagues, which enabled me to have difficult conversations at the earliest opportunity, address things early, and promote healthy and honest conversations when supervising and managing staff. This can support staff to be promoted early in their organization.

Internationally recruited staff nurse

5.3.4 CONFLICT MANAGEMENT

Conflict management can be challenging within healthcare organisations. Conflict can be due to gaps in communication, individual behaviour, organisational structures or intergroup conflicts, leading to failure in working practices (Al-Sawai, 2013). Healthcare leaders must use suitable approaches for addressing conflict at all levels within the organisation to create positive outcomes for staff. Strategies to address conflict include competition, avoidance, compromise, accommodation, collaboration, bargaining/negotiation, mediation, facilitating effective communication, seeking consensus and engendering vision to aid in conflict resolution.

The **language** of **leadership** in educational and healthcare organisations along with team leaders, reinforcing and encouraging collaboration and contribution with staff is important. Effective communication includes understanding the message, which requires both active listening and active talking (Van Diggele et al., 2020). This process requires clear communication with clarity of purpose; ensuring stimulating message delivery in a powerful, inspiring and dramatic manner; using congruence to lead by example ('walking the talk'); using active listening by acknowledging what is

TABLE 5.10 ■ Reflection Task

Organisational leadership
Reflect on **models** of **leadership** in your current workplace and educational institutions that you have been part of.
What stood out to you the most?
What did most people respond to well?
How were the organisational goals best achieved?
Individual leadership
What leadership competencies (Table 5.9) do you believe you already possess?
What qualities do you need to further develop?

communicated; using questioning and feedback; and showing that staff and their contributions are valued.

Leadership in healthcare and education may face unique issues and challenges (Van Diggele et al., 2020), because both are delivered across professional disciplines and organisational boundaries, including universities, hospitals and other healthcare services. These organisations have their own systems, structures, policies, cultures and values (Table 5.10). Opportunities within organisations should be used to contribute to addressing these challenges throughout staff members' careers, e.g. by matching the required experiences with capabilities (McKimm & Swanwick, 2011).

5.3.5 DEVELOPMENT OF LEADERSHIP SKILLS

Development of leadership skills includes the use of workforce data to determine the necessary experience among clinicians and healthcare educators (Van Diggele et al., 2020). Effective succession planning and leadership training are necessary (Matthews et al., 2017), to increase the number of emerging leaders moving into leadership roles. Staff can be supported and nurtured by their educational or healthcare organisations to become effective leaders (Northouse, 2011). Relevant strategies include leadership development, training, assessment and feedback as part of the education and training of health staff. 'Talent spotting' should be used to identify and develop aspiring and current leaders through embedding formal leadership development programmes/courses and supportive organisational cultures, e.g. by providing opportunities for leadership practice, and promoting professional networks within and beyond the organisation. Mentorship and coaching are key within healthcare and education settings, because they enhance leadership and engagement within the workforce (Burgess et al., 2018). Developing leadership skills is part of life-long learning (Van Diggele et al., 2020). Therefore, further resources and opportunities should be considered to aid in the development of leadership skills, e.g. through reading about leadership styles and theories; attending leadership workshops; participating in mentorship programmes as mentees or mentors; joining small group seminars on leadership development; and accepting more responsibilities as required or when opportunities arise.

The process of effective leadership may occur in daily duties in collaboration with other professionals within education and healthcare systems, such as in leadership, teaching, administration and research, to ensure excellence in clinical practice.

For leading and delivering effectively, various tools can be used to organise and manage busy schedules, and to practise effective delegation to share the work required for new projects.

Shared leadership is team-level management and leadership that empowers staff in the decision-making processes to improve practices (Burgess et al., 2014). Shared leadership provides opportunities for staff to develop within a team, thereby contributing to job satisfaction and improving the work environment, including effective teamwork and a focus on team values (Burgess et al., 2014). Multiple studies have indicated that autonomous highly qualified healthcare professionals with direct responsibility for their patients and services respond well to effective collaborative leadership (Al-Sawai, 2013). This leadership includes support and task delegation. The shared leadership model should be used more widely within healthcare settings, because it promotes shared governance, continuous workplace learning and development of constructive working relationships (Al-Sawai, 2013). Shared leadership enables staff to use leadership behaviours, have greater autonomy and achieve improved patient care outcomes (Al-Sawai, 2013). However, a poor team ethos, high workload and staff turnover, uninteresting work, lack of responsibility and insufficient goal setting can hinder the development of shared leadership and therefore must be addressed.

Shared leadership is an ongoing and fluid process that requires continuous evaluation to respond to ever-changing healthcare challenges, as well as a good working relationships between managers and staff (Al-Sawai, 2013). When organisational and group interrelationships are developed and fostered to achieve defined goals, the practices of groups and individuals outside the core team may be influenced, thus increasing the standing of the group within the organisational hierarchy (Al-Sawai, 2013).

Distributed leadership is increasingly important with globalisation and requirements for broader distribution of responsibilities and initiatives. Many large corporations, recognising this aspect, have become less hierarchical and more collaborative in their leadership approach. Distributed leadership includes the use of four key characteristics (Al-Sawai, 2013): sense making, which includes understanding the continually changing professional environment and adjusting to changes within the organisation; relating, which includes building trusting relationships, balancing advocacy with inquiry and cultivating networks of supportive confidants; visioning, which includes creating credibility and the aspiration for a future that staff in the organisation can work towards; and inventing, which includes creating new ways of working and overcoming seemingly insurmountable problems. These characteristics of distributed leadership throughout the organisation allow staff to complement one another's strengths and offset one another's weaknesses (Al-Sawai, 2013).

Ethical leadership refers to practising effective leadership, thereby substantially affecting the working lives of healthcare staff, patient outcomes and the fate of the organisation. This leadership may include influencing group members through enthusiasm for innovative strategies and encouraging changes in underlying beliefs and values (Al-Sawai, 2013). A good and ethical leader has intentions, values and behaviours that intend no harm and respect the rights of all parties.

Functional results-oriented healthcare leadership refers to addressing the challenges faced by professionals leading within complex modern healthcare settings and services, which include diverse changing needs, increasing patient expectations and high costs of new interventions and treatments. Professionals must consider the needs of the wider patient population; make decisions that make the best use of resources and simultaneously deliver clinical quality; and implement clinically led service improvements that are likely to succeed (McKimm & Swanwick, 2011). Therefore, the leadership role is important in facilitating effective and efficient healthcare provision, while delivering the desired outcomes (Al-Sawai, 2013).

Leadership style summary: Numerous theories and models have influenced the leadership strategies currently used by staff in healthcare settings. Effective leadership should focus on the dynamic relationships among leadership values, culture, capabilities and the organisational context. A leader's developmental journey must operate within this dynamic, supported by high levels of self, team and organisational awareness. Leadership development is important in the role of the leader and a ready supply of replacement leaders should be ensured to support continued organisational progress in the ever-changing healthcare environment through succession planning. This planning includes the use of leadership competencies as part of leadership development programmes provided across all health professions, including allied health, nursing, pharmacy, dentistry and medicine, to meet the needs of healthcare in the 21st century (Al-Sawai, 2013). With the increase in interprofessional teams and emphasis on collaboration, more effective outcomes can be achieved (Clarke, 2015). Healthcare and education leaders must work effectively and collaboratively across professional groups and organisational boundaries, as titles of staff are not always associated with leadership roles but are part of everyday work. Good leadership also includes supporting others in their personal and professional journeys at the right time, including the provision of opportunities for leadership development in education sectors and health services, thereby supporting change and staff progression. Healthcare and education leaders who demonstrate excellence in teamwork, clinical skills and patient-centred care, and who responsibly balance accountability with autonomy, will be the leaders of the future. Internationally recruited staff should access resources early, to progress in career development and achieve happy working lives in health and care service.

5.3.6 KEY MESSAGES FOR STAFF

Key messages include the following:
- Titles are not always associated with leadership roles.
- Today's leaders must step forward, collaborate and contribute.
- A good leader is a good team player who values and seeks the opinions of others.
- Leadership requires clear, respectful communication that acknowledges the input and achievements of others.

The Career Development guide (Indeed, 2022b) also describes additional characteristics for effective leadership in healthcare (Indeed, 2022b), including information to guide staff through their career journeys (Indeed, 2022b), such as leadership development in health and care, and contributing to delivering high-quality care. The use of effective leadership skills improves the workplace and leads to better patient outcomes; these skills apply to staff in administrative roles and management positions, senior practitioners and clinical staff in the NHS (Indeed, 2022c).

TABLE 5.11 ■ **Features of Highly Effective Organisations**

A Guide to Operating Systems for Team and Service Management

Effective Engagement and Commitment to Shared Vision	**Effective Problem Solving**
Team shared and agreed-upon vision Aligning team vision with organisational objectives Visible visions and goals Using successful indicators to convert to objectives	Problem identification and solving Understanding root cause Options appraisals Resolving problems at the right level Stakeholders' engagement in problem solving
Effective Performance Management	**Effective Process Management**
Clear performance indicators Understanding baseline performance Tracking performance (daily, weekly or monthly) Stakeholders' engagement in kep performance indicator (KPI) setting Sharing/visible performance results Celebrating success Positive performance feedback Avoidance of problems by using early warning systems	Identifying and solving process problems Ideas for improvement Multidisciplinary input Integrated teamwork New ways of working and role redesign Addressing efficiency and flow Capacity and demand management
Effective Teamwork and Communication	**Effective Workload Management**
Shared reflection on performance Understanding teams' roles and responsibilities Visibility of team's achievement, performance, commitments and competence Joint problem solving Workload management and redesign Identifying risks, issues and problems Multidisciplinary teamwork Prioritisation of tasks and duties according to urgency	Workload visibility Task clarity Workload allocation and delegation Responding to variable demand Prioritising urgent tasks to achieve KPIs Multi-tasking, task transfer and use of support workers
Effective Managers and Leadership Support	**Effective and Efficient Use of Resources**
Visibility Feedback on positive performance Accountability for delivery Problem solving and resolution of issues Understanding of risks Understanding frontline issues and experience Listening and acting on concerns Communication and engagement	Task and comparative productive analysis Assessing capacity and demand Matching resource with demand Skill mix analysis: matching skills and tasks to maximise results Volume added analysis: what values do tasks and roles add?

Healthcare leadership is an important professional skill in directing teams in healthcare organisations to achieve desired outcomes. Such leadership can be undertaken by any team members, regardless of whether they are in supervisory positions. Leadership ensures that all team members understand their roles and work together to reach their goals, by using skills such as analytical thinking to assess complex situations and develop effective strategies for resolution. Healthcare management (Indeed, 2022d), aligned with leadership for effective service delivery is detailed in Table 5.11 listing the features of highly effective organisations.

Identifying and accepting opportunities for **professional development** for growth is important for healthcare leaders to demonstrate their initiative and dedication to their careers. Professional development opportunities may include training sessions, conferences, continuing education, or voluntary or paid activities and duties in other organisations. These opportunities facilitate the development of excellence in new skills that benefit staff and teams.

Promoting opportunities by creating learning opportunities for others may include training and development sessions supported by guest speakers, to ensure that staff and team members grow, acquire skills and apply their abilities in the workplace. Funded CPD options should be included. CPD can be gained through short courses; study days; workshops; modules; and postgraduate training in advanced and specialist practice, leadership, management, professional education, public health and community, midwifery, physiotherapy and rehabilitation, and social work (Indeed, 2022b).

5.3.7 MENTORING

Mentoring is a personal development relationship involving a knowledgeable and experienced individual (mentor) offering guidance and advice to someone else (mentee), thereby enabling mutual learning. Mentorship roles help leaders guide and support others, particularly those who are new to a healthcare environment, by working directly with junior staff to support them in gaining the skills needed to excel in their roles, after assessment of their strengths and weaknesses. Mentoring allows individuals to work with identified staff, model expected behaviours, answer questions and provide encouragement, to achieve professional and personal goals, as staff move into their new jobs.

5.4 Career Conversations and Reviews

Measures of performance, potential, aspirations and readiness, as well as indications of the support and or development required for staff to sustain or enhance their performance, are important in effective talent conversations and succession planning. All leaders and managers responsible for undertaking talent conversations should be trained and developed to do so, thereby ensuring a focus on maximising the potential of all staff (NHS Leadership Academy, 2023k). Career conversations, options and means of progression should be included (NHS Leadership Academy, 2023l).

5.4.1 CAREER CONVERSATION RESOURCES AND TEMPLATES

The following resources and templates provide more information on career conversations (NHS Leadership Academy, 2023l).

The review and career conversation framework (NHS Leadership Academy, 2023l) includes appraisal, career conversations and a review of health and well-being and personal development planning as part of a combined conversation, which provides a structure for staff and managers to explore talent management opportunities.

The review and career conversation implementation guide (NHS Leadership Academy, 2023l) is for managers and describes the steps involved in implementing the review and career conversation framework; preparation; reviewing objectives and behaviour; measuring potential; and discussing aspirations, readiness and development.

The review and career conversation user guide (NHS Leadership Academy, 2023l) provides information for briefing staff regarding what they should expect from their review and career/talent conversations, how their information will be used and their responsibility for preparing and taking ownership of any actions.

The review and career conversation briefing materials for staff: slide deck (NHS Leadership Academy, 2023l) provides content for staff briefing sessions, which should be used with the facilitator guide described later, to guide staff through the organisation's approach.

The review and career conversation briefing materials for staff: workbook (NHS Leadership Academy, 2023l) supplements the briefing slides for staff and the review and career/talent conversation document and is aimed at further supporting preparation and self-reflection to help staff maximise the value of conversations.

The review and career conversation briefing materials for staff: facilitator guide (NHS Leadership Academy, 2023l) is designed to accompany the briefing agenda and slides and to cover the key points that should be relayed to ensure that staff are fully prepared for their review and career and talent conversations.

Further support regarding career conversations includes the following:

The Talent management toolkit promotes a culture of talent management; equality, diversity and inclusion; identifying, managing and retaining talent; developing and mobilising talent; connecting talent interventions across local systems; and use of diagnostic tools (NHS Leadership Academy, 2023l).

Having a career conversation (NHS Professionals, 2023a) facilitates discussions with staff regarding their current and future professional development, progression, support and health well-being needs. Although this process is voluntary, it provides opportunities to explore healthcare career options, where trained professional leaders encourage staff to explore possibilities, focus their attention and identify their next steps. The career conversation tool (Table 5.12) and features of highly effective organisations (Table 5.11) facilitates useful reflection in preparation for career conversations (Table 5.13). The questions regarding career aspirations (Table 5.14) provide the general career conversation structure that is usually followed to help staff understand what to expect.

Preparing for the career conversation includes key items to consider before the conversation itself, as well as key areas to guide staff through the conversation, as described below.

Know oneself: Staff should consider their ultimate goals for both the meeting and their current and subsequent roles in the health and care setting, including their strengths, operational technical skills, soft transferable skills, work values and areas of interest.

Explore possibilities: Staff should commence exploring options that might suit them best and use the career conversation meeting to provide confirmation and identify possibilities.

TABLE 5.12 ■ **Career Conversation Tool**

Employee	Stage	Coach
	Opening	
Who am I? My past experience. My skills and strengths. My aspirations and motivations.	Exploring	**Exploration:** Clarify purpose. Question and listen.
What are my options? What roles am I suitable for? What training would I need? How can you support me?	Focusing	**Discuss possibilities:** What are the options? What is possible now and later? Provide realistic options.

Personal development:
How do I get there?
What can I do to make myself
    more employable?
	Taking
	action
		Encouraging action:
		Discuss possible strategies and immediate
		    actions.
		Direct to appropriate training and
		    resources.

	Closing	

Modified with permission from NHS Professionals. (2023a). *NHS Staffing Pool Hub - Getting Started – Having a career conversation.* https://www.nhsprofessionals.nhs.uk/nhs-staffing-pool-hub/getting-started. Accessed 25 March 2023.

TABLE 5.13 ■ **Useful Reflections to Help Prepare for Career Conversations**

Which roles interested you during your exploration?
Do you have all skills/experience required for these roles?
What transferable skills do you have?
What did you gain from your experience as a vaccinator?
What can you do to boost your employability?
What must you do to be promoted into a new role?
What can the organisation/coach and mentor do to support me to be promoted into a new role?
What development do I need? How can I be supported to achieve that development?

Modified from NHS Professionals. (2023a). *NHS Staffing Pool Hub - Getting Started - Having a career conversation.* https://www.nhsprofessionals.nhs.uk/nhs-staffing-pool-hub/getting-started. Accessed 25 March 2023.

Making career choices: Staff should assess themselves to determine their development needs. The process may include reviewing career websites to determine the potentially necessary skills and qualifications and the that is support is available in gaining the required skills and qualifications.

Making it happen: Staff should consider their key development needs and then focus on gaining skills, experience and knowledge to fulfil those needs, through secondments, stretch assignment, acting up (working in a higher role temporarily), or new roles and duties.

TABLE 5.14 ■ Career Aspiration Questions

Questions to Help Determine Current Career Position and Future Career Aspirations

Current status: e.g. developing competence in current role

Current aspirations: e.g. looking for a change in role

Primary motivator: e.g. ready to broaden skill set

Aspiration progression status:

Staff:	Manager:	Date:	Time:

Why do I want to work in the NHS?
What was my background before being part of the COVID-19 response?
On the basis of my research, what roles would I be suitable for?
What have I enjoyed most about the work I have been doing?
What setting do I want to work in?
What are my opportunities for employment?
How will I be supported?
What do I want my working hours to be?
Will I need training?
What are my aspirations?

Describe how the motivation for a change in career direction can be achieved in the current role.

E.g.: Staff member has expressed a desire to become a director at board level.
Manager agreed to shadowing at different corporate and board level meetings.
Manager discussed changes to her job, which could mean taking a managerial as ward manager, matron, head of nursing or maternity or deputy chief nurse, on the basis of her current career level.
Staff member asked about rotation in managerial positions across surgery, medicine, maternity and the corporate team to gain varied experience, which was agreed upon by her manager.
Staff member was also sign-posted to speak to the general managers and divisional directors in these areas, to gain additional support.
These actions are particularly important, because the staff member's career trajectory to date has comprised specialised roles (IPC, continence and TVN).

If you are seeking a different role, what kind of role are you looking for?

E.g.: Looking to work in an operational role trust-wide or in a divisional role involving wider trust issues, in which I can contribute to improvement by using my transferable experience from my specialist role.

Future career aspirations:

Aiming to work at **executive board** level:

Career aspirations comments:

Comments:
Agreed completion by (SMART objective format):
Date: .... Time:...
Staff:.................................... Manager:......................................
NB: SMART: specific, measurable, achievable, relevant and time-bound objectives.

Modified from NHS Professionals. (2023a). *NHS Staffing Pool Hub - Getting Started - Having a career conversation*. https://www.nhsprofessionals.nhs.uk/nhs-staffing-pool-hub/getting-started. Accessed 25 March 2023.

5.4.2 NHS STAFFING POOL HUB

Other resources, such as the NHS Staffing Pool Hub (NHS Professionals, 2023a), provide more information about working in the UK healthcare system and how to get started with a career in the NHS. The NHS Staffing Pool Hub (NHS Professionals, 2023a) includes details on working in healthcare, opportunities, healthcare careers, career conversations, apprenticeships and applying for a job. Staff are provided with further information on how to reflect on and discuss potential future roles in health and social care, and the options and opportunities that might be available to them (NHS Professionals, 2023a). Staff should spend time considering where they are currently situated in their career and what they want to achieve in the future, by using the questions below as a guide for thinking about roles in health or social care settings. Many career roles are available, including nursing and midwifery; medical, scientific and engineering roles; healthcare support or HCA roles; AHP roles; social care roles; and support professional roles. Moreover, apprenticeship pathways are available for people at all stages of their careers (NHS Professionals, 2023a).

5.4.3 CAREER ASPIRATIONS

Regular conversations should be held between staff and their line managers regarding career aspirations (Table 5.14). Career aspirations may include developing competencies in a current role or changing career direction, according to defined internal or external motivation. Individuals changing direction relatively late their career journeys or pathways may face challenges including a lack of demonstrated experience in the new chosen specialty. Therefore, career destinations are best planned as early as possible (Box 5.4).

Resources to help staff embark on their career journeys include information and guidance regarding working in health; who works for the NHS; exploration of career options; and career planning.

Further resources to help staff can be found by exploring careers in specific healthcare roles, social care and other NHS job opportunities, including Skills for Care and the National Careers Service.

Resources to provide staff with information and an overview of healthcare support workers (HCSW) and HCA roles include the following:

- Healthcare support worker overview (NHS, 2022h), describing a crucial role ensuring smooth service delivery.
- HCA overview and careers resource for nursing support workers (Royal College of Nursing, 2023j).
- Career paths for nursing support workers (Royal College of Nursing, 2023h).
- HCSW2020 Accelerated Care Certificate (NHS England, 2022i).

BOX 5.4	**Career Conversation Testimonial**

I found career conversations with my manager very useful in agreeing my strengths and weaknesses, and then using these to create my personal development plan (PDP) which has helped me progress in my career.

Matron in a hospital

5.4.4 THE CARE CERTIFICATE

The care certificate standards define the knowledge, skills and behaviours expected in specific job roles in the health and social care sectors. A minimum of 15 standards should be covered for new HCSWs and those new to care, and should form part of a robust induction programme including HCAs, assistant practitioners, care support workers and adult social workers. The standards can be completed by staff working in noncare roles, e.g. cooks or maintenance personnel.

Assistant practitioners (usually band 4) roles can be applied for by individuals who have completed a foundational degree and have theoretical knowledge in a particular subject area. Assistant practitioners can undertake roles in areas including ambulatory care; assessment of patients, including history taking and application of the Wells score; and following a strict pathway working with the clinical team. This is on the basis of specific job description and workbooks, where assistant practitioners can escalate items when necessary, while working as part of a multidisciplinary team, supported by training and competencies in the area of practice.

The **care certificate assessor document** includes the qualifications, onboarding programme learning and mapping document for all 15 standards for HCSWs, including the following care certificate standards:

- Understand your role.
- Your personal development.
- Duty of care.
- Equality, diversity and inclusion.
- Work in a person-centred manner.
- Communication.
- Privacy and dignity.
- Fluids and nutrition.
- Awareness of mental health, dementia and learning disabilities and autism.
- Safeguarding adults and children.
- Basic life support.
- Health and safety.
- Handling information.
- IPC.

(Skills for Care, 2023a, 2023b).

5.4.4.1 Care Certificate Workbook Sample

Care certificate workbooks and training modules are usually provided internally to each organisation, to help healthcare support workers understand their roles and the requirements to undertake their duties. As many as 15 standards may apply, including standard 1 (Table 5.15): (HCSW tasks, behaviours and standards of work), according to the main duties and responsibilities outlined in specified job descriptions. The code of conduct for HCSWs and adult social care workers is also included (Skills for Care, 2023c).

HCSWs or adult social care workers in England (Skills for Health, 2023c) must be accountable by being able to answer for their actions or omissions. Self-awareness regarding how previous experience, attitudes and beliefs affect the role is necessary.

TABLE 5.15 ■ Care Certificate Workbook: Progress Log, Mapping and Sign-Off Document: Standard 1

Care certificate Progress Log, Mapping and Sign-Off Document: The Roles of Health and Social Care Workers

An introduction to this document: This document provides an outline of the suggested mapping of outcomes and criteria within standard 1 (understand your role) of the care certificate to the recommended Qualifications and Credit Framework (QCF) unit, the National Minimum Training Standards for Healthcare Support Workers and Adult Social Care Workers in England, and the Common Induction Standards. This document does not necessarily indicate direct mapping of criteria; therefore, assessors and/or managers should follow the guidance below. Of note, the term 'assessor' throughout this document may refer to the manager, supervisor or assessor, as decided upon by the employing organisation.

This document should always be used in conjunction with the guidance provided in the Care Certificate Framework Technical Document.

Guidance for assessors.

Assessors must ensure that learners have demonstrated valid, authentic, reliable, current and sufficient evidence for each assessment criterion. Assessors must not assume that if the mapping document indicates that a criterion could have already been achieved, the mapped criteria within the QCF unit should automatically be awarded. Learners and assessors are responsible for ensuring that the outcomes and criteria within the QCF unit and the standards below have been achieved to the required standard. For reference, within the column referring to coverage of the relevant QCF unit, a P indicates partial coverage of the relevant criteria within the QCF unit, whereas an F indicates full coverage.

This assessment method is used by assessors to provide evidence of the type of assessment method used to assess the care certificate criteria. This assessment process is likely to be noted as part of the care certificate workbook in organisations. However, further information might include professional discussion, observation, question and answer, e-learning or witness testimony. This document can also be completed to provide evidence of competence by using these example assessment methods.

The evidence location column is included to provide a clear signpost indicating where the learner's evidence can be found, e.g. within a portfolio of evidence, a CPD file, or electronically via e-learning or an e-portfolio.

Care Certificate Standard 1 Outcome	Care Certificate Standard 1 Criteria	Knowledge/Competence	Question Within Workbook	QCF Unit: The Role of the Health and Social Care Worker (P = partial; F = full)	National Minimum Training Standards: Standard 1 (Roles of Healthcare Support Workers and Adult Social Care Workers)	Common Induction Standards: Standard 1 (Roles of Health and Social Care Workers), Standard 2 (Personal Development) and Standard 5 (Principles for Implementing Duty of Care)	Assessment Method Used	Evidence Location	Sign-Off Initials	Date
1.1 Understand their own role	1.1a Describe their main duties and responsibilities.	K	1.1a			S2 – 1.1				
	1.1b List the standards and codes of conduct and practice that relate to their role.	K	1.1b			S2 – 1.2				
	1.1c Demonstrate that they are working in accordance with the agreed-upon ways of working with their employer.	C		AC2.3 – P						
	1.1d Explain how their previous experiences, attitudes and beliefs might affect the way in which they work.	K	1.1d			S2 – 1.3				
1.2 Work in ways agreed upon with their employer	1.2a Describe their employment rights and responsibilities.	K	1.2a		1.3.1					
	1.2b List the aims, objectives and values of the service in which they work.	K	1.2b		1.3.2	S1 – 2.1				

(Continued)

TABLE 5.15 ■ **Care Certificate Workbook: Progress Log, Mapping and Sign-Off Document: Standard 1—cont'd**

		1.2c	AC2.1 – P	1.3.3	S1 – 2.2
1.2c Explain why working in ways agreed upon with their employer is important.	K	1.2c		1.3.3	S1 – 2.2
1.2d Demonstrate how to access full and up-to-date details of agreed-upon ways of working that are relevant to their role.	C		AC2.2 – F	1.3.4	S1 – 2.3
1.2e Explain how and when to escalate any concerns that they might have (whistleblowing).	K	1.2e Part i 1.2e Part ii		1.3.5	
1.2f Explain the importance of honesty, identifying where errors might have occurred and telling the appropriate person.	K	1.2f			
1.3 Understand working relationships in health and social care					
1.3a Describe their responsibilities to the individuals whom they support.	K	1.3a		1.2.1	S1 – 1.1
1.3b Explain how a working relationship differs from a personal relationship.	K	1.3b	AC1.1 – F	1.2.2	S1 – 1.2
1.3c Describe different working relationships in health and social care settings.	K	1.3c	AC1.2 – F	1.2.2	S1 – 1.2

1.4 Work in partnership with others	1.4a Explain why working in teams and in partnership with others is important.	K	1.4a and b	AC3.1 - F	1.4.2	S1 – 3.2
	1.4b Explain why working in partnership with key people, advocates and others who are significant to an individual is important.	K	1.4a and b	AC3.1 – P	1.4.1	S1 – 3.1
	1.4c Demonstrate behaviours, attitudes and ways of working that can help improve work in partnerships.	C		AC3.2 – F	1.4.3	S1 – 3.3
	1.4d Demonstrate how and when to access support and advice regarding: Partnership work and conflict resolution.	C		AC3.4 – F		S5 – 2.2

Declaration of completion

I confirm that the evidence provided by the employee meets the full requirements for **Standard 1: Understand Your Role in the Care Certificate.**

Employee signature: ....

Name of assessor: ....

Assessor signature: .... Completion date: ....

The Assessor can be a manager, supervisor, or someone else authorised by the employing organisation. This individual provides confirmation that all learning outcomes and assessment criteria for the care certificate standard identified above have been completed and signed off by and authorising person.

Modified from Skills for Care. (2023d). *The Care Certificate Standards*. https://www.skillsforcare.org.uk/resources/documents/Developing-your-workforce/Care-Certificate/The-Care-Certificate-Standards.pdf. Accessed 31 October 2023)

Employment rights and responsibilities relating to the role, including health and safety, IPC, confidentiality, working times, and pay and wages, are important to understand.

The internal care certificate standard 1 progress log, mapping and sign-off document sample are described in Table 5.15. This document provides an overview of the outcomes and assessment criteria for standard 1 (understand your role) and identifies the criteria within the standard (Skills for Care, 2023d).

Further resources to help staff assess which roles are right for them include the following:

- Find a health career in the NHS.
- Step into the NHS careers test.
- Exploring adult social care careers.
- National Careers Service: skills assessment.

(NHS, 2022i).

5.4.5 SKILLS FOR CARE RESOURCES

Resources to help ensure a capable, confident and skilled workforce by using a workforce development strategy include the following:

- Workforce intelligence and research.
- Workforce redesign, innovation and community skills development.
- Carers.
- Autonomous professionals for registered managers and social workers.
- Standards, learning and qualifications (induction, apprenticeships and qualifications).
- Recruitment and retention.
- Leadership and management.
- Employer engagement.

Skills for Care helps create a well-led, skilled and valued adult social care workforce, providing various practical tools and support to organisations and individuals (Skills for Care, 2023e).

The NHS People Plan (NHS England, 2021) contributes to ensuring that processes are in place to make the NHS the best place to work; improve the leadership culture, including through supporting equality and diversity; support the present and future healthcare agenda, including for nursing and midwifery and the wider workforce; deliver healthcare to meet growing population needs; and develop a new operating model for the future.

Career conversations with trained professionals enable staff to discuss their learnings. These tools and resources help staff make career choices, given that choosing among the more than 350 careers available in the NHS, including clinical and nonclinical jobs, may be daunting (NHS, 2022j).

5.4.6 THE NHS CAREER MANAGEMENT FRAMEWORK

The **NHS Career Management Framework breaks career planning** into four stages:

1. **Self-assessment**, involving discovering staff's values, skills and interests, to gain an understanding of the desired outcome from career and work.

2. **Exploring the options**, involving identifying available roles and narrowing down all options.
3. **Decision-making**, including evaluating the available options and deciding which roles to apply for.
4. **Applications** and interviews, including how to make a submitted application stand out and how to impress an interviewer.

Staff can undertake several exercises to help decide on a career, as detailed below. Additional information for helping individuals make career choice decisions can be gained from the following tools available at the NHS Working in Health website, under career planning (2022i):

- The values exercise (NHS), which helps staff identify their work-associated values to help them set their career goals.
- SWOT analysis (NHS), which helps staff identify the strengths, weaknesses, opportunities and threats associated with the roles under consideration.
- The life-line exercise (NHS), which helps staff review significant decisions that they have made in the past to help them decide on their future career.
- The factors exercise (NHS), which helps staff compare a variety of roles under consideration and identify which job factors are most important to them.
- The benefits and drawbacks exercise (NHS), which helps staff weigh the positives and negatives of a particular job option.
- The force field exercise (NHS), which helps staff identify the forces for and against a career option.

(NHS, 2022i).

Additional resources for maximising staff chances of success in applying for jobs in the NHS include tools to use transferable skills and maximise value from every contact, among other helpful resources (NHS Professionals, 2023a).

Further information on career conversations in the NHS, including supporting people in early and late career stages is available from the NHS Leadership Academy (2023l).

5.4.7 THE CAPITAL NURSE DIGITAL CAREER FRAMEWORK TOOL

HEE (2023e) provides additional information for use in career conversations and succession planning, which can occur at any time but can be part of one-on-one or clinical supervision sessions.

5.4.8 SPONSORSHIP FOR CAREER DEVELOPMENT

Professional development can be supported and sponsored through various means, at forums such as breakfast meetings, working lunches or dinners, speaking at staff awards ceremonies, professional or annual dinners, receptions and conferences.

Examples of previous sponsors of these events include the following:

- Royal colleges such as the Royal College of Psychiatrists.
- Restaurants such as Jamie Oliver.

- Journals such as the British Medical Journal.
- Newspapers such as The Mirror.
- The NHS Partners Dinner.
- Departments such as the Cambridge Centre for Science and Policy.
- Forums such as the Founders Forum.
- Independent charities such as The King's Fund.
- Organisations such as foundation trusts and private hospitals.
- The Healthcare Financial Management Association (HFMA) (2023), the professional body for finance staff working in healthcare.
- The National Association of Primary Care (NAPC) (2023), a membership organisation representing the interests of primary care professionals.
- RCNI.
- One CPD, Salford Professional Development.
- Association of the British Pharmaceutical Industry.
- NHS Confederation.
- Association of Optometrists.
- Klynveld Peat Marwick Goerdeler.

5.4.9 SPONSORSHIPS FOR FUNDING OF DEVELOPMENT

Sponsorships, including the following, are also a means of funding development work:

- **Ponsonby Travel Scholarship,** which can be internal to organisations, and provides funding for travel and performing leadership work.
- **Florence Nightingale Award**, including the Florence Nightingale Foundation (2023b) Scholarships for midwives and health visitors.
- **Mary Seacole Nursing Development and Leadership Award** (Post Graduate Funding, 2023).
- **General Florence Nightingale Foundation** (2023a) Leadership Scholarship.
- **Aspiring nurse director leadership scholarships**, such as the New Digital Leadership Scholarships for nurses and midwives (NHS, 2022k).
- **Young Professionals Programme** (United Nation (UN) Careers, 2023), a recruitment initiative for talented, highly qualified professionals to start careers as international civil servants with the UN Secretariat; includes an entrance examination and professional development after the successful start of a career with the UN.
- **Young Professionals Programme**, **World Trade Organization** (**WTO**), which provides opportunities for qualified young professionals from developing and least-developed countries that are members of the WTO to enhance their knowledge regarding WTO and international trade issues, and improve their chances of being recruited by the WTO and/or other regional and international organisations; part of the Secretariat's efforts to increase diversity and broaden the representation of the membership (WTO, 2023).
- **Young Professionals Program**, World Bank: an inspirational pathway into the World Bank Group, in which young professionals are recruited worldwide with various academic and professional backgrounds relevant to the World Bank (2023) Group; applicants must demonstrate a passion for international development, graduate education, relevant professional experience and the potential to grow into impactful leadership roles across institutions (World Bank, 2023).

5.5 Summary of Strategies for Coping and Flourishing in Healthcare Staff Roles

This chapter covered leadership and management; career conversations; organisational insights; working in multi-professional teams; and addressing daily and long-term challenges. These communication approaches cover elements specifically from the viewpoint of internationally recruited nurses. The content in this chapter should also be helpful for all nationally/UK qualified nurses (newly qualified nurses). The career and study pathways available in the UK healthcare system were also covered in this chapter, to guide staff through the various processes.

CHAPTER 6

Accelerating Staff Development and Progression in the Workplace

6.1 Introduction

This chapter details further elements, processes and areas required for accelerating the development and progression of staff in the health and care workplace setting, including nurses, midwives, allied health professionals (AHP) and various other staff, accelerating their progression into more senior leadership and management roles in the health and care workplace. Political and media astuteness, the development and advancement of personal and team needs, and using determination and resilience are explored in terms of how they promote staff success, job satisfaction and progression. Self-confidence is important for staff to progress in their careers, and this is influenced and supported by role modelling; staff from an international and diverse background who are appointed to senior roles provide encouragement to others who 'look like them'. This chapter also covers career development and planning for nurses, midwives, AHPs and various other staff. Compassionately and inclusively leading teams by example to overcome challenges is discussed and specific skills and tips to support staff are provided.

Additional information on ways to improve and accelerate personal leadership; life-long personal and career development; and gaining support and advice from others who have successfully done these things before are detailed in this chapter, as well as reflections from the author. Advice is also provided to support staff in delineating their personal and professional path, including how their skills can be used to further benefit them. Guidance is provided for creating a timeline for development and comparing development opportunities and additional advice is provided for learning and success.

Information is also provided on how to start the career development process at an early stage using internships, secondments, contracts, agencies and consultancies; by undertaking extracurricular learning; by making time for relaxation; and by accessing skills and offers. Additional references for further learning, guidance and resources are also provided in this chapter, pertaining to the National Health Service (NHS) Leadership Academy and leadership competence, for example. The elements of this chapter aimed at accelerating staff development and progression in the workplace are detailed under relevant headings.

Ways to gain access to presentations and panel discussions on key strategies that can be used to accelerate the progression of nurses, midwives and other staff into leadership positions in the workplace are also described in this chapter.

6.2 Political and Media Astuteness

The health and care service can be complicated by informal politics, titles, positions, entitlements and organisational norms, including competing interests and priorities. Staff from an international and diverse background need to be aware of these elements and spot them as they arise, drawing on support and experience to succeed and thrive in their roles and careers. This includes adopting and developing leadership styles that make use of political savvy and astuteness (Waring et al., 2018), such as:

- **Personal skills** to exercise self-awareness and self-control.
- **Interpersonal skills** to influence the thinking and behaviours of others, even without formal authority.
- **Reading people** and situations and thinking about the dynamics that can occur when groups of staff come together, supporting the wider health and care system and processes.
- **Fostering alignment** and alliances, promoting collaboration when there are different interests and motives.
- **Strategising** and scanning, having a sense of the organisation's purpose and thinking about the long-term factors that may impact the organisation.

6.3 Developing and Advancing Clear Personal and Team Needs

Compassionate leadership, as detailed in Section 4.3.7.14 on compassionate and inclusive leadership, is key for meeting the development and advancement needs of individual staff and the team. Leading a team involves leading by example and using inclusive leadership to overcome challenges. This involves participating in the corporate culture, as well as creating and establishing your own rules. Teamwork is an important part of successful leadership. Staff can create a list of professional and leadership development needs in alignment with current and future job plans, as these are useful for both career progression and daily life.

6.3.1 DEVELOPMENT OPTIONS

Development opportunities provide highly capable staff with challenging and interesting opportunities where they can learn and develop (Box 6.1). These include experiential learning opportunities that provide a means for development not accessible through conventional training or learning interventions.

This gives staff the opportunity to:

- Gain first-hand experience of working in a complex political environment.
- Develop a better sense of commercial decision-making and leadership.
- Experience a different perspective on accountability and transparency.
- Increase understanding of the challenges faced in various parts of the healthcare system.
- Learn more about national health and care system drivers and constraints.
- Broaden and deepen professional networks.

BOX 6.1	Leadership and Career Development Testimonial

My learning journey has not been easy, having both positives and negatives.

But someone invested in and sponsored me, helping me to progress.

Sponsorship will benefit others by supporting progression, including as part of leadership development programmes. Sponsors can provide support with interviews, the writing of a CV, job applications, creating a personal development plan (PDP), coaching and mentoring based on knowing what needs to happen, signposting sideways moves and role modelling. A diverse interview panel is also important to ensure equity in the process and boost confidence, which will support the recruitment of international nurses. It is important to ensure staff who sit on interview panels are trained and have confidence to make the right decision as panel members.

Head of Midwifery

- Consider how national bodies across health and care can collaborate more for improved public services and business growth.
- Experience different ways of leading, managing change and delivering services.

In this way, staff have opportunities to find a new working environment with new stakeholders, thereby accelerating learning, acquiring knowledge and ideas that can be used in organisations to improve ways of working and making a greater contribution to the health and care system as a whole.

6.4 Reflection From the Author

Expanding on the introduction and preface, this section reflects on the unique professional experiences of the author, who is an internationally educated nurse. The author has been a director of nursing (DON) for professional and system development, a DON for direct commissioning and a director of infection prevention and control (DIPC), and she has worked in all healthcare settings. This section includes knowledge based on the author's own experience as an internationally educated and recruited nurse, forming the 'heart' of the book.

6.4.1 OVERCOMING CHALLENGES AND OBSTACLES

Progression up the career ladder presents its own difficulties. Examples of common challenges and obstacles, and solutions that have been proven to work are outlined in Table 6.1.

A **job appointment** does not always result from the first interview, for various reasons. Many interviews occur prior to successful progression to a more senior role. Therefore keep applying and accessing the professional services, coaches and mentors available to support interview success.

Working in roles such as matron, senior staff nurse or clinical nurse specialist (CNS) in areas such as infection prevention and control (IPC) or tissue viability can be key to success and progression up the career ladder. This is outlined in Fig. 6.1, which shows the career ladder and timeline to success.

TABLE 6.1 ■ Common Challenges and Obstacles and Their Solutions

Examples of Common Challenges and Obstacles	Common Solutions
Informed you do not have the management skills for the role.	Complete an MSc in management or other courses.
Informed you do not have the management experience for the role.	Continue applying for the role you want with the support of a mentor and coach.
Broad management role and duties: informed your approach was too theoretical ('by the book').	Maintain confidence in your ability and shadow others to aid development.

It can be difficult to move to broad leadership from a specialist role; hence, thinking about the desired future career in advance and selecting early career jobs that will allow for a natural progression into senior roles is beneficial (Fig. 6.1).

Training, development and health and wellbeing support are available across healthcare services to support staff to overcome setbacks, bounce back from uncertainty and progress in their roles. Refer to the further information section for more resources on staff development and progression in the workplace.

6.4.2 DETERMINATION, RESILIENCE AND CONFIDENCE

Determination, resilience and self-confidence help drive progress and success as staff progress in their career. Resilience in healthcare requires access to resources and programmes to support staff to thrive in their role. Resilient nurses display distinctive qualities such as intelligence, self-confidence, resourcefulness and flexibility (Ramalisa et al., 2018). Role modelling of staff who have progressed in their role and made an impact encourages other internationally recruited (IR) staff to succeed and is thus important. Additionally, confidence based on successes and failures, observations and verbal feedback from others can influence self-efficacy and behaviours (Hecimovich, 2009). Self-esteem, self-compassion and psychological resilience among staff nurses and other staff, including when dealing with crises during and after the COVID-19 pandemic, are needed now more than ever, especially to aid the recovery process for staff (Joy et al., 2023).

6.4.3 WAYS TO IMPROVE AND ACCELERATE LEADERSHIP IMPACT

Following on from Chapter 5, further information on leadership development is provided below, including ways to improve and accelerate leadership in the health and care setting.

6.4.4 LIFELONG PERSONAL DEVELOPMENT

Lifelong personal development is key to success in your career. There are many resources included in this book, as well as links to other resources, which will ensure that staff succeed in their role.

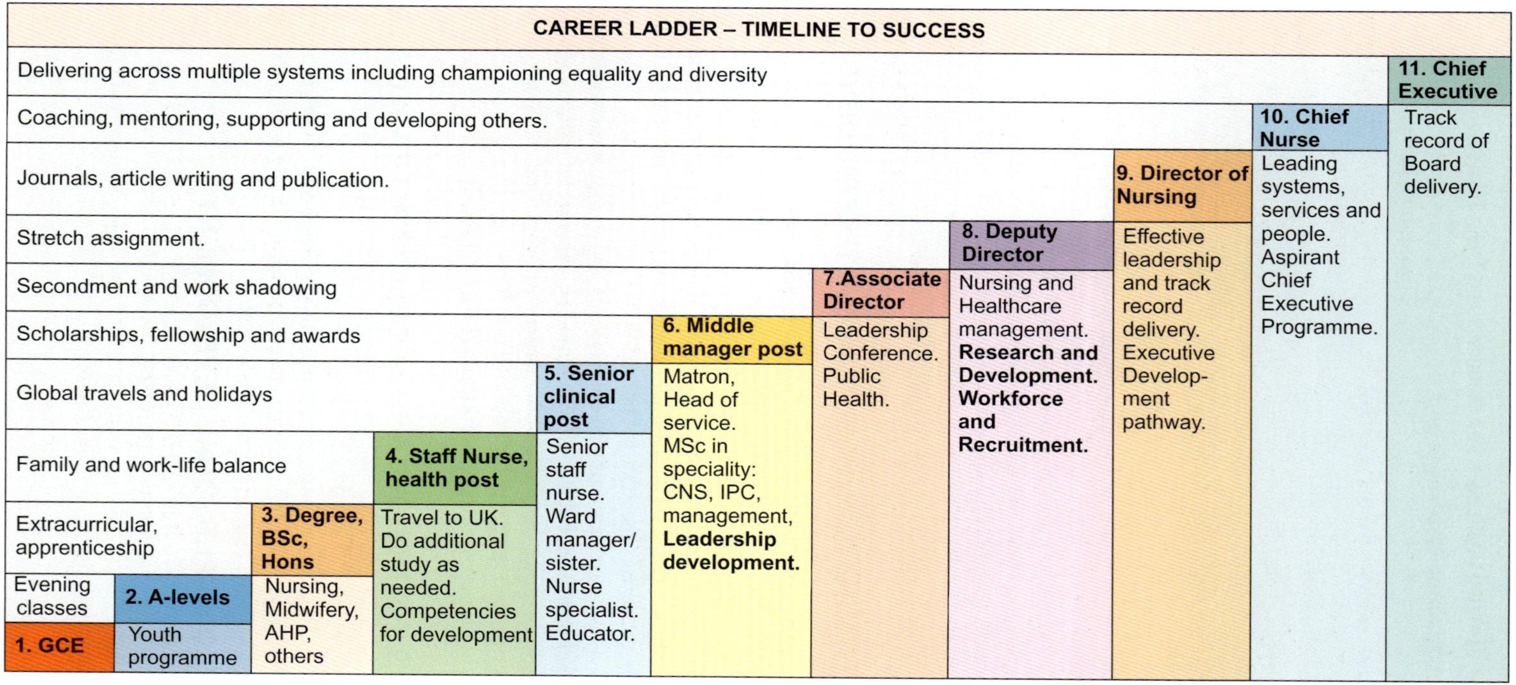

CAREER LADDER – TIMELINE TO SUCCESS

1. GCE	
2. A-levels	Youth programme
3. Degree, BSc, Hons	Nursing, Midwifery, AHP, others
4. Staff Nurse, health post	Travel to UK. Do additional study as needed. Competencies for development.
5. Senior clinical post	Senior staff nurse. Ward manager/sister. Nurse specialist. Educator.
6. Middle manager post	Matron, Head of service. MSc in speciality: CNS, IPC, management, **Leadership development.**
7. Associate Director	Leadership Conference. Public Health.
8. Deputy Director	Nursing and Healthcare management. **Research and Development. Workforce and Recruitment.**
9. Director of Nursing	Effective leadership and track record delivery. Executive Development pathway.
10. Chief Nurse	Leading systems, services and people. Aspirant Chief Executive Programme.
11. Chief Executive	Track record of Board delivery.

Cross-cutting themes (ordered from entry level to senior level):

- Evening classes
- Extracurricular, apprenticeship
- Family and work-life balance
- Global travels and holidays
- Scholarships, fellowship and awards
- Secondment and work shadowing
- Stretch assignment.
- Journals, article writing and publication.
- Coaching, mentoring, supporting and developing others.
- Delivering across multiple systems including championing equality and diversity

Fig. 6.1 Career ladder.

6.4.5 SPECIFY YOUR PATH: YOU AND YOUR SKILLS

Based on your interests and skills, specify your career path such as nursing, midwifery, nursing associate, healthcare support worker or AHP. Staff with other healthcare roles, such as medical doctors, scientists and healthcare technologists, engineers, lawyers, educators, lecturers and business managers can also use these tips and advice.

Narrow down your area of interest and make sure you have a good understanding of its career options and prospects. Seek to develop key skills and interests, ensuring they are suitable for a particular job. Then, seek and prioritise opportunities. Refer to 'Annesha Archyangelio's career ladder: Timeline to success' (Fig. 6.1) for guidance on career planning.

6.4.6 STARTING CAREER DEVELOPMENT EARLY

Workplaces, universities and conferences are good places to make many helpful contacts. Creating your own network enables you to broaden your career opportunities. Keeping in touch with these colleagues can help you find your dream job.

6.4.7 CREATE A TIMELINE FOR YOUR DEVELOPMENT

Planning how to get that dream job involves creating a personal development timeline. It is also helpful to have this ready for interviews, as employers sometimes ask you where you want to be in life in 5 years. You are not expected to share all your dreams but need to demonstrate sound knowledge of your plans. Refer to Fig. 6.1 for an example of a career timeline.

The career development and progression ladder in Fig. 6.1 is a very important tool, helping to increase the banding of international nurses and supporting international staff to progress through the Agenda for Change (AfC) banding. This timeline to success will help international nurses overcome some of the challenges and successfully move into senior roles at an early stage. It is important to reflect on the reasons for success, what the barriers are and how to overcome them. The author has navigated some of these challenges, with varying degrees of success, and has described what was done well and what did not go so well. Efforts are being made to address these challenges as part of recruitment strategies, such as starting IR staff at band 6 or promoting them soon after recruitment. This tool gives hints and tips on how others can climb the ladder and resolves some of the issues that limit career progression among IR staff. The author herself, having climbed the ladder, provides advice from a personal point of view to assist with this journey. Some staff may require more career moves than others to advance into senior roles and some may need to take sideways career moves to acquire the authentic experience required for career progression. The career ladder in Fig. 6.1 was specifically created to allow people to match themselves against it, identifying things that they can do to get to the top in their career.

6.4.8 PROMOTION INTO HIGHER BANDINGS AFTER INTERNATIONAL RECRUITMENT

What is needed to be promptly promoted to higher bandings after being recruited as an international staff member (Table 6.2)?

TABLE 6.2 ■ Promotion Into the Higher Bandings After International Recruitment

Helpful steps include:
Completing preceptorship.
Effective induction.
Knowing the job role and performing the duties very well using the relevant competencies.
Building a network of support, including relevant staff associations, for example.
Completing the relevant clinical skills, leadership and management training courses.
Applying for a new job when confident regarding readiness for the desired role.
Continuing to believe in oneself and not being discouraged.
Getting a coach and mentor to provide support and signposting.
Writing a 'winning' job application, curriculum vitae (CV) and cover letters.
'Acing' the job interview using the resources for preparing for a mock interview, and the
    actual interview, using the Situation–Task–Action–Result (STAR) technique.
Please note: refer to the relevant sections of this book for guidance on these elements.

6.4.9 CAREER DEVELOPMENT ACTION PLAN

It is important to create a career development action plan early on in your career. This can be in the form of a 5-year plan; an example is outlined in Table 6.3.

6.4.10 CAREER PLANNING

The points in the 5-year plan for career development (Table 6.3) assist staff in thinking about what they really want to achieve in their career and to identify and understand what they are good at, what motivates them and what their values are. It also helps staff to set themselves career goals and aspirations. Other factors that can help staff recognise their preferences as they pertain to specific areas of their career/job include:

- Technical and functional competencies.
- Managerial competencies.
- Autonomy/independence.
- Security/stability.
- Entrepreneurial creativity.
- Dedication to a cause.
- Pure challenge.
- Lifestyle.

6.4.11 CAREER STORIES

Career stories (Box 6.2) are provided by staff who are happy to share their stories and experience in relation to attaining senior roles, such as DON and head of service. This includes describing the most rewarding and challenging parts of their job, who inspires them, what helped them achieve their career goals and what advice they have for aspirant directors and heads of service.

TABLE 6.3 ■ A 5-Year Plan for Career Development

5-Year Plan Action Points	Actions to Complete to Move Forward	Date Completed
Aims: I want to achieve completion of this plan to help me fulfil my career potential and reap the rewards of my continuous programmes of study and skills development. To become a senior healthcare staff (above band 9) in the NHS.	1.Attend/utilise all of the leadership coaching programmes, including: a.Top Talent programme. b.Coaching programme. c.Top management programme competition. d.Masterclass training. Attend the National Leadership Conference to network and develop.	_/_/_
5-year timeline starting at band 5:		_/_/_
In the first 6 months: to have a full-time band 6 clinical specialist, senior staff nurse, midwife or AHP job.	Review the job description of these roles to identify what skills and knowledge I need to develop.	_/_/_
Year 1: to have a band 7 clinical specialist, senior staff nurse, midwife or AHP job.	Attend training to develop the skills and knowledge that I need.	_/_/_
Year 2: to become a band 8a/b clinical specialist nurse, ward manager, ward sister, midwife or AHP.	Engage in media activities and public speaking.	_/_/_
Year 3: to become a band 8c/d nurse, midwife, AHP consultant, matron or advanced practitioner.	Present papers at large conferences. Develop skills related to providing inspiration and showing genuineness and presence.	_/_/_
Year 4: to have a band 9 NHS/healthcare deputy director job.	Write a new policy from scratch.	_/_/_
Year 5: to have a very senior management (VSM)/executive senior management (ESM) NHS/healthcare job.	Lead the management of all services in hospitals, including executive on-call services. Chair executive and board meetings.	_/_/_
Year 6 onwards: to have a higher-level executive VSM NHS/healthcare job.	Search for opportunities using various methods. Create a network list and speak to those people for help. Keep my CV and cover letter updated to reflect my skills.	_/_/_

BOX 6.2	Career Stories

Career summary: A staff member shared her story of progressing to the DON role in the fields of substance misuse and health and justice. She ran her own company, providing management and consultancy services, including operational delivery of substance misuse contracts in third-sector organisations in relation to specific systems.

Career commencement: I started working in my local hospital as a nursing assistant. I loved it and decided I wanted to become a nurse, even though my initial plan was to become an occupational therapist.

Becoming a DON: After qualifying as a nurse, I realised that I needed to be in a position of power to make significant changes in my area of work and challenge practice regarding standards of care. This inspired me to become a DON, as did another DON who showed clarity and humility in delivering strategic and transformational change through compassionate leadership and good people management. This enabled me to make important decisions about the direction and practice of my services, focusing on valuing the patient and staff populations I serve.

Rewards and challenges: It is rewarding to support people dealing with difficulties and help, encourage and inspire staff to progress to the top in their careers while also leading and improving patient care quality. However, the slow pace of effecting change in some aspects of health and care is challenging.

Advice for aspirant directors of nursing: Be assertive and never give up on trying to do things better. Lead by taking staff with you, and be visible, accessible and approachable.

Enjoy your job and advocate for quality patient care and staff professionalism while also dealing with the demands of care delivery.

Key to career goals success: Resilience, determination and innovation.

Aim for the top role in your profession. Have out of work activities to rejuvenate!

6.4.12 MEDIA AND PUBLIC SPEAKING

Media and public speaking training is provided to develop skills related to television (TV), media interviews, presentations, press release writing, media awareness and broadcasting, including on the radio, to help senior staff with political issues. Support is provided to deal with new media stories, audio and video modalities, hostile audiences, integrated marketing, reputation and organisation status management, crisis management, podcasting, blogging and vlogging.

6.4.13 TRAINING AND PRESENTATION SKILLS

Training and presentation skills are important to support staff as they progress through their career. This includes techniques such as 'breaking the ice' at the start of a session; use of a systematic presentation approach to identify the audience's needs; setting objectives; preparing to provide training, monitoring and support; transferring learnings in the workplace; and evaluation and additional steps. Teaching methods include brainstorming, collaboration, teamwork and using clear instructions.

6.4.14 DEVELOPMENT AND ADVANCING

Being clear on individual needs and being bolder in the face of adversity are vital for career development and advancement. Women have additional challenges in career progression as they are often the family supporter and sometimes the only source of household income. IR and ethnic minority staff have challenges regarding equal access to opportunities and promotion in the workplace. Other disadvantaged groups also have their own challenges. Ways to address these as part of the career progression timeline should be considered. In addition, never be shy to suggest ideas or ask for a job promotion or salary increase, based on the level and type of work being undertaken, as described in Section 6.4.12. on media and public speaking and in Table 6.4 on media messaging reminders.

6.4.15 GAINING SUPPORT FROM OTHERS WHO HAVE GONE BEFORE YOU

Gain support from others who have gone before you by noticing and emulating key role models within your organisation and interact with other industry and company leaders who can help you. Follow key influencers on social media to learn about pitfalls and successes in their work. Network, network, network! And never stop trying!

6.4.16 STUDY AND COMPARE CAREER OFFERS

Make an appointment for career advice with individuals, organisations and services that can help you. National, regional and local career seminars and conferences are useful places to study and compare career offers. As noted in Section 5.3 on professional leadership in healthcare and Section 5.2 on career and study pathways available in the United Kingdom (UK) healthcare system, coaches and mentors are essential in supporting staff throughout their careers.Section 5.2

Searching for a job and preparing for the interview is another area that requires careful preparation. Setting up job alerts, creating a 'winning' curriculum vitae (CV) and gaining job application support are important to succeed in being called for an interview and getting the job.

6.4.17 ADVICE AND LEARNINGS FOR SUCCESS BASED ON LIVED EXPERIENCE

Some additional advice and learnings for successful career progression, based on lived experience, to help you move up the career ladder include:

- **career progression**Develop yourself by accessing all the opportunities available.
- Apply for jobs along the desired career pathway.
- Ask for the development support that you want and need.
- Do not forget the things you did not achieve in your last job.
- Ask for the help needed for career progression.
- Shadow, work with and learn from others.
- Use your experience as a steppingstone.
- Write a career 'to do' list.
- Compare yourself to the greatest.
- Dream big with regard to your career aspirations.
- Keep on trying to achieve your desired career goals.

Please note: Even if you have a great plan and it works, a career advisor is something like a personal therapist.

TABLE 6.4 ■ **Media Messaging Reminders Tool**

Topic	Building a Private Wing in a Hospital Example Answers
Who is your audience?	The audience include the public, healthcare staff, local campaign groups and members of parliament (MPs).
What do you want them to do?	Accept the proposal.
Key message	Potential opportunities to treat private patients in hospital to increase income, which will contribute to the treatment of more NHS patients. Safe and sustainable service for the future.
Key point 1	Generate income: Bring in more income to support NHS services. Contribute to the recruitment of more staff for the hospital. Continue to provide access to high-quality service at different sites.
Point 2	Reinvest in healthcare facilities. Designate local elective sites.
Point 3	Increase service delivery capacity. Contribute to protecting the future of the hospital. Enhance postoperative recovery services closer to home.
Memorable phrase or case study	Bring in income. Expand service delivery. Designate local elective care with reduced wait times.
Other notes *This area can be used to describe three extra points if you are listing both pros and cons.*	This service model is already provided elsewhere. Units runs well elsewhere. Takes more money to provide more services. Groups of clinicians are in favour of this. Increases clinician numbers and leads to quicker elective care and treatment.
Presentation reminders Energy!	Increase income to provide more NHS services. Patient stories: a large number of patients are waiting for this routine service; reduce wait times and demonstrate local services in action.
Notes	**Key points for media interviews:** Do not take phone calls in interviews.**interviews** Work closely with the comms director. Attend the interview along with the communications director. Be calm and authoritative.

6.4.18 STRATEGIES FOR PROGRESSING IN YOUR CURRENT ROLE

These include fellowships, internships, shadowing, secondments, contracts, use of agencies and consultancies, apprenticeships (Box 6.3), volunteering, graduate schemes and other jobs in hospitals and the NHS for young individuals. Strategies for progressing in

I have grown in confidence, learned a lot of new skills and feel really happy in my apprenticeship.

A business apprentice

your current role apply to staff who are interested in a different career pathway; additional courses and experience can support this. You can learn about your dream job from your colleagues or the internet. Career experience gives insights to shape your future goals.

Strategies applicable to over 350 NHS careers are also open to the 14 to 16, 16 to 18 and over 19 years age groups and include:

- **Apprenticeships**: individuals can apply for jobs and apprenticeships at an early stage (aged 16 years and over); these offer routes into the NHS (health careers) through a mix of classroom and on-the-job training at various levels.
- **Work experience** in the health and care sector provides the opportunity to experience what it would be like to work in the NHS and learn about the roles and responsibilities of different healthcare professionals, while also giving strong insight into the different career pathways.
- **Royal College of Nursing (RCN) cadet scheme**.
- **Volunteering** (NHS, 2022j).

6.4.18.1 Secondments

Secondments are among the resources that can be used to develop employees and encourage skills exchange between staff, building capability and capacity. This helps to support high-potential individuals to progress and reach their optimum potential.

6.4.18.2 Work Shadowing

This is on-the-job learning, a career and leadership development intervention involving one staff member working with another who might be performing a different role or working in a different setting, and who has knowledge to share regarding specific leadership behaviour and competencies. This intervention allows learning of new aspects related to one's work in organisations and systems, reaching across borders.

6.4.18.3 Stretch Assignments

Stretch assignments are roles, programmes, projects or tasks given to individuals by an organisation that extend beyond the staff member's current knowledge or skills, thus stretching them developmentally. This is achieved by challenging the individual through placing them in an unfamiliar situation or setting.

6.4.18.4 Extracurricular Learning

Additional extracurricular learning may be required depending on the career path you choose to follow. Ongoing study is part of continued professional development and lifelong learning as part of career progression and can include conference attendance, project management and other similar activities. This should be aligned with national priorities, professional trends and learning. Many extracurricular activities provide the added skills and knowledge needed and look good on your CV. Participating in these activities gives you time for yourself, saves you from burning out and keeps up your motivation. This gives you an advantage over the competition.

6.4.19 ACCESSING SKILLS AND SUPPORT OFFERS

Accessing the right skills and support offers increases productivity in the healthcare setting. Helping others to grow by supporting them with their career and developmental needs is also important. Job satisfaction, personal power and happiness in your job can be achieved by finding and doing a job you love. Therefore spend time to find the job that is right for you.

6.4.20 PROJECT MANAGEMENT SHORT COURSES

Additional project management short courses, which can support career progression, include Prince2 and other project management courses.

Prince2 can be a helpful qualification for project management office (PMO) roles and jobs such as project manager, service manager, operations manager and performance manager.

Prince2 courses including Introduction, Foundation, Practitioner and Agile provide theoretical knowledge of how to plan, manage and deliver projects from start to finish (Axelos, 2023).

6.4.21 QUALITY IMPROVEMENT TRAINING

The Institute for Healthcare Improvement (IHI) (2023a) provides quality improvement (QI) training that focuses on improvement science and patient safety to advance and sustain better outcomes in health and healthcare, including via improvement of capabilities, person- and family-centred care, patient safety, quality, cost and value and delivering on the triple aim of improving population care and population health while also reducing costs and improving value (IHI, 2023a).

QI as part of clinical leadership is important and is detailed in the following paragraph and bullet points.

QI contributes to improving the quality of outcomes for patients, supported by clinical and system leadership, and commissioning of care, using knowledge and understanding of patients care needs. This is supported by clinical networks of experts on specific conditions and services and by clinical senates comprising a range of clinical voices in specific areas of the country.

Examples of areas requiring QI and clinical leadership include:
- Ambulance response programme.
- Operational performance and emergency care.
- Innovation, digital technology, systems and interpreting data using run charts, control charts and other tools.
- Finance and use of resources.
- Shared decision-making.
- Strategic change using methods such as Plan, Do, Study, Act (PDSA).

- IPC
- Palliative and end-of-life care (PEoLC).
- The experience of care, covering winter resilience, patient care, the Friends and Family Test (FFT) and frailty.
- Workforce programmes and safer staffing for acute, district and community nursing and AHPs.
- Quality and safety, which could be improved by reducing errors and harms, responding to adverse events and instilling a safety culture based on human factors, team work and communication.
- Mental and physical health.
- Learning disabilities and autism (LDA).
- Safeguarding
- Clinical auditing.
- Seven-day service.
- Health visiting.
- Patient-Led Assessments of the Care Environment (PLACE).
- Heart disease care.
- Pathology services.
- Medicine management.
- Diabetes care.
- Cancer care.
- Midwifery supervision.

Achievement of these aims is supported by resources such as the Quality Improvement Hub (QIHub) resource pack for health and social care staff. QIHub uses QI approaches as a core part of their work (AHSN Network, 2023), empowering teams to make safety improvements.

QI is supported by NHS IMPACT (IMproving Patient Care Together), which, through a unified approach creating the right conditions for continuous improvement and high performance, helps organisations to respond to healthcare challenges, delivering better care for patients and better outcomes for communities (NHS England, 2023y). These elements contribute to strengthening leadership in the clinical environment.

Aspirant director talent programmes are offered by various organisations, for aspiring directors and other senior staff, to help staff identify their development needs and acquire support with leadership development to enhance quality and navigate change. This can be achieved by shadowing others, undertaking a stretch assignment, participating in an action learning set or online learning activities, working in pairs and groups, performing peer reviews, going on a secondment, or working as an interim consultant to transition into executive director roles. Help in accessing coaches and mentors, reverse mentoring, and CV drafting for leadership development and the transition into executive director roles is also provided. Staff also get the opportunity to identify what type of director they would like to be, such as an operational DON supervising staff on the frontline, which contrasts with a strategic or academic role focusing on developing practice and engineering new ways of working. These programmes, which support staff to learn and use political skills as they progress into senior roles, include assessments and simulated executive board meetings.

6.4.22 TALENT MANAGEMENT RESOURCES

The provision and use of specific talent management resources is important for developing both leadership and leaders. There are talent management resources to help staff take leadership actions and create ideas that change healthcare, including in the key areas of recruiting, developing, retaining and deploying talent, as well as succession planning, as detailed later (NHS Leadership Academy, 2023a).

6.4.23 RECRUITING TALENT

Although technical skills, competencies, knowledge and qualifications are important to do the job, communication, consultation and relationship development skills are more important considerations than ever before when recruiting talent to an organisation at both junior and senior levels. Staff with the right values, traits, behaviours and motivation to drive high-quality service delivery should be recruited. Given the high level of complexity of healthcare, staff should be adaptive, resourceful and able to thrive in an uncertain and ever-changing environment. Diversity is vital to success in a high-performing organisation and there should be ongoing efforts to ensure that staff recruited including at senior and board level, represent the population they serve. 'Talent spotting' should be done, internally and externally, to move staff, including those from a diverse background, from clinical managerial roles to senior leadership roles in the organisation.

6.4.24 DEVELOPING AND RETAINING TALENT

Identifying and retaining the type of talent that is most critical to leading and implementing an organisation's strategy is important and individuals should be recruited and developed in line with that. Care should be taken to ensure not only that talent management is applied to all but also to use a collective leadership approach to benefit the whole organisation. Board and senior leaders should ensure that talent management is applied to high-potential staff as well as staff at all levels to deliver its business strategy and objectives and ensure that everyone knows that the organisation cares for and invests in them. The human resources (HR) culture should value the contribution and personal growth of staff, foster relationships in alignment with the organisation's goals and show vision and commitment to problem-solve and deliver high-quality, safe and innovative care.

6.4.25 DEPLOYING TALENT

The continuous deployment of talent enables an organisation's leadership to be agile, future-focused and responsive to changing needs. As staff become more senior, the organisation should support them to make the shift from broad leadership skills to specific leadership roles, and from technical functionality and business know-how to strategic and conceptual thinking, which requires the ability to deal with complex and ambiguous clinical and healthcare situations and enhanced decision-making authority. This may require experimental learning and opportunities to work in a more integrated and collaborative way, such as through secondments, to meet strategic and system-level challenges. Many top-performing organisations followed this process, including for filling director posts, which has contributed to their ongoing success given that staff can hone their leadership skills in less familiar areas of clinical practice.

The diversity of staff, in terms of their potential, within the talent pool needs to be identified and recognised, treating staff as individuals rather than homogenous groups. Leaders needs to be coached on having more effective conversations about talent at all levels in the organisation. Talent conversations include two key elements, i.e. a 'hard' and 'soft' side; the use of different strategies focused on innovation, patient/user needs and QI; as well as a skills and knowledge base to achieve the desired outcomes. It is also important to focus on interpersonal and intrapersonal activities to create the right employee value position to keep talented individuals engaged. Talented individuals are vital to fill the high number of executive-level vacancies across organisations, reduce staff turnover and ensure organisational stability.

6.4.26 TALENT MANAGEMENT CONVERSATIONS

All staff should be offered a talent management conversation and develop a talent management plan, focusing on building capacity, continuous improvement, transformation, commercial and system leadership and building a diverse and inclusive workforce reflecting the diverse population we serve (NHS England, 2019b). Talent management is about considering everyone as an individual and the development that is right for them, making them feel rewarded and able to do good. The first part of the talent management toolkit covers definitions, why we need talent management and how you can strengthen the workforce (NHS Leadership Academy, 2023a).

6.4.27 SUCCESSION PLANNING

Succession planning includes the identification of vital job roles that may become vacant due to retirement, attrition, business growth, innovation, change or promotion, as well as strategic consideration of where and how internal candidates might fill those roles.

Succession planning also includes identifying and developing future leaders to increase their potential and performance outcomes in these roles. This impacts on the engagement levels among staff, preserves organisational memory and enables the organisation to stay viable.

Succession planning involves asking key questions to identify staff who are approaching retirement; determining whether staff can be supported to work elsewhere in the system; and determining whether there are new innovation and business ideas in the strategic plans that could create new positions for talented staff to contribute to fulfilling the vision, values and objectives of the organisation. Changes and trends occurring within the organisation, health system, services and wider market can create these opportunities. A diverse staff group should be considered for these opportunities. Succession planning should not focus on targeted individuals but rather develop capacity, capability and marketability to ensure there is a pool of potential applicants who have the right skills in the right areas for key vacancies that may arise.

These strategies help to support recruitment, development, deployment and retention of talent to ensure an agile and mobile workforce. Successful talent management is an ethos and is key to developing a safe, compassionate culture (NHS Leadership Academy, 2023a).

6.4.27.1 Leadership and Leadership Development in Healthcare

The delivery of continuously improving, high-quality, safe and compassionate healthcare is supported by additional elements of leadership including;

- The leadership task.
- Individual leadership in health services.
- Team leadership.
- Leadership of organisation.
- National-level leadership.
- Leader and leadership development.

A culture of high-quality care:

- Inspiring visions operationalised at every level.
- Clear, aligned objectives for all teams, departments and individual staff.
- Supportive and enabling people management and high levels of staff engagement.
- Learning, innovation and QI embedded in the practice of all staff
- Effective team working.

Leadership theory and research—personality and leader effectiveness:

- High energy level and stress tolerance.
- Self-confidence.
- Internal locus of control.
- Emotional maturity
- Personal integrity.
- Socialised power motivation.
- Achievement orientation.
- Low need for affiliation.

Leadership competencies (see also Section 5.3.3):

- Leader behaviours.

Leadership theory and research in healthcare:

- Theories of leadership.
- Nurse leaders.
- Medical leaders.
- Board leadership.
- Team leaders in healthcare.
- Organisational leaders

Leadership, culture and climate in healthcare:

- Organisational culture in healthcare.
- Organisational climate in healthcare.

Leader and leadership development interventions:

- Multisource (360-degree) feedback using questionnaires.
- Developmental assessment centres.
- Job rotation

- Action learning.
- Mentoring.
- Executive coaching.

Leaders and leadership development in healthcare:

- National-level leadership.
- Reflections on leaders and leadership development in healthcare.

(NHS Leadership Academy, 2023a).

6.4.28 NHS INTERIM MANAGEMENT AND SUPPORT TALENT POOL

NHS Interim Management and Support (NHS IMAS) offers NHS organisations that need short- or medium-term support the means to access the management expertise that exists throughout the NHS. Resource management and creating an effective workforce requires an evidence-based workforce plan integrated with finance, activity and performance plans. By providing high-level NHS expertise to NHS organisations with no fee, staff can put patients first (NHS, 2022 l). Attracting, recruiting, developing and retaining talented people from all backgrounds is a key commitment in our NHS People Promise.

6.4.29 THE GOLDEN RULE OF RELAXATION

Hard work pays off! However, 'workaholism' doesn't always lead to success. A proper regime of work and rest keeps your mind and body in good working order, making you more creative and ultimately a better person. The key is quality, not the quantity of hours spent working. Have a strategy, ask experts for advice and build plenty of relaxation time into your work and career progression routine, as supported by Section 6.4.17 on advice and learnings for success based on lived experience and Box 6.4 on progression to a senior career role.

6.4.30 OTHER PROGRAMME AND PATHWAYS

These can support career progression and staff development and include:

6.4.30.1 The Operation Black Vote Leadership Programme

The Operation Black Vote (OBV) programme aims to improve the representation of Black, Asian and minority ethnic (BAME) communities in civic and political roles in the UK. Further information is provided by Lord Simon Woolley Commander of the British Empire (CBE), who established OBV in 1996 (OBV, 2023).

6.4.30.2 The UK Parliament

The Backbench Business Committee holds regular debates at Westminster Hall, on matters such as IPC standards in the NHS, which are open to the public to attend. Individuals can sign up to receive the UK Parliament Newsletter and book to attend a public parliamentary session (UK Parliament, 2023).

6.4.30.3 International Engagement Work

Volunteering at the World Health Organization (WHO) or International Council of Nurses (ICN), and engagement with other professional bodies such as the Commission on Graduates of Foreign Nursing Schools (CGFNS), can contribute to the development of senior healthcare leaders.

6.4.30.4 The World Health Organisation

Networking with the WHO enables international collaboration and sharing of knowledge globally, as well as the opportunity to provide input regarding the WHO's policies and strategies. There are various global development programmes that staff can participate in, such as programmes aimed at increasing vaccination uptake and reducing vaccine hesitancy to improve the health of the global population; surveillance to monitor disease trends; tuberculosis control; antimicrobial resistance reduction; and support of lower-to-middle income countries. There may even be opportunities to shadow/observe delegates who attend the World Health Assembly (WHA) to understand the workings of the WHO. The WHO EURO Internship programme is another avenue through which staff can participate in engagement work with the WHO.

6.4.30.5 The International Council of Nurses

The ICN, which is the global voice of millions of nurses worldwide, is a federation of more than 132 national nursing associations. The ICN uses its position statements to address various areas related to health, wellbeing and nursing professional advancement. Staff can participate in the work of the ICN, including by presenting at the ICN Congress along with other activities (ICN, 2023).

6.5 Additional Resources and Guidance to Support Healthcare Staff

Special roles that staff can apply for in addition to their jobs include:

6.5.1 NURSING NOW CAMPAIGN AMBASSADORS

Nursing Now was a global campaign to improve health by raising the profile and status of nursing worldwide (WHO, 2023a).

6.5.2 THE NURSING NOW CHALLENGE

The Nursing Now Challenge is a programme of the Burdett Trust for Nursing Charity to protect the Nursing Now name and logo (Nursing Now Challenge, 2023).

6.5.3 CAVELL NURSES' TRUST

The Cavell Nurses' Trust, which works with its members throughout the year, is committed to supporting the UK nursing profession through dedicated resources; welcome packs; press and media launches; collaborations, surveys and reporting; and events and fund raising (Cavell Nurses' Trust, 2023).

6.5.4 AWARDS

Awards ensure that the work that is undertaken in healthcare and other capacities to deliver high-quality care is recognised, including voluntary and community services. This help to build a supportive network and provides a means for sharing success with others. Awards that staff can apply for include the following:

6.5.4.1 Royal College of Nursing and Royal College of Nursing Institute (RCNI) Awards

Entries are distributed among RCN members, providing a chance to make an impact (RCN, 2023 l).

6.5.4.2 Royal College of Nursing Fellowship

Staff can be nominated for the RCN Fellowship and Honorary Fellowship, which recognise practitioners, researchers, educationalists and leaders who share the RCN's commitment to advancing the art and science of nursing and improving healthcare (RCN, 2023 m).

6.5.4.3 Queen's Nurse Award

The Queen's Nursing Institute (QNI) offers various awards to community nurses for past service that are distinct from grants and other forms of financial and personal assistance (QNI, 2023a).

6.5.4.4 Queen's Nursing Institute Grants

The QNI provides resources that help community nurses give excellent patient care. This includes the Queen's Nurse Leadership Programme, funded by the National Garden Scheme and delivered by The Leadership Trust in collaboration with the QNI. This is a leadership programme for Queen's Nurse (QN) health visitors, educators and managers working in the community setting (QNI, 2023b).

Resources for community nurses (QNI, 2023b) include:

- Educational grants: QNI.
- The Community Nurse Executive Network (CNEN).
- The Executive Nurse Leadership Programme.

QNI resources to support the transition to community nursing and care home nursing include:

- Free QNI supporting carers (a new development).
- The QNI/Queen's Nursing Institute Scotland (QNIS) voluntary standards for community children's nurse education and practice.
- Guidance on general practice nursing in the 21st century (a time of opportunity) covering patient care, long-term conditions, family support, promoting good health, prescribing, community service and other areas.
- A report on district nurse education in the UK (5-year review).

- Guidance on assessing the health of people who are homeless including a health assessment tool.
- Guidance on discharge planning, including best practice in the transition of care, identifying barriers and challenges that affect discharge and sharing areas that have led to workable solutions. The discharge planning process includes looking at who is affected; informing community teams about the discharge, including the timing and day of discharge; liaison; working in a multidisciplinary team (MDT); home visits prior to discharge; contact with family; assessment; discharge coordinators and key workers; discharge planning; social care packages; medication; equipment for the home; the effectiveness of discharge planning; actions to improve discharge planning; and examples of best discharge planning (QNI, 2023b).

6.5.4.5 Fellowship of the Institute of Health Visiting

Honorary Fellowships of the Institute of Health Visiting (FiHVs) are awarded at the iHV's annual celebration event held each year in recognition of contributions to both the institute and the health visiting profession. An honorary fellowship is a mark of the high esteem in which the awardee is held by the institute's board (IHV, 2023b).

6.5.4.6 Additional Nursing Awards

There are other nursing awards that staff can apply for. These include:
- NHS parliamentary awards.
- Health Service Journal (HSJ) awards.
- Nursing Times awards.
- Health and social care awards.

6.5.4.7 Doctoral Awards

Individuals can study for a PhD at a university to receive the award of Doctor of Philosophy, using different methods of study including PhD by completing a thesis, PhD by publication, Professional Doctorate, Integrated or Online PhDs (Prospects, 2023).

Doctoral awards are also supported by the National Institute for Health and Care Research (NIHR), such as the Oxford Biomedical Research Centre.

Doctoral awards usually cover the salary, tuition fees and research costs of staff while they are studying for a doctorate. Awards cover either 3 years (full-time) or 5 years (part-time). There are plenty of external providers who provide funding, including the following:
- **The NIHR Doctoral Fellowship** for PhDs undertaken in an area of NIHR research.
- **The NIHR Clinical Doctoral Research Fellowship**, awarded so that healthcare professionals can undertake a research PhD aiding professional development and clinical practice.
- **Medical Research Council for Clinical Research Training Fellowships** (CRTFs), which support clinicians including nursing, midwifery and allied health professionals (NMAHPS) to undertake a PhD or other higher research degree.
- **Wellcome PhD Training Fellowships** allowing clinicians to undertake a PhD within a structured environment including mentoring.

- **British Heart Foundation PhD programmes** for both clinical and nonclinical cardiovascular researchers.
- **Cancer Research UK PhD scholarships** for research to be undertaken in the UK.
- **Versus Arthritis offers PhD scholarships** for basic scientists and nonmedical healthcare professionals to embark on a research career in any discipline relevant to arthritis and related musculoskeletal diseases.
- **The Multiple Sclerosis (MS) Society offers PhD Fellowships** for those wishing to embark on a research career focusing on MS.
- **Diabetes UK offers PhD studentships** for research projects relevant to the aims of their research strategy.
- **The British Geriatrics Society (BGS) and the Dunhill Medical Trust (DMT)** offer frontline health professionals doctoral training fellowships to undertake research on diseases and frailty. The Grand Union Economic and Social Research Council Doctoral Training Partnership offers studentships for training in domains including health and wellbeing.
- **Biotechnology and Biological Science Research Council**: The Oxford Interdisciplinary Bioscience Doctoral Training Programme supports research on molecular mechanisms and cellular bioscience, transformative technologies, bioscience for health, industrial biotechnology and pharmaceuticals (NIHR, 2023b).

6.5.4.8 The British Federation of Women Graduates

The British Federation of Women Graduates (BFWG) offers a range of awards and competition prizes each year to female doctoral students, thus providing financial support (BFWG, 2023).

6.5.4.9 UK Honours System and Awards Applications

Individuals can nominate someone who has gone above and beyond for a British Empire Medal (BEM), Member of the Order of the British Empire (MBE), Officer of the Order of the British Empire (OBE), CBE, Damehood or Knighthood award. This could include work where staff identified gaps in hospital procedures, went out of their way to address them and rolled out their process across the organisation, thereby having a positive impact on health and patient care. This may include staff who sit on a local or regional board, thus having local reach, and who go out into the **community** to make an impact and a difference.

6.5.4.10 Excellence in Healthcare Science Awards

The Chief Scientific Officer (CSO) Excellence in Healthcare Science Lifetime Achievement award (NHS England, 2022j) supports the work of professionals in healthcare science and applied science who support diagnosis and treatment to improve patient care outcomes.

6.5.4.11 Institute of Electrical and Electronics Engineers Biomedical Engineering Award

This prize includes Institute of Electrical and Electronics Engineer (IEEE) Medals, Recognitions and Technical Field Awards for outstanding contributions to the field of biomedical engineering. The award consists of a bronze medal, certificate and cash honorarium (IEEE Awards, 2023). The award can be granted for work that impacts the profession and/or society; makes a significant technical or other type of contribution; demonstrates leadership in the accomplishment of worthwhile goal(s); leads to publications, patents or other types of achievement; and demonstrates high quality.

6.5.5 CLINICAL NETWORKS AND CLINICAL SENATES

Clinical networks and senates bring together individuals who use, provide and commission services to improve outcomes in complex patient pathways using an integrated whole-system approach. Key areas posing major health and wellbeing challenges include cardiovascular diseases (including cardiac disease, stroke, renal disease and diabetes), maternity care, children and young people, mental health (MH), dementia and neurological conditions and cancer. Clinical senates are a source of independent, strategic advice and guidance for commissioners and other stakeholders, assisting them in making the best decisions about healthcare for the populations they represent (NHS England, 2022k).

6.5.6 NHS EVENTS AND NEWS

The events, activities and news that staff can participate in help people to celebrate the NHS, giving them the opportunity to mark the NHS's 75th birthday, for example. The NHS and other organisations organise exciting nationwide events that help staff learn more about the NHS, including its history and plans for the future, and provide an opportunity to meet the staff who make the NHS what it is (NHS England, 2022l).

6.5.7 CALENDAR OF NATIONAL CAMPAIGNS

This includes national campaigns, awards and awareness days to help staff plan activities for the year (NHS Employers, 2023f).

6.5.8 INTERNATIONAL NURSES' DAY: 12 MAY

International Nurses' Day (GOV.UK, 2023q) is an important day that is celebrated by nurses across the world on 12 May every year. Activities and events can include fundraising and charitable work, territorial army nursing, digital innovation in clinical practice, workforce recruitment and retention, adult and paediatric education, local academy work, the retire and return programme, RCN events, tissue viability and pressure ulcer management, medicine management and nutrition services and resources. The celebration also encompasses health and wellbeing, mind and body, occupational health, staff benefits, community nursing and health visiting, women's services, and specialities such as haematology and oncology, clinical imaging and medical physics, medical and surgical services, and ambulatory and cardiovascular care. Other areas are covered including safeguarding, integrated and perioperative services, discharge and flow, research and development, IPC and sterile services, continuous professional development (CPD) and free resources for staff including cakes, sweets, stationery and prizes. International Nurses'

Day is also an occasion to celebrate nurses and midwives and provide them with many awards, including for poster competitions as well as an executive director award, senior leadership award, nursing and midwifery award, chief nurse award, student awards, fellowship awards and awards for the nurse, midwife, care assistant and team of the year.

6.5.9 SETTING UP A JOURNAL CLUB

A journal club comprises a group of people with common interests who gather together to discuss a journal article. These clubs are often linked with the local library and involve hearing and learning about others' viewpoints; this can contribute to Nursing and Midwifery Council (NMC) revalidation.

Journal clubs make the following contributions:
- Support learning and improve critical appraisal skills.
- Encourage evidenced based-medicine.
- Promote awareness of research skills.
- Keep members abreast of new literature.
- Encourages use of research.
- Provide an opportunity for networking, peer learning and the sharing of experience.
- Provide continuing education and opportunities for professional development.
- Stimulate debate and improve understanding of current topics.

(Nursing Times, 2023).

6.5.10 BULLETINS AND NEWSLETTERS

Sign-up for bulletins and newsletters in your organisation.

Bulletins and newsletters may be in the form of a monthly team brief providing a summary of key messages that everyone in the organisation needs to know about, sponsored by an executive or director such as the Chief Executive Officer (CEO), Chief Nursing Officer (CNO)/DON or director of human resources (HR) and organisational development (OD). The newsletter may include content such as the flu campaign (#GiveItASHot); Restart a Heart Day; free hospital partnerships or memberships; performance in cancer and 52 waiting times; mortality and morbidity; emergency department (ED) performance referral to treatment (RTT); new harms; Friends and Family Test (FFT) results; and winter planning. There may also be updates on finance, budget, savings and fund raising, as well as hospital environment redevelopment plans including limitations, funding, modelling, governance, and strategic outline cases (SOCs), as well as progress with timescales for site completion, strategic, public and clinical engagement, evaluation and feedback. Newsletters may also include Care Quality Commission (CQC) updates including guidance and a quality checklist, the organisation's quality commitments regarding care, culture, learning, improvement, leadership and clinical pathways, IT services or new apps, parking, mandatory training, staff surveys where staff can have their say (the 'big 5') and recruitment (e.g. of new CEOs or directors). The newsletter can include information on new career networks, career coaching, mentoring, buddying and new intranet sites; talking about healthy interests; understanding stress; MH first aid; delivering excellence in care; equality, diversity and inclusion (EDI) (Equality Act, 2010); and delivering on the nine protected characteristics of race, age,

BOX 6.4	Progression to a Senior Career Role

Senior career role success stories include:

Progression to national director roles for specific clinical pathways (covering urgent and emergency care, acute care, patient and public participation, commissioning, community, MH, maternity and other specialities).

Provided national leadership in the delivery of care in these areas.

Drove major improvements in key areas such as cancer, MH and primary care across the whole health system in line with the NHS long-term plan (2019) and operation plan (2023) for health (these are updated regularly).

Successful performance in the delivery of health and care across portfolios.

Provided leadership oversight for specified services across the country, e.g. commissioning and Emergency Preparedness, Resilience and Response (EPRR).

Completed work for the WHO and established an international track record in relation to patient safety:

Commissioning of MH care, social care, community safety and education.

Director General at the Department of Health, leading the Cabinet Office health team.

Commenced career as a graduate management trainee, chair of national societies and trusts and panel chair.

Ongoing **career development** and support helped me to achieve the above.

National senior manager

disability, gender reassignment, marriage and civil partnerships, pregnancy and maternity, religion or beliefs, sex and sexual orientation.

6.5.10.1 Chief Nursing Officer Bulletin

Subscribe for this bulletin from the CNO for England. It provides key information for nursing, midwifery and care staff with a focus on the workforce, leadership, key news and updates. It details good practice, describes events and provides a host of resources designed to support the delivery of patient-focused, evidence-based, high-quality care. Staff can also submit an article or contact us about the CNO bulletin (NHS England, 2023z).

6.5.11 COLLABORATING CENTRES

There are more than 800 institutions in over 80 countries that support WHO programmes (WHO, 2023b). These include organisations such as research institutes, universities and academies, which undertake activities to support the WHO's programmes.

6.5.12 PUBLIC HEALTH LOCAL PRACTICE

Public health (PH) local practice examples are used to celebrate successes and demonstrate the work that staff has undertaken. Although not formal research, PH local practice makes an invaluable contribution to knowledge translation and learning or research generation (UK Health Security Agency (UKHSA), 2023b).

6.6 Summary: Accelerating Staff Development and Progression in the Workplace

The additional elements and processes required for accelerating staff development and progression in the health and care workplace setting were detailed in this chapter. These additional elements include gaining access to presentations and panel discussions on key strategies that can accelerate the transition of nurses, midwives, AHP staff and various other staff into more senior leadership and management roles in the workplace; political and media astuteness; the development and advancement of clear personal and team goals; and using determination and resilience to support staff success, job satisfaction and progression. The chapter also covered ways of building self-confidence, which is important for staff to grow in their careers along with role modelling, being appointed to senior roles, encouraging other staff who are from an international and diverse background 'that look like us', and career development and planning activities for nurses, midwives, AHP staff and various other staff. Compassionately and inclusively leading teams by example to overcoming challenges was discussed and specific skills and tips to support staff were provided. Additional details on ways to improve and accelerate personal leadership, lifelong personal and career development, and gaining support and advice from others who have been successful were provided in this chapter. Advice was also provided to support staff in specifying their personal and professional goals and using their skills for their own benefit. Moreover, guidance was offered regarding the creation of a development timeline and comparing development offers. Additional advice and learnings for success were also detailed and information was provided on how to start developing one's career at an early stage; using programmes and resources such as internships, secondments, contracts, agencies and consultancies; undertaking extracurricular learning; making time for relaxation; and accessing skills and support offers, with reflections from the author. Finally, additional resources and guidance to support health and care staff through further learning were provided in this chapter, including the NHS Leadership Academy competencies.

CHAPTER 7

Competencies and Tools for Use in the Healthcare Setting

7.1 Introduction

This chapter covers competencies and tools for use in healthcare, including new induction tools; clinical supervision competencies; preceptorship competencies; clinical competencies; specialist competencies for infection prevention and control (IPC), tissue viability nursing (TVN), central venous catheters (CVCs), venous access devices (VADs) and urinary catheter care. Further discussion covers orientation and competencies for theatre support workers; the Core Competency Framework for Anaesthetic Practitioners; band 5 staff competencies; patient observations; fundamentals for care plans; skin care assessment; safety huddle records; documentation; and coaching competencies. This information is cross-referenced to Chapter 6 on staff development, Table 5.1 on personal development plan (PDP) competencies and Chapters 4 and 5 on leadership competencies. This chapter also includes the mentor portfolio of evidence for nurses; applying for jobs (see also Section 2.2.7 on applying from overseas to work in the UK); and job applications, curriculum vitae (CV), cover letters and interviews.

7.2 Competencies and Tools for Use in Healthcare

7.2.1 NEW INDUCTION TOOLS

An effective induction for new staff is crucial for becoming familiar with the staff, people and processes in a new organisation. An example induction tool is outlined in Table 7.1. This checklist covers the essential elements of an organisation's local induction programme, which should be used for new staff members on their first day/shift and completed within the agreed-upon timeframe (1 to 6 weeks, depending on the items).

TABLE 7.1 ■ **Local Induction Checklist (within the healthcare setting)**

Name:	**Role/position:**
Ward/department:	**Directorate:**
Line manager/supervisor:	**Site base:**
Start date:	**Completion date:**

CONTENTS
Section 1: Introduction to the workplace.
Section 2: Introduction to the post and department.
Section 3: Policies and procedures.
Section 4: Learning and development.
Section 5: Health, safety and security.

Introduction and instructions: The checklist is designed for all new starters in the trust and all departmental transfers.
After full completion, place a copy of the checklist in the employee's file. The checklist will be required for audit purposes.

Responsibilities: The manager is responsible for ensuring that the checklist is completed and signed.

Timescale for completion/compliance: The manager is responsible for ensuring that the checklist is completed within 6 weeks of commencement of employment.

New starter details: Please note that all areas must be completed.

Section 1: Introduction to the Workplace:

	Line manager/ supervisor initials	Inductee initials	Date
1.1 Before starting: Introduction to the organisation:			
• Call new employee to confirm the start date and time, where to report and special requirements.			
• Book welcome meetings with the line manager.			
• Complete and submit on boarding form to the team.			
• Attend corporate induction.			
1.2 Workplace and department introduction:			
• Welcome meeting with line manager.			
• Introduction to team/key people: manager/ colleagues/clients, etc.			
• Location of facilities, e.g. domestic facilities, toilets, beverage facilities, restaurant and offices.			
• Lunch breaks.			
• Accessing trust computer systems.			
• Trust values: commitment, care and quality.			
• Outline department health and safety.			
• Hours of work/shift patterns.			
• Key duties/responsibilities and objectives.			
• Dress code and uniform.			
1.3 Department/base orientation:			
• Local fire safety including evacuation (see section 3), fire instructions and raising the alarm; walking tour of local work area and fire exits/escape routes.			
• Infection prevention and control (IPC), including hand hygiene and COVID-19-related information/ considerations.			

(Continued)

TABLE 7.1 ■ Local Induction Checklist (within the healthcare setting)—cont'd

- Work arrangements; workstation, lockers, refreshments, etc.
- Orientation to the ward/department.
- Immediate point of day-to-day reference/support (supervisor).
- Meet other key individuals in ward/department.
- Orientation to other areas in the organisation relevant to role.

Section 2: Introduction to Post and Department:

2.1 Explanation of the work of the department, client group and services provided:

- Corporate values and behaviours.
- Department/directorate business objectives and priorities.
- Duties/roles and expectations for new member.
- Clarification of job description.
- Code of conduct, if appropriate.
- Structure of management, department and directorate: areas of responsibility.
- Activation of email account and access to shared folders.
- Colleague orientation: 'who's who'.
- Orientation to relevant equipment.
- Arrangements for practice supervision and mentorship, if appropriate

2.2 Manager responsibilities (as appropriate):

- Leadership and management: basics of good people management.
- Sickness management, how to report absence and whom to call; refer to employee relations toolkit on local intranet.
- Appraisal: overview of current process.
- Statutory and mandatory training compliance: ensure all staff are up to date with training as required.
- Management of performance responsibilities.
- Explanation of probationary period and arrangement of monthly progress meetings:
  - Book mid-probation review for 3 months.
  - Book final probation review for 6 months.

2.3 Terms and conditions of the job:

- Confidentiality.
- Additional employment.
- Supervision and support systems.
- Allowances and enhancements.
- Opportunities for improving working life.
- Departmental systems and processes.

2.4 Other information:

- Meet with employee regarding progress and training needs.
- Provide feedback regarding induction.
- Evaluate job description (JD).
- Meet with employee regarding feedback on employment to date.

TABLE 7.1 ■ **Local Induction Checklist (within the healthcare setting)—cont'd**

Section 3: Policies and Procedures:

3.1 Understanding role and safe practice:

Key duties/roles/responsibilities:
Role expectations/boundaries; including trust values
and behaviours.
Familiarisation with critical policies (general):
- Internet and email usage.
- Confidentiality.
- Data protection/data sharing.
- Dignity and respect at work.
- Trade union representative.
- Freedom to Speak Up (FTSU) guardian: raising
  concerns.
- Lone worker guidelines.
- IPC.
- Other trust representative and lead.

Key ward/department specific policies

Corporate policies: awareness and discussion:
How to find trust policies and procedures online:
- Location of policies on intranet.
- Local or job specific policies and procedures, e.g.
  nursing.
- Equal opportunities; whistleblowing; grievances;
  disciplinary action; sickness; study leave; special
  leave; equality, diversity and inclusion (EDI);
  zero tolerance; smoke-free trust; major incident
  procedure; finance policies; and complaints
  procedure.
Other related work policies:
Blood collection:
- Clinical staff.
- Patient group directives and medication common
  to specialities.
- Blood collection and administration procedure.
- Local relevant policies and procedures not
  covered above.

3.2 Communication and staying informed:
- Communication systems/bleeps.
- How to use telephone/switchboard and bleep
  system.

Information technology (IT) training:
- How to access/use trust IT, the organisation's
  intranet, email and relevant policies.
Contact information for IT helpdesk.
Information governance and security.
Data protection and confidentiality.
- Email etiquette guidance, including Freedom of
  Information request and wording for out-of-office
  messages.
- Use of emergency contact numbers, e.g. fire and
  cardiac arrest.

(Continued)

- Current team/trust updating arrangements (including those associated with IPC, COVID-19 and outbreaks).

3.3 HR and well-being-related items:

Occupational health notification:

- Email trust occupational health team with 'New Starter Notification' as subject header.
- Process for referrals for occupational health/stress management.
- Important contact information/next of kin details.

3.4 Working arrangements, including hours and/or shift pattern:

- Discuss any adjustments associated with COVID-19, including consideration of outcome of prerecruitment risk assessment for staff in vulnerable groups.
- Reporting/e-rostering/time sheets.
- Shift systems/breaks.
- Arrangements for additional hours.

Travel arrangements:

- Travel to work and parking; signpost to information and check understanding (as appropriate)
- Arrangements for car parking/travel across site: car parking permits, restrictions, scratch cards, shuttle bus.

Absence management:

- All staff are informed of the process for reporting absence/sickness.
- All staff have received an information pack and key fob with contact details.

Sickness and absence (general and short term):

- COVID-19-related considerations.
- Testing and isolation.
- Reporting and return to work procedures.

Signpost towards sickness absence and other HR policies and leave arrangements:

- Annual leave and bank holiday entitlement/special leave: importance and how to request, and booking process.
- Employee online familiarisation/training (as appropriate).

Check pay arrangements covered / understood Electronic Patient Record (ESR) self-service (as appropriate)

Creating a culture of civility and respect, including:

Values and behaviours:

- Identifying the appropriate behaviour set.
  - Dignity and respect at work (including no excuse for abuse campaign and bullying and harassment contacts).
  - Raising concerns (including FTSU): video and trust materials on the local intranet and ambassadors).
  - Importance of incident reporting or raising concerns

TABLE 7.1 ■ Local Induction Checklist (within the healthcare setting)—cont'd

Wellbeing check-in completed, including:

- Importance placed on wellbeing at individual, team and trust levels.
- Wellbeing/rest areas across trust premises; importance of breaks and regular annual leave.
- Opportunities to be physically active at work.
- Range of support provided by the trust, and as part of national health and wellbeing programmes, including psychological support.
- Going home checklist.
- Health and wellbeing team and bulletins.
- Ongoing health and wellbeing discussions.

3.4 Emergency policies, procedures and arrangements:

Resuscitation/first aid procedures:

- Cardiac arrest.
- Equipment location.
- Emergency telephone number and procedure.
- Ward/departmental first aiders' roles and duties.

Local fire safety and evacuation procedures:

- Awareness of fire evacuation procedures and fire safety aspects of the area (fire alarm system, fire doors, fire extinguishers, alarm call points, etc.).
- Local means of escape, evacuation arrangements and firefighting equipment.
- Local risks present (e.g. chemicals and oxygen cylinders).
- Employer/employee responsibilities: keeping fire exit routes clear, methods for opening doors, keeping fire doors shut, reporting defective equipment, 'break glass' call points, etc.
- Key roles: Health and safety officer, fire warden and fire officer.

Emergency preparedness resilience and response:

Understand, in the event of an emergency (major incident/business continuity):

- Role of the department/ward, including critical functions and equipment, and how they are maintained in an emergency (e.g. power failure).
- Location of emergency plans and how to access them on the local intranet.
- Own role and responsibilities (including winter weather and communicable disease outbreaks).
- Use of trust emergency bleep system.

(Continued)

TABLE 7.1 ■ Local Induction Checklist (within the healthcare setting)—cont'd

Section 4: Learning and Development:

4.1 Education, induction training and appraisal:

Induction training (booked or completed):
- Trust induction; check clarity of content and any follow-up items.

Core skills mandatory training:
- Check potential learning transfer and signpost to staff development as appropriate.
- Self-registration with e-learning for healthcare (eLfH). (Register fully with nhs.net or drs.org mail for reporting purposes).
- Signpost to core mandatory training guidance on the local intranet.
- Support with protected time/roster.
- Adjustment to ensure booking of training, attendance and completion of e-learning.

Note: additional information/guidance is provided in the eLfH COVID-19 folder

Corporate induction: statutory and mandatory training attended and completed:
- Child protection (safeguarding children).
- Safeguarding adults (included in clinical staff induction only).
- Equality, diversity and inclusion (EDI).
- Resuscitation, including use and maintenance of the resuscitation trolley.
- IPC (including clinical induction).
- Patient handling (including clinical induction).
- Fire safety.
- Risk management and health and safety.
- Complaints.
- Dementia awareness.

Core skills mandatory training:
- Check potential learning transfer and signpost to staff development as appropriate.
- Self-registration with eLfH.
- Register fully with nhs.net and organisation email for reporting purposes.
- Signpost to core mandatory training guidance on the local intranet.
- Support with protected time/roster.
- Adjustment to ensure booking of training, attendance and completion of e-learning.

Note: additional information/guidance is provided in the IPC and COVID-19 folders

E-learning details

System/IT training (as appropriate):
- Organisation's electronic patient record management system.
- Integra user setup and training via procurement team.

TABLE 7.1 ■ **Local Induction Checklist (within the healthcare setting)—cont'd**

Additional role-specific training:

Information of how and where to contact key training providers:

- Trust learning and organisational development team contact number and email.
- Signpost towards practice development nurses (PDN) and/or clinical or medical education.
- Study leave policy and procedures.
- Learning and organisational procedures
- Development training programme, access and information.
- Statutory and mandatory training policy and checklist for role.
- Discussion and planning of statutory and mandatory training requirements for the year.
- Completion of all statutory and mandatory training; checklist signed by manager and signed.
- Explanation and demonstration of the internal training and development system.

Any other job-specific learning and development identified

Continuing professional development (CPD):

- Set early one-to-one dates plus probationary review (as appropriate).
- Outline trust appraisal process and arrange meeting dates.
- Outline trust commitment to developing staff, including via apprenticeships and a broad in-house education programme.
- External training and study support (as appropriate).

Section 5: Health, Safety and Security:

- **Health and safety policy** and procedures, including trust level and individual duties.
- Signpost to the slide deck on the trust induction (interim guidance) page on the local intranet; additional to e-learning.
- Health and safety considerations specific to ward/department.
- Waste disposal (as appropriate to role/area), including medications, particularly controlled drugs for relevant staff.
- Workstation setup (as appropriate) and display screen equipment assessment.
- Home working arrangements and support (as appropriate).
- **Security procedures** for patients' personal property/belongings.

(Continued)

TABLE 7.1 ■ Local Induction Checklist (within the healthcare setting)—cont'd

Specific risks to which staff might be exposed:

- Harmful substances (Control of Substances Hazardous to Health (COSHH)).
- Moving and handling procedures.
- Electricity.
- IPC.
- Food poisoning.
- Display screen equipment workstation user.
- Slips, trips and falls.
- Fire.

Infection prevention and control procedures (as appropriate to role):

- **Hand hygiene procedures (all staff)**, including hand hygiene practice.
- Personal protective equipment (PPE) (access and training; view video on PPE hub, local intranet), including donning and doffing.
- Fit testing (see PPE hub for current guidance on how to arrange).
- Inoculation injury procedures.
- Infection status of clinical setting.
- Location of IPC folders and documents.
- Additional/priority COVID-19-related guidance.
- IPC key performance indicator (KPI) monitoring/auditing including for HCAIs such as *Clostridioides difficile* or MRSA, COVID-19 and other infections.

Security for each department:

- Photo identification card/badge: cards, security pass and access codes.
- Access control card, and keys.
- Personal security/lockers.
- Intruder alarm codes/access codes for community settings.
- Department locking/unlocking procedure.
- Security staff contact details.
- Local security management specialist (telephone or email).
- Security of information, including confidentiality and information technology (IT).
- Provision of uniform and protective clothing, or department/ward dress code, as appropriate.

5.1 Patient care (as appropriate to role):

Medicine safety procedures (as appropriate):

- Provide information on pharmacy and local protocols.
- Ensure that staff sign to confirm they have read and understand relevant policies.
- Ensure that specimen signature has been obtained for Controlled Drugs (CD) register.
- Provide a copy of *Key Messages for Medications Safety* (on the local intranet).

TABLE 7.1 ■ Local Induction Checklist (within the healthcare setting)—cont'd

Incident reporting procedures:
- How to report incidents, near misses, risk assessments and safe working.
- Patient identification policy.
- Reporting risks.
- Use of Datix incident reporting on the local intranet.
- Raising serious concerns (whistleblowing): ensure that staff are aware of how to raise and document concerns.
- Duty of candour requirements.
- Freedom To Speak Up (FTSU) Ambassadors.
- Staff bullying and harassment contacts.
- Reporting methods for hazard and faults.
- Reporting of Injuries, Diseases and Dangerous Occurrences Regulation (RIDDOR), including location of RIDDOR forms.

Please sign and retain a copy to be placed in the individual's personal file:
Declaration: I can confirm that my local induction has taken place.
Name of new starter: .... Signature: ....
Name of Manager: ....Signature: .... Date: ....

Local Induction Confirmation Form for Learning and Organisational Development Team:
NHS Trust Name:
This form provides confirmation that the staff member is comfortable with the range of induction information and support provided, and that the line manager or nominated individual has verified that a robust local induction process has been completed.
Staff member name: ....Role: ....
Staff member start date: ....Staff member signature: ....
Line manager name: ....Line manager signature: ....
Ward/department: ....Directorate: ....
Local induction checklist completed on: ....
Please return this page to the Staff Development and Education Department in the hospital.
Alternatively, staff may complete the **Local Induction Online Confirmation Form** on the local intranet.
Local Induction Checklist

This checklist is intended to support structuring of the local induction and ensuring that new staff receive key information as they settle into the work setting. When completing this checklist, staff should consider the organisation's values, for example (e.g.), commitment, care and quality.

The local induction checklist (Table 7.1) **should be completed and kept in the staff member's personal file**. All items should be confirmed by both the individual completing induction and the party responsible for supporting the staff member's induction (usually the line manager/supervisor/point of day-to-day reference). Each component of the local induction checklist should be initialled after its completion and the final page should also be completed, signed and dated.

Line managers are responsible for ensuring that all staff whom they supervise have access to the organisation's policies and procedures and are supported in understanding their implications.

Any factors that might affect an individual's ability to access and/or understand guidance (e.g. a disability or health condition) must be identified, and appropriate adjustments and/or assistance must be provided. The team's HR business partner should be contacted for further advice. The local induction provides an opportunity for managers to support and welcome new starters to the team. The quality of the local induction demonstrates care and commitment to ensuring new starters' success in their roles. All items in the local induction checklist must be covered and the final page of the checklists should be sent to the staff development team (or confirmed online on the organisation's intranet).

7.2.2 E-ROSTERING

E-rostering is an important duty for managers including ward manager, nurses in charge, and other leaders and managers. E-rostering covers important items, such as skill mix; annual leave entitlement; sick leave and study days; bank holidays; rostering staff for duties; revalidation completion; recording overtime; documenting bank and agency shifts; and roster monitoring using systems such as safe care, which includes input acuity data and printing reports.

7.2.3 CLINICAL SUPERVISION COMPETENCIES

Clinical supervision brings skilled supervisors and practitioners together to reflect on practice, increase understanding of professional issues, undertake case reviews, identify solutions to problems, ensure lifelong learning and evaluate experiences, to develop and improve clinical practice and the standard of patient care.

7.2.4 PRACTICE SUPERVISION AND ASSESSMENT FOR PREREGISTRATION LEARNERS

Internal organisational policies for practice supervision and assessment for preregistration learners supports students by providing the supervision that they require to complete their practice placement and become familiar with the clinical environment. The purpose of this guide on practice supervision and assessment for preregistration learners (Section 7.2.4) is to establish best practices; ensure the highest-quality learner experience; and align the organisation's management of learners with standards and quality frameworks. The guide includes the roles of practice placements, practice supervisors, practice assessors, academic assessors, clinical facilitators, educators, mentors, mentorship, learners, work-based learners, triennial reviews, return to practice, nursing associates, apprentices, sign-off mentors, and preregistration students and nurses. The guide (Section 7.2.4) additionally covers responsibilities including induction and support for learners; written guidance for learners; guidance for placement staff and mentors; monitoring of learners' attendance in placement; ensuring learners' quality experience; preparation for the mentors' role; the mentors supported by Section 7.10 on mentor portfolio of evidence for staff; and assessment of learners in practice. Practice supervision and assessment for preregistration learners are supported by the Nursing and Midwifery Council (NMC) (2023r).

The **NMC standards** outline the roles and responsibilities of practice supervisors and assessors, to ensure that students receive the proper support and practice learning, with flexibility in developing and innovating care.**assessors**

Practice supervisors support learning in practice, to help students achieve proficiencies, programme outcomes and skill acquisition.

Practice assessors are **registered nurses (RNs)** with appropriate experience who assess students in line with the relevant field of practice.

Academic assessors collate and confirm students' achievement of proficiency and programme outcomes in the academic learning environment, through several activities.

7.2.5 PRECEPTORSHIP COMPETENCIES

Preceptorship is an important part of the Standard for Student Supervision and Assessment. Preceptorship equips individuals to teach, supervise and assess learners in clinical practice, including preregistration NMC candidates, those returning to practice, apprentices, nursing associates, work experience students, specialist practitioners, postregistration students and newly qualified staff. Preceptors support staff who are newly registered with the NMC, providing them with professional guidance to identify learning needs; an introduction to staff; and support for navigating the learning environment, preparing to meet with their line managers and escalating concerns as appropriate. See also Section 5.2.12.7 on preceptorships for newly qualified staff and the preceptor support testimonial in Box 7.1. The preceptorship programme (Table 7.2) contains key items regarding preceptorship.

7.2.6 CLINICAL COMPETENCIES

Key clinical competencies (Box 7.2) for staff in healthcare settings include aseptic technique; care for patients with a peripheral vascular access device; urethral catheterisation; patient assessment; assessment of vital signs; administration of emergency oxygen in adult patients; maintaining fluid balance; maintaining optimal nutrition; neurological observations; medications management; patient discharge; and pressure ulcer prevention (PUP).

These **RN clinical competencies** educate staff and enable a competent workforce capable of promoting safety and delivering quality care to patients by performing duties meeting the required standards. These competencies also support personal development,

---

BOX 7.1	**Preceptor Support Testimonial**

*With the preceptor support, every day I became the nurse I dreamed of being. I learn so much from the preceptor's programme and feel enthused to continue to learn.***preceptor support**
It made me confident to teach junior staff, enabling them to develop their clinical skills, and become a competent, confident and proud nurse.

Preceptor lead nurse

TABLE 7.2 ■ Sample Preceptorship Programme

Programmes	Comments	Date Completed
Induction to preceptorship: • Expectations and fears. • Medicine management. • Documentation workshop.		
Clinical skills: • Medical devices. • Venepuncture and cannulation. • Handover workshop.		
Nutrition and hydration: • Dietician and enteral nutrition. • Stomach care. • Diabetes.		
Discharge study day: • Acute Life-threatening Events Recognition and Treatment (**ALERT) course** management of deteriorating patient (refer to ALERT section)		
Emotional intelligence and resilience: • Principles of emotional intelligence and resilience. • Workshop on difficult situations.		
Intravenous medication administration: • IV therapy complications. • Pharmacokinetics. • Practical skills workshop.		
Skin care: • Pressure ulcer care and wound assessment. • Continence. • Urinary catheterisation workshop.		
Pain management study day: • Pain therapy and physiology. • Assessment and management. • Patient scenarios.		
Cancer and palliative care: • The cancer journey. • Chemotherapy and oncological emergencies. • Palliative and end of life care.		
Cardio-respiratory study day: • Anatomy and physiology (A&P), heart, arrhythmias and heart failure. • Care of respiratory patients. • Skills station, simulation and clinical scenarios.		
Acute care study day: • Acute kidney injury sepsis. • Scenarios workshop.		

TABLE 7.2 ■ **Sample Preceptorship Programme—cont'd**

Programmes	Comments	Date Completed
Neurology study day: • Neurological assessment. • Care of patient with neurological deficit. • Workshops.		
Leadership and human factors		
Staff preceptee: Preceptor: Date completed:		

BOX 7.2 **Clinical Competencies**

These clinical competencies are important in supporting RNs who are accountable to follow the NMC Code (NMC, 2023e) and are personally responsible for the delivery of safe and competent care to patients.. The interpretation, decision-making and planning of care remain the responsibilities of the RN, even when elements are delegated to HCA who are competent to undertake the delegated duties.

NMC (2023e)

---

learning and career progression, by helping staff acquire and develop the skills necessary to deliver their duties in the clinical setting. The learning delivery for these competencies occurs in various ways, including activities such as workshops, reading, observation, discussion, online resources, feedback sessions and reflection, to contribute to the quality of care.

The NMC Code (2023e) states that all nurses must be professionally accountable and use clinical governance processes to maintain and improve nursing practice and standards of healthcare (NMC, 2023e).

Other competencies can be accessed through the internal organisational learning and development team for RNs and midwives, including mental health, paediatric care, women's health, neonatal care, critical care, perioperative care, radiology, medical care, surgical care, haematology and oncology, organ transplantation, urology, cardiovascular care, emergency medicine and other competencies relevant to the area of practice, to further develop skills, knowledge and expertise in these areas.

7.2.7 SPECIALIST COMPETENCIES

The specialist competencies for IPC, TVN, CVC, VAD and urinary catheter care are detailed in the following sections.

7.2.8 INFECTION PREVENTION AND CONTROL COMPETENCIES

Key elements of the IPC competencies (Box 7.3) are detailed here, to ensure a clean and safe environment in health and care settings, in accordance with the requirements of the Health and Social Care Act 2008: Code of Practice on the Prevention and Control of

BOX 7.3	**IPC Competency Testimonial**

IPC competence for compliance is supported by the IPS (2022), which ensures that IPC is effectively delivered by supporting and informing service planning, workforce development, and management at strategic and operational level. This assists staff appraisals, PDP (IPS, 2022), other CPD requirements, and support in the developing team structures and the IPC role requirements. These competencies are important to ensure that IPC is embedded in everyday practice and that IPC is everyone's business.
Director of Infection Prevention and Control

Infections (GOV.UK, 2022). The role of IPC includes cleanliness, optimising antimicrobial use and preventing antimicrobial resistance (GOV.UK, 2022). Competencies for IPC are provided by organisations such as the Infection Prevention Society (IPS) (2022) and the European Network, to promote infection prevention for patient safety, as supported by IPC competencies internal to organisations.

Key IPC competencies include the following domains:

Leadership and management: providing supervision and supporting the development of junior staff.

Clinical practice: collecting, understanding, interpreting and reporting surveillance data; educating, monitoring and reviewing the effectiveness of the decontamination process and equipment, and the clinical and built environment; maintaining patient safety by recognising and managing incidents and outbreaks; and improving quality and safety by developing and implementing evidence-based policy and guidance for IPC.

Quality improvement (QI) in **IPC practice**: using improvement methods, considering human factors and the need for behaviour change; using risk assessment in IPC practices; and embedding research in clinical practice.

IPC QI programmes may cover areas including urinary tract infection, *Clostridioides difficile* (*C. difficile*) and methicillin-resistant *Staphylococcus aureus* (MRSA).

IPC education: developing one's own knowledge, skills and practice; educating patients, carers and all staff working in health and social care settings; developing and implementing learning opportunities by using evidence-based practice; and developing, implementing, evaluating and embedding IPC within workforce development strategies. These efforts support the development of expert IPC practitioners through reasoning, critical thinking, reflection and analysis, to inform assessment and decision-making.

The **elements** of the **IPC competency framework** include the following:

- **Specialist knowledge** of microbiology, immunology, epidemiology, IPC practice and decontamination.
- **Evidence-based practice**, including research in practice and auditing to improve quality.
- **Clinical research** interpretation and conduct.
- **Teaching and learning**, including facilitating learning in others, self-directed learning and professional development.
- **Management and leadership** including that of the IPC service across organisations (IPS, 2022).

Additional IPC core competencies (IPS, 2022) include the following:

Programme development: elaborating on and advocating for an IPC programme and managing an infection control programme, as well as work plans and projects. QI in IPC involves the key domains of managing (implementation, follow-up and evaluation) a surveillance system, as well as identifying, investigating and managing outbreaks.

Surveillance and investigation of healthcare-associated infections (HCAIs): contributing to quality management; contributing to risk management; performing audits of professional practices and evaluating performance; providing IPC training for employees; and contributing to research.

IPC activities and interventions: implementing IPC healthcare procedures; contributing to decreasing antimicrobial resistance; and advising on appropriate laboratory testing and use of laboratory data, decontamination and sterilisation of medical devices, and controlling environmental sources of infections (European Centre for Disease Prevention and Control (ECDC), 2023).

The **World Health Organization (WHO)** also has core competencies for IPC, including ensuring dedicated training of IPC team members in areas such as hand hygiene, surgical site infections, injection safety, IPC and antimicrobial resistance, sepsis and basics of IPC in health and care settings (WHO, 2016).

7.2.9 TISSUE VIABILITY NURSE AND PRESSURE ULCER PREVENTION COMPETENCIES

These competencies include completing TVN audits, which cover important documentation and other assurance processes. Items include pressure ulcer checking and scoring and ensuring that the proper pressure relieving equipment is in place for patients at risk, for example, mattresses for beds and cushions for chairs.

PUP covers key elements including the following:

- Supporting people at risk of pressure ulcers, including neonates, children younger than 16 years and adults.
- Embedding the use of PUP strategies in the clinical setting and ensuring correct documentation and communication, including through policies and leaflets.
- Ensuring the correct use of foam and dynamic mattresses and profiling beds to reduce pressure.
- Providing assurance through auditing and Datix aligned to the new Patient Safety Incident Response Framework (PSIRF) process, verification by TVNs, and leadership development supported by the TVN nurse.

Improvement evidence identified elements that are vital for PUP and management, including the following key strategies:

- Effective communication among TVNs, trusts, local authorities, systems, commissioners, regions, and national staff and teams.
- Appropriate management of safeguarding concerns by using safeguarding pressure ulcer protocols.
- Transparent processes regarding investigations and outcomes for patients, including duty of candour.
- Contributing to reducing the incidence of healthcare acquired pressure ulcers, including through pressure ulcer panels.

- Sharing of learning from analysis and investigations, to ensure continuing improvement in PUP strategies and practices, e.g. pressure area care and prevention training programmes for staff, including nurses and midwives (N&M), nursing associate's and AHPs, regarding risk identification and assessment.
- PUP and management, and care bundle and plan.
- Skin care study days, including skin tear, documentation, wound management, wound dressing formulary, bed and mattress management, link nurse development, and preventing leg or diabetic ulcers and surgical site infections.

PUP governance processes include the following:

- Organisation's PUP policy, including safeguarding pressure ulcer tools.
- Pressure ulcer identification and reporting through the trust incident management systems (Datix/PSIRF).
- Use of Waterlow and risk assessment tools.
- Trust-wide pressure ulcer panels, working groups and champions.
- Investigation of all category 2, 3 and 4 pressure ulcers, learning identification and reporting to the trust board.
- Regular training programmes for staff, ensuring early identification to facilitate PUP.
- Auditing, including prevalence, incidence, bed days and occupancy.
- Pressure ulcer monitoring of patients by ward and TVN teams, including pressure ulcer risk assessment.
- Incident reporting (with a trust system, such as Datix/PSIRF).

7.2.10 CENTRAL VENOUS CATHETER DEVICE COMPETENCIES

Key elements regarding central venous catheter device (CVAD) competencies are summarised in the CVAD competencies in Table 7.3. A CVAD is a long, thin and hollow plastic tube called a 'catheter' or 'line', which is placed in a vein to provide a route for administering intravenous (IV) medications (British Society of Interventional Radiology, 2023). The various CVAD types include short-term (nontunnelled) devices, such as central venous catheters (CVCs), tunnelled (Hickman) devices, and implanted ports. Dialysis catheters, such as Vascath, are used in dialysis; peripherally inserted central catheters (PICCs) are used for drug therapy, IV fluids, blood, total parenteral nutrition (TPN) and other fluids (British Society of Interventional Radiology, 2023).

7.2.11 URINARY CATHETER CARE COMPETENCIES

Key elements of urinary catheter care competencies are summarised in Table 7.4. These competencies include ensuring auditing of urinary catheter care and ensuring that catheter resources and packs are provided in wards and relevant departments. Patients with catheters require a VIP for the specific type of catheter to be completed, as monitored through clinical auditing.

7.2.12 ORIENTATION AND PROBATION

Orientation and probation policies and procedures help staff new to organisations achieve success, by providing advice and guidance regarding the organisation, probation, reviews, conduct and attendance, to improve staff and patient experience, thereby ensuring the quality and safety of care.

TABLE 7.3 ■ **CVAD Competencies**

CVAD Competency Area	Compliance Area	Date Completed
Insertion	National Institute for Health and Care Excellence (NICE) guidelines for ultrasound, MRSA screening, aseptic non-touch technique (ANNT)/aseptic technique, skin antisepsis and preparation.	
Care and management	Infection prevention and control, line patency and assessment, complication prevention and aftercare.	
CVAD workbook completion	Assessment, management, theory, practical, competency and resources.	
PICC/mid line care and IV therapy	Care and use, including flushing, dressing, cleaning, asepsis, competency, guidance lines compliance and MRSA screening.	
CVAD: PICC/mid line, CVC, Hickman and peripheral line care plan	Assessment, line length and check, patency, consent, ANTT, IPC, Visual Infusion Phlebitis score (VIP) score, resources, dressing, rationale for insertion, removal, unblocking, hand hygiene, barrier precaution, documentation, saving lives care bundle use, device management and maintenance, multidisciplinary team (MDT) review, personal protective equipment (PPE) and ensuring ongoing care of other devices.	
CVAD service provision	CVAD referrals, IV access, study day, Patient Group Directions (PGD), teaching, healthcare at home, community and Outpatient Parenteral Antibiotic Therapy (OPAT) service, blood sampling, auditing, incident investigation, risk management, governance, evaluation and safeguarding.	
CVAD CNS routine duties	Service management and leadership, postinsertion chest X-ray (CXR), reviews, administration and checks, equipment, microbiology results review, clinical visits, teaching, data input and administration, patient follow-up, troubleshooting and report writing.	

Related policies: Central venous access guideline; high impact interventions (HII) for CVC care; NICE guideline by Loveday, Wilson, Wilcox; Royal Marsden CVAD policy.

Related polices: ANTT, MRSA, hand hygiene (HH), CVC, blood culture collection, venepuncture and parenteral feeding (TPN)

Staff name:
Signed off by:
Date completed:

7.2.13 ORIENTATION AND COMPETENCIES FOR THEATRE SUPPORT WORKERS

Orientation and competencies are important to support theatre support workers in doing their job to the best of their abilities.

Competencies for theatre support workers include assessment of the following (NHS, 2022m):

- Cleanliness of the perioperative theatre between cases and at the end of the day.
- Maintenance of stock levels and stock rotation in the theatre.

TABLE 7.4 ■ Urinary Catheter Care Competencies

Urinary Catheter Competency Area	Compliance Area	Date Completed
Insertion	National Institute for Health and Care Excellence (NICE) guidelines for ultrasound, MRSA screening, ANNT/aseptic technique, skin antisepsis and preparation.	
Care and management	Infection prevention, line patency and assessment, prevention of complications and aftercare.	
Urinary catheter workbook completion	Assessment, management, theory, practical, competency and resources.	
Urinary catheter care	Care and use, including flushing, dressing, cleaning, asepsis, competency, guidance line compliance and MRSA screening.	
Urinary catheter care plan and pathway	Assessment, line length and check, patency, consent, Aseptic Non-Touch Technique (ANTT), IPC, Visual Infusion Phlebitis score (VIP) score, resources, rationale for insertion, removal, hand hygiene, barrier precaution, documentation, saving lives care bundle use/HII, device management and maintenance, Multidisciplinary team (MDT) review, personal protective equipment (PPE), drainage bag position and ensuring ongoing care. Continence management care including skin care.	
Urinary catheter service provision	Urinary catheter referrals, study days, Patient Group Directions (PGD), teaching, urine sampling, auditing, incident investigation, risk management, governance, evaluation and safeguarding.	
CNS routine duties	Service management and leadership, post insertion review and checks, equipment, microbiology results review, clinical visits, teaching, data input and administration, patient follow-up, troubleshooting and report writing.	

Related policies: urinary catheter guideline; HII for urinary catheter care; NICE guideline and organisation policy for urinary catheterisation.

Related polices: e.g. ANTT

Staff name:
Signed off by:
Date completed:

- Safe use of medical devices, instrument trays and supplementary items used in the preoperative environment.
- Effective performance of role.
- Measurement and recording of patients' body fluid outputs, blood loss and wound drainage.
- Promotion and maintenance of a clean, safe perioperative environment in the theatre and the corridor.
- Safe positioning of patients undergoing surgery.
- Safe use of the operating table and attachments.

- Receipt, handling and dispatching of clinical specimens.
- Safe transportation of patients to the theatre.
- Receiving patients in the theatre holding bay and recovery area.
- Completion of theatre support worker orientation and competency checklist.
- Theatre sign-off sheet and action plan.
- Code of conduct for healthcare assistants (HCAs).
- Mandatory training for HCAs.
- Essential readings.

7.2.14 CORE COMPETENCY FRAMEWORK FOR ANAESTHETIC PRACTITIONERS

The Core Competency Framework for Anaesthetic Practitioners covers the 'valuable role that anaesthetic practitioners play within the theatre workforce, contributing to delivery of safe, effective and person-centred care', including the following:

- Recovery and theatre sterile surgical unit orientation.
- Preoperative preparation of the environment.
- Preoperative preparation of patients, including airway management.
- Perioperative care of patients, including positioning, equipment management and fibreoptic scopes.
- Postoperative care of patients.
- Emergency care and treatment.
- Anaesthesia in remote and isolated locations.
- Anaesthesia and obstetrics.
- Anaesthesia and paediatrics.
- Record of signatories.
- Theatre sign-off sheet and action plan.
- List of preceptors.
- Essential readings.

(Association for Perioperative Practice (AfPP), 2023).

7.2.15 ORIENTATION AND COMPETENCY PACK SCRUB STAFF COMPETENCIES

Relevant competencies include: introduction; clinical profile; clinical shifts; orientation; theatre skills; scrub skills; specialist equipment; spines; emergency objectives; anaesthetics; recovery and theatre sterile surgical unit; record of signatories; theatre sign-off sheet and action plan; list of preceptors; and essential readings.

7.2.16 BAND 5 STAFF COMPETENCIES

All trained nurses need to be well equipped to lead and manage their own areas of responsibility effectively. They also need to make an effective contribution to the future direction and ongoing performance of the trust. Specific core nursing competencies have been developed to support the trust values and to set out clear expectations in relation to behaviour, knowledge and the skills required to fulfill the role and responsibilities of a trained nurse/midwife.

The band 5 competency includes, but is not limited to, IPC, falls prevention, continence, tissue viability (pressure ulcer), manual handling, patient observation (vital signs), nutrition and hydration, personal care, emergency response, medication safety, pain management, dementia, communication, end-of-life care, organisational aspects of care, action planning and assessments. These competencies support band 5 nurses to develop their knowledge and skills to be confident and competent professionals, thus enabling staff to function effectively in health and care settings. Not all competency assessments and skills are detailed herein. Additional competencies relevant to each clinical department are usually provided locally in each organisation and ward, including by helping staff evaluate their performance and identify their learning needs and areas to develop in their role. This use of band 5 competencies in conjunction with the preceptorship document are supported by the ward manager, senior sister or designated ward assessor. The band 5 competencies include, but are not limited to, assessments for medicine management, aseptic technique, peripheral IV administration, nasogastric tube insertion, the Mental Capacity Act (MCA) 2005 and Deprivation of Liberty Safeguards 2009.

The NMC (2023e, q and 2024b) states that all nurses, midwives and nursing associates must uphold the **code**, including their knowledge and skills for safe and effective practice when working. This includes ensuring nurses, midwives and nursing associates can demonstrate competencies across the areas of effective practice; professional and ethical practice; developing individual staff; and achieving quality care through evaluation and research. The NMC (2024) Code also presents the professional standards that nurses, midwives and nursing associates must satisfy for registration to practise in the UK. Other competencies in each organisation cover the relevant speciality of practice, such as community, mental health, learning disabilities and autism, paediatrics, and maternity and neonatal services. The competencies and self-assessment for each level of professionally qualified staff differ, ranging from band 5 to executive level, and are supported by career and leadership development pathways covering key pillars of practice, including the following: (1) clinical practice, (2) facilitation of learning, (3) leadership and (4) evidence and research development (NMC, 2023e). A testimonial on how others have competencies and self-assessment is presented in Box 7.4.

7.2.17 PATIENT OBSERVATION COMPETENCIES

Related competencies include ensuring that observations are performed according to the frequency of the National Early Warning Score (NEWS) 2 and escalation of NEWS2 score above zero (0) at all times (consistently).

7.3 Fundamentals for Care Planning

Relevant fundamentals are detailed in the following sections.

7.3.1 BREATHLESS PATIENTS WHO MAY REQUIRE AN OXYGEN CARE PLAN

This care plan is used to ensure that oxygen is administered safely to patients and to prevent patients from developing pressure ulcers behind the ears because of oxygen devices, by using the steps and actions required for oxygen administration.

7.3.2 PAIN MANAGEMENT CARE PLAN

This care plan is used to keep patients comfortable by adequately managing acute and or chronic pain, by following the steps and actions required for pain management to be initiated when a patient consistently reports pain, with a score exceeding 1, or a care plan is triggered according to the nursing assessment pro forma.

7.3.3 FALL RISK CARE PLAN

This care plan is used to reduce patients' risk of slips, trips or falls in hospital, according to the policy for the prevention and management of inpatient slips, trips and falls, and the use of bed rails with adult patients. This care plan includes general safety precautions, including those for patients identified to be at particularly high risk.

7.3.4 PRESSURE ULCER PREVENTION AND MANAGEMENT CARE PLAN

This care plan is used to address the problems and needs of patients at risk of developing new and or further pressure damage, according to the organisation's PUP policy and the equipment selection guidance, as required. The aims and goals of this care plan include assessment, the skin, surfaces used, keeping the patient moving, incontinence management, nutrition and hydration, provision of information and medical device management.

7.3.5 SKIN CARE ASSESSMENT

Skin assessment charts are used in some clinical settings for daily pressure area checks, to determine whether the skin is intact or whether signs of pressure ulcers, such as redness or blanching, deep tissue injury or moisture lesions, are present. Skin assessment charts should be completed daily and after intentional rounding notes, for use of devices such as nasogastric tubes, oxygen masks including non-invasive ventilation masks, antiembolic stockings, oxygen saturation probes, percutaneous endoscopic gastrostomy/gastrostomy tubes, urethral catheters, orthopaedic casts/braces/splints, cardiac monitors, endotracheal tubes, tracheostomy tubes, cannulas, IV lines and cervical collars.

7.3.6 URINARY CATHETER CARE PLAN

The aims and goals of this care plan are to ensure safe insertion and ongoing care for patients with catheters, while referring to the urinary catheterisation policy for further advice. Aspects include ensuring that catheters are reviewed and removed at the correct intervals for short- and long-term catheters. This care plan includes general safety precautions of determining whether a catheter is needed or whether alternatives exist to catheter insertion, such as trials without a catheter or discharging patients home with a catheter.

BOX 7.4	Competencies and Self-assessment Testimonial

These competencies and self-assessment are supported by the NMC (2023e) Code and standards which states that all nurses in all four fields of nursing must demonstrate competencies across the four areas: professional values; communication and interpersonal skills; leadership, management and team working; and nursing practice and decision-making.

Practice development lead

7.3.7 RISK OF MALNUTRITION MANAGEMENT CARE PLAN

The aims and goals of this care plan are to reduce patients' risk of malnutrition and maximise their nutritional intake when patients are at risk of malnutrition, unintentional weight loss, minimal or no oral intake for 5 consecutive days or other clear incidents of weight loss. This care plan includes general safety procedures for patients identified as being at risk of malnutrition, such as referral to a dietician and starting a food chart for documenting all oral intake. Designated trays should be used at all mealtimes. Patients should be assessed for their ability to feed themselves and the presence of swallowing problems. Referral to speech and language therapy (SALT) and modified food and fluid intake should be recommended and oral nutrition supplements should be prescribed by a dietician, as required. Patients must be weighed and the Malnutrition Universal Screening Tool (MUST) should be completed for patients at risk. Patient nutrition is monitored through clinical auditing.

7.3.8 BOWEL CARE PLAN

Patients' bowel motions must be recorded and monitored through clinical auditing.

7.3.9 MOUTH CARE PLAN

The aims and goals of this care plan are to reduce the risk of patients developing mouth-related problems, dental diseases and general health problems, and to provide patients needing support with mouth care activities to achieve good oral health and be as independent as possible. Clinical judgement should always be applied in implementing actions to help maintain good oral hygiene. Mouth care is monitored through clinical auditing.

7.3.10 SAFETY HUDDLE RECORDS

A safety huddle record book may be kept in wards and departments to document regular discussions. These huddles include short briefings to help teams stay informed, review work, make plans and make progress in achieving team goals, including key values of commitment, care and quality. The safety huddles are usually led by the charge nurse in the morning, and documentation tools, as described in the competencies in Table 7.5, can provide support. The goals include identifying patients at risk, including the most ill patients in the clinical area each day; improving staff engagement in giving clinical and bedside care; increasing opportunities for gathering information, making decisions and strategising; and maintaining the ward and unit momentum. Additional benefits include checking workload balance; keeping abreast of issues and being proactive in anticipating issues; providing regular updates to staff; improving patients' and families' experiences; and continually improving quality and safety daily. Safety huddles promote awareness of activities in the unit/ward and organisation-wide; decrease staff isolation; and improve teamwork.

Key topics discussed at safety huddles may include the following:

- Do not attempt cardiopulmonary resuscitation (DNACPR) orders and treatment escalation plans (TEPS).

- Deprivation of liberty safeguards.
- MCA and safeguarding issues.
- High risk patients, according to measures such as the NEWS.
- Waterlow score and falls risk assessment.
- MUST (nutrition issues) including body mass index (BMI) calculation.
- Pressure ulcers.
- Nasogastric tubes.
- Infection risks such as SARS-CoV-2, MRSA, *C. difficile* and catheter-associated urinary tract infection (CAUTI).
- Venous thromboembolisms and CVCs.
- Medicine management.
- Verification that patients are ready for discharge (medications to take out (TTOs) and step down to discharge lounge).
- Workload and ward activities (high acuity in one bay, junior staff, high number of patient investigations, reassessment of where help is needed).
- Patients' and relatives' issues.
- Any other business.

7.4 Documentation Competencies

A documentation group is often used to develop documentation processes. The documentation competencies in Table 7.5 provide a guide to support these efforts. The key elements of best practices in nursing and midwifery documentation (NMC, 2021c; NMC, 2023c) are summarised in the sample competencies in Table 7.5.

This documentation competency is aligned with the NMC (2021c) record keeping guiding principles and the NMC Code (2023c), which states that individuals must keep clear and accurate records relevant to practice. This competency promotes a just culture, through having clear policies and procedures, and following best practice guidance locally (NMC, 2021c, 2023c).

7.5 Ward and Department Manager Leadership Development Programme

The ward and department manager leadership development programme are often sponsored by the chief nurse/director of nursing (DON) and the director of IPC of the organisation, to deliver excellent, kind, responsible and respectful care to patients and service users. Delivery of the programme may include collaboration with training and development, QI, leadership academy, finance, corporate nursing, wards and departmental managers. The roles of ward and department manager are important in engaging, inspiring and equipping staff, and developing people and organisations in the present and future.

- This programme is pivotal in the management of services and improving patient outcomes and experience.
- Effective leadership directly affects patient safety incidents.
- This programme sets the tone and culture of a ward/department, thereby affecting staff morale, sickness and turnover.

TABLE 7.5 ■ Documentation Competencies

Best practices in nursing and midwifery documentation:

Good record keeping is a crucial part of skilled and safe nursing, midwifery and specialist and community public health nursing practice, to ensure that risks and problems are documented and shared with others for actioning.

Key principles of documentation include the following:

- Records should be clear, factual, consistent and accurate.
- Abbreviations, jargon, phrases, speculation, and offensive or subjective phases should be avoided.
- Records should be accurately dated, timed and signed.
- Entries in the patient records should be easily understood.
- Documentation should use terms that the patient/client can easily understand.
- Records should be audited to identify areas for staff training and development.
- Patient/client should have the right to access their records.
- Confidentiality of patient/client records should be protected, in line with ethics.
- All relevant information should be added to patients' records according to professional judgement.
- A clear process should be in place for updating or correcting patient records.
- Records may be subject to scrutiny or presented in evidence.
- Good record keeping helps protect patient welfare.

Competency areas:	Description and notes relating to charts and care plans: Understand and use the following appropriately.
Staff should be competent in documenting use of the following charts and care plans.	
Drug chart	Inpatient medication, prescription and administration (per the British National Formulary (BNF) and NMC Code, 2023c) records, including regular, antimicrobial, thromboprophylaxis, subcutaneous, anticoagulant, venous thromboembolism (VTE) prophylaxis and other prescriptions, as well as documentation of allergies, sensitivities and adverse reactions.
Patient 'This is me' record	Used for patients with dementia; completed by relatives and carers, to help staff better understand patients.
Patient risk assessment	Documentation of patient risks, covering falls, bed rails, pressure ulcers, continence, manual handling, Malnutrition Universal Screening Tool (MUST) and hydration assessment, according to the related flowcharts.
Nursing Assessment Proforma (NAP)	NAP form completed at admission to assist with the planning of care.
24-hour intentional rounding	24-hour intentional rounding document, including assessing, checking and repositioning patients at set intervals.
Observation/National Early Warning Score (NEWS)	NEWS chart and 24-hour fluid balance chart completion at agreed-upon intervals, including neurological observations.
Breathing	For breathless patients who may require oxygen, ensuring that bedside oxygen, suction and air flow metres are verified at every shift.
Pain	Pain assessment and management care plan use for patients with pain scores of 1 or above.
Falls	Fall risk assessment and management, including use of bed safety rails in line with the agreed-upon time frame, to reduce slips, trips and falls.
Manual handling	Moving and handling completion according to trust policy.

TABLE 7.5 ■ Documentation Competencies—cont'd

Eating and drinking	Eating and drinking: nutrition and hydration, including MUST and hydration chart completion.
Sleep	Sleep hygiene completion per trust policy, commencing the appropriate plans for patients with difficulty sleeping, including the offer of ear plugs.
Confused patients	Confused patients' behaviour observation and management care plan, including deprivation-of-liberty safeguarding and Mental Capacity Act (MCA) assessment.
Self-care	Self-care assessment and hygiene care, including mouth care and personal hygiene interventions.
Individualised care plan for dying patients	Individualised care plan for dying patients, including medication management, comfort care, daily senior clinical review and referral to palliative care teams as required; should include allowance for open visiting, refreshments, bedding, washing and parking, in line with local policy.
Diabetes	Blood glucose and ketone monitoring and management of medically deteriorating patients.
Pressure ulcers	Pressure ulcer assessment and treatment, including wound assessment, negative pressure wound therapy, management of deterioration and improvement in skin condition, and referral to the tissue viability nurse (TVN) as required.
Infection prevention and control (IPC)	Peripheral intravenous (IV) access (VIP scores), surgical site infection, MRSA, *C. difficile*, glycopeptide resistant enterococcus (GRE), vancomycin-resistant enterococci (VRE), carbapenemase producing Enterobacteriaceae (CPE), COVID-19 assessment and management, ensuring cleaning and HH; refer to the IPC competencies in Section 7.2.8 and the IPC competencies testimonial in Box 7.3
Bladder and bowel function	Stool chart, continence, and urinary catheter and stoma assessment and management.
Venous thromboembolism (VTE) risk	VTE intermittent pneumatic compression and anti-embolic stocking (AES) assessment and care planning, ensuring prevention of blood loss.
Personal property	Property and indemnity form use, completion on admission and in line with local policy to manage patients' personal effects safely
Accountability and responsibility	Accountability and responsibility in signing sheet use, for all patient care delivered, confirming that all documentations, care plans and assessments have been updated.
Miscellaneous	Use of additional documents relevant to clinical care, such as blood transfusion, and renal and heart failure plans.

Staff Name:.....................
Manager's name:.....................
Date completed:.................

- This programme influences others across professional boundaries to work towards shared values.
- This programme helps deliver the organisations' objectives and recovery plan to meet the Care Quality Commission (CQC) Key Lines of Enquiry (KLOEs), including quality, performance and finance.

- The service provided is monitored and evaluated.
- This highly complex and challenging role can be rewarding.

This ward and department manager leadership development programme may include study days; teaching modules covering the leadership domains including (1) leading the ward, (2) leading self, (3) leading the service, (4) leading the organisation and (5) working with others; action learning sets; QI projects; course presentations; 360-degree feedback; passport to management course; and congratulations and certificate presentation to staff in each ward for successful completion of the programme.

Details of the five leadership domains include the following:

1. **Leading the ward** includes developing the team, managing the authority/approachability tension and becoming a visible and strong clinical leader in providing safe effective and high-quality care.
2. **Leading self** includes exploring one's own personal qualities, developing self-confidence and understanding different leadership styles, e.g. knowing when and how to coach, and understanding resilience and behaviours to sustain improvements.
3. **Leading the service** includes identifying, advancing and following through on ideas for service improvement; being a change champion; and understanding wider context, including the effects of decisions on quality, performance and finance.
4. **Leading the organisation** includes connecting with the organisations' strategy and vision and building on the organisation's objectives, to assess one's own services and identify service improvement goals.
5. **Working with other staff** collaboratively to ensure duties and responsibilities are completed, leading peers and colleagues; setting and giving direction; providing feedback; influencing skills; and having difficult conversations.

The testimonial in Box 7.5 reflects on the ward manager/sister role.

7.6 Staff Development/Personal Development Plan Competencies

Key elements regarding staff development/PDP competencies are summarised in the staff development/PDP competencies in Tables 7.6, including a band 6 and 7 development programme, which is supported by the Appraisals and Personal Development Plan tool in Chapter 5.

Table 7.7 contributes to this Section 7.6 on staff development/PDP competencies and the band 6 to band 7 staff development programme outlined in Table 7.5.

BOX 7.5   Ward Manager/Sister Testimonial

On a daily basis, I take pride in the running of my ward, including the care delivery, monitoring the cleanliness, how staff provide care, and interaction with patients and visitors. It is my responsibility to provide the high standards of care which the public expects, whilst treating patient and staff with respect and dignity during their stay, and meeting their basic needs such as eating and drinking. I do this through good leadership and staff education and development.

Ward mana

The passport to management programme (Table 7.8) supplements the band 6 and 7 development programmes in Tables 7.6 and 7.7, thereby contributing to effective management at middle management levels.

TABLE 7.6 ■ Staff Development/PDP Competencies

Adult senior registered nurse professional development pathway and clinical education. These are (but not limited to) the essential and desirable competencies that band 6 to 7 staff may require. Individuals can assess themselves against these competencies and the assessment to help with career progression and or accessing further development.

Band 6 to band 7 ⟶		Band 7 ward manager
Junior band 6 nurse, up to 9 months in role	Senior band 6 to newly appointed band 7 ward manager	Established band 7 ward manager
Essential	**Essential**	**Essential**
Completed the following: • Leadership, managing people, building teams. • Supervised management in ward areas. • Student nurses and preceptor assessor. • Undertaking audits, presentation and teaching. • Senior link nurse role. • Senior registered practitioner study day attendance. • Senior registered practitioner development programme. • Further study including degree or MSc. • Multiprofessional simulation. • Mandatory training and competencies for: • Medication. • IV administration. • Phlebotomy and cannulation. • Yearly appraisals.	Completed the following: • Senior nurse development programme: • Senior registered practitioner study day attendance, plus: • Appraisal skills. • Investigation of adverse clinical incidents. • Recruitment and selection training. • Supernumerary shift with matron and site manager. • Participation in recruitment and selection. • Management of department/team with supervision. • Mandatory training and competencies for: • Medication. • IV administration. • Phlebotomy and cannulation. • Yearly appraisals.	Completed the following: • Leadership foundation programme (5 days). • Powerful conversation workshop. • Active promotion and management of practice development in line with local objectives. • Supernumerary shift with senior nursing team (e.g. ADON). • Management of team, ward and department (unsupervised). • Professional management and development of team members: • Lead recruitment and selection. • Complaints/conflict management. • Incidents and investigation management. • Active involvement in quality improvement projects for department and organisation. • Mandatory training and competencies for: • Medication. • IV administration. • Phlebotomy and cannulation. • Yearly appraisals.

(Continued)

TABLE 7.6 ■ Staff Development/PDP Competencies—cont'd

Adult senior registered nurse professional development pathway and clinical education. These are (but not limited to) the essential and desirable competencies that band 6 to 7 staff may require. Individuals can assess themselves against these competencies and the assessment to help with career progression and or accessing further development.

Band 6 to band 7 ➡		Band 7 ward manager
Desirable	Desirable	Desirable
Completed the following: Leadership foundation programme (2 days). • Charted management degree apprentice. • Communicating effectively in the clinical environment study day. • QI techniques in healthcare SD. • Schwartz round participation.	Completed the following: Leadership foundation programme (5 days). • Communicating effectively in the clinical environment study day. • QI techniques in healthcare SD. • Further studies such as degree or MSc, including leadership modules at an institution of higher learning.	Completed the following: • Further module study to attain master's degree. • Level 7 leadership and management apprenticeship.

Completed by:...........................
Signed off by:...........................
Date:...................

TABLE 7.7 ■ Band 7 Development Programme

To develop knowledge, skills and confidence in leadership.

A 5-day programme for new and experienced band 7 nurses, midwives and AHPs.

Day 1	Quality assurance; improvement methods; patient experience/safety; prevention.
Day 2	Workforce; recruitment and resources; employee management.
Day 3	Supervision and coaching.
Day 4	Clinical effectiveness; productivity and innovation.
Day 5	Finance and workforce data.

Reflection on the programme:
Completed by:...........................
Signed off by:...........................
Date:..................

The band 7 and above nursing competency self-assessment (Table 7.9) is an important part of self-assessment, to apply an effective leadership development and competency framework in ensuring service delivery.

The site night senior sister development programme (Table 7.10) focuses on key areas of knowledge and experience for middle managers who must run and manage hospital sites during night shifts and outside usual working hours.

TABLE 7.8 ■ **Passport to Management Programme**

Programme introduction and overview:

Day 1:

Engagement and climate setting.

Leadership and management.

Effective communication.

Coaching.

Reflection on the programme:

Day 2:

Budget and finance.

E-rostering for managers.

Leading and managing in the organisation.

Incident and risk management.

Understanding human factors.

Complaints management.

Creating a positive environment for staff.

Raising concerns: freedom to speak up.

Reflection on the programme:

Day 3:

Having difficult conversations.

Sickness and leave management.

Working with occupational health to create a positive environment for staff.

Objective setting.

Performance management.

Managing investigations.

Programme summary and evaluation:

Completed by:...............................

Signed off by:........................

Date:....................

Reflection on the programme:

7.7 Ward and Department Assessment and Accreditation Framework

The standard operating procedure for the assessment and accreditation framework for wards and departments is usually sponsored by the executive Chief Nursing Officer (CNO)/DON. This sample ward accreditation programme is used organisation-wide by clinical staff, including nurses, physicians, AHPs, HCAs, domestics and housekeepers, to advance quality and safety in the organisation, and ensure patient-centred care. This type of ward and department assessment and accreditation framework is used along with other documents and policies for admission, safe discharge planning, bed escalation, patient transfers, medical teams, aseptic nontouch technique (ANTT), bed rails, blood transfusion, capabilities and capacities, uniform attire and pain management including epidural and early warning systems. Other policies and procedures supporting ward assessment and accreditation include record management; patient identification; deprivation of liberty; MCA; safeguarding; whistleblowing; consent; medicine administration and management; DNACPR; resuscitation; e-rostering; palliative and end-of-life

TABLE 7.9 ■ Band 7 and Above Nursing Competency Self-Assessment, including mental health:

Complete this self-assessment as part of the leadership development and competency framework for band 7 staff, indicating where individuals' own competencies are situated. This baseline measurement can be used to identify individual personal development plans (PDPs), wherein goals can be achieved through specific activities including clinical supervision, training, e-learning, shadowing, buddying, action learning sets, mentoring, **coaching** and annual appraisal.

Name: Role: Length of time in post:

Competency: Skills and development area	Select: Novice, advanced beginner, competent, proficient, or expert	Notes/PDP actions
Patient safety and quality.		
Risk assessment and care planning.		
Regulatory compliance, e.g. CQC.		
Medication administration including intramuscular injection (IM), subcutaneous (SC), insulin, CDs.		
Therapeutic engagement and observation.		
Rapid tranquilisation and seclusion.		
Patient group facilitation.		
Supervision and appraisals.		
E-roster, safe care, safe staffing, skill mix review.		
Clinical skills.		
Performance support and management of attendance.		
Experience and understanding of patient flow.		
Ward finance and budget management.		
Shift and care coordination.		
Delegation of duties.		
Management of complaints and compliments.		
Conflict resolution.		
Patient experience.		
Experience in service user engagement and involvement.		
Use of medical devices.		
NEW2.		
Mental Health Act (MHA), MCA, Section 132 rights.		
Safeguarding.		
De-escalation, personal safety.		

TABLE 7.9 ■ Band 7 and Above Nursing Competency Self-Assessment—cont'd

IPC, personal hygiene.

Leadership, mentoring and coaching.

Strategy development.

Team building.

Time management and organisation skills.

Communication skills, influencing, and networking.

Professional standards, conduct and behaviour.

Safe ward: ward accreditation and audit.

Quality improvement (QI).

Change management.

Recruitment and retention.

People management, and human resources.

Personal impact.

Talent management.

Research and development.

Student/apprenticeship framework.

Clinical incident investigation.

Incidents review: Datix, Ulysses, PSIRF.

IT/computer skills.

Refer to the ward leader's handbook for additional elements on general band 7 competency assessment, as detailed in Chapter 5 providing further information regarding strategies for staff to use in coping and flourishing in their roles.

Self-assessment reflection:

Completed by:...........................

Signed off by:........................

Date.......................

care; and food hygiene and safety. Ward assessment and accreditation also relate to policies for the critical care pathway and management of patients who are acutely ill/deteriorating; blood transfusion; patient flow and management of patients in accident and emergency; theatres; recovery; urethral catheter care plan; IPC including diarrhoea and vomiting/hand hygiene/cleaning; patient equipment management; interpretation and translation; manual handling; nutrition and hydration; prevention of slips, trips and falls; tissue viability/PUP/wound care; long-term conditions including diabetes; privacy and dignity; and care and treatment of patients with learning disability and autism. Assessments of leadership and professionalism, people management, mentorship and coaching, clinical governance,

TABLE 7.10 ■ Site Night Senior Sister Development Programme

Topic Area	Training Delivered by
Emergency planning.	Head of emergency management.
Site team role.	Site manager.
Paediatrics at night.	Paediatric matron.
Pastoral support.	Site pastor.
Outreach role.	Acute medicine matron.
Roles and responsibilities.	Head of nursing for medicine.
Matron's handbook/IPC.	Matron's handbook author/deputy director of IPC.
Safe care/e-roster.	Safe care lead nurse.
Completed by:............................	
Signed off by:..........................	
Date:..........................	

BOX 7.6   Personal Development Testimonial

It is an NMC Code (2023c) requirement that all nurses maintain their competencies for the role they undertake. I have completed PDP competencies in Tables 7.5 to 7.8, which has contributed to my revalidation; my manager noted that it is one of the most comprehensive revalidation documents she has come across.

Senior nurse

---

learning from incidents/investigation and experience, risk management, Patient Advice and Liaison Services (PALs), complaints and serious incident (SIs) (aligned to PSIRF) are performed. These aspects support recognition and retention of the ward accreditation status and achievements, including the use of audits and ward score cards. Ward accreditation may use platinum, gold, silver and bronze awards, and a recognition system to reward staff for their work. Box 7.6 provides a personal development testimonial regarding the benefits of the various PDP tools and competencies in this chapter.

7.8 Ward Audit Tool

The ward audit tool (Table 7.11) is available in many formats, including hard copies, and can be accessed through mobile devices, applications, telephones or computers. This tool automates the inspection and audit process, and can be used for monthly performance and progress monitoring/compliance, including identifying and addressing issues and raising standards of care.

7.9 Coaching for Leadership

Coaching for leadership (Table 7.12) is a crucial part of career development, progression and management to lead and progress. Key elements of coaching are summarised in coaching for leadership in Table 7.13.

Staff can register for coaching on the NHS Leadership Academy (2023d) website, which includes various types of coaching such as a linguistic coaching programmes or career coaching. Coaching training programmes are also available, such as Ignite

TABLE 7.11 ■ **Ward Audit Tool**

Type of Audit Inspection	Description
Safeguarding	MCA, Deprivation of Liberty Safeguards (DOLs).
Finance/use of resources	Ensuring cost savings, efficient and lean processes.
Health and safety	Risk assessment, moving and handling.
IPC	Diarrhoea and vomiting, hand hygiene and cleaning.
Skin integrity/pressure ulcer (PU).	Checking for moisture lesions.
Training and education	Staff knowledge.
Human resources	Health and wellbeing, leadership, management.
Patient and user experience	Friends and Family Test (FFT), engagement.
Medication	Pharmacy, medication rounds.
Care records and documentation	Handover, care plans, do not attempt cardiopulmonary resuscitation (DNACPRDs), NEWS chart.
Nutrition and hydration	MUST.
Environment	Clinical departments, treatment/medications rooms.
Quality and safety	SI, complaints, harm free care, quality performance and actions.
Staffing	Satisfaction, professional development, workforce, vacancy rate, sickness, shift coverage, acuity, ratios.
Patient observation	NEWS.
Falls	SWARM, risk assessment.
Ward accreditation programme	Supported by the wards and departments assessment and accreditation framework in Section 7.7.

Completed by:..........................
Signed off by:.............................
Date:.....................

leadership coaching training, delivered by multinational coaching agencies, and a level 7 leadership coaching course (NHS Leadership Academy, 2023d). These courses provide transformational skills for leadership through teaching of coaching skills such as listening, questioning, reflection and support; follow-up seminars; and coaching in practice. Leadership coaching enables leading with excitement, thereby inspiring best practice in healthcare and excellent quality of care every day.

Executive coaching helps with the following:

- Goals.
- Preparation.
- Leadership.
- Use of qualifications in practice.
- Feeling good enough.
- Having courage.
- Being the best one can be.

Refer to the style of leadership, including transformational, transactional and trait-based leadership, as part of coaching programme delivery.

Inspirational leadership is also a key part of coaching for leadership, including the following:

- Being personally successful and enabling success in others.
- Personal: belief in oneself.
- Team: belief in the team as part of organisation.
- Organisation: belief in the organisation as part of society.
- Society: making people well and doing good.

Table 7.12 lists detailed elements of using coaching for leadership.

TABLE 7.12 ■ Coaching for Leadership

What skills, attributes and abilities do client need to develop to grow as a leader?

Coaching enables effective leadership through the following:

Clarity of vision: enrol people with their vision/take people with them.

Having a role model.

Approachable, kind, fair, calm, cool and transparent.

Receptive context.

Team player.

Prove yourself as a leader.

Survivor.

Strong communicator with confidence: spread my word and influence others.

Make the best of given situations.

Empower and influence others.

Inspirational.

Charismatic.

Controversial.

Heroic.

Determined.

Self-sacrificing.

Authentic.

Trust and empathy.

Build relationships/get to know people Connect with colleagues.

Proactive/disruptive, challenge the normal and change the status quo for improvement.

Self-belief, awareness of self.

Personal growth.

Good listener.

Lead on a larger scale.

Complete recognised qualifications.

Develop service in one team.

Fairness, firmness and understanding.

Say thank you.

Coaching to lead: leadership style supporting people to lead, succeed and achieve, without doing tasks for them or telling them what to do.

Achieve personally and professionally, and via others.

Impact on others' improvement and progress.

Emotional intelligence.

Engagement and relationships.

What must change in order for me to respond in a more coach-like way:

The professional leadership coaching model:

The skills (to use as a coach): listening, supporting and questioning.

The steps: determine the purpose, reality, plans, and activities of the clients goal and review the progress of these.

The field PIES/location: where coaching occurs: environment: resources (physical, emotional, intellectual and social), structure (lesson plan) and domain (the model).

The principles: where coaching starts.

Using coaching skills and approach:

Coaching skills: presence, listening, supporting reflection, questioning

Regarding the challenged journey (difficulty with career progression):

Give coachees space to talk.

Listen to coachees.

Explore the qualities of the person being coached.

Caring manager.

Allow coachees to guide themselves in the conversation.

TABLE 7.12 ■ Coaching for Leadership—cont'd

Coaching questions: follow the proper steps:	Coaching questions: (reality, open, closed)
Purpose/vision: What is the client's purpose? What does the client/coachee want to bring to the world? Leadership, values and ideal-self vision How can the proposed activities and actions be undertaken? Where does the client want to get to in their career? **Vision:** what does the person want to achieve with coaching? Plan, action and review can develop a plan to refine the vision. **What do** the client **want to achieve: vision?** **What do** the coachee **want to create?** **Where do** the client **want to go in their career?** **Articulate** the client **vision in two sentences** **Where do** the client **see themself in 5 years' time?** E.g., to be good at what the client is doing at present	What would the client (the individual being coached) like to talk about? What methods have the client tried to resolve the issues? What other options are the client able to try? What would the client preference be? What steps might the client take? Are there any options the client have not tried? What do the client need to do now/next? How do the client feel now? Have the client spoken to other people who have successfully done this work? How are the client getting on with doing this work? What would the client like to do now, having explored so many options? What do the client feel are missing with this method? **What have you explored in the area described?** Have the client tried anything else? How did that go? What do the client need to do to get to the next level of their career? What are the barriers to doing that, by when? By what date can the client do that?

Coaching using principles of trust and possibilities, in which clients take control of their own problems:
Coaching cycle:
purpose (vision); **reality** (possibility); **plan** (chosen action); **action** (review stage).
Describe the personal situation.
What personal shift must you make to become more coach-like?

Listening techniques:	Feedback:
Active listening by: Listening with respect, the ears, heart and eyes, and perceive, sense, observe the client to gather information about them during the coaching session. **Listen** without judgement. **Listen** to what the client is saying and not saying. **Listen for the field PIES resources/ structure/resources:** **Physical.** **Intellectual.** **Emotional:** feelings, mood, values/ beliefs: Excited, proud, enthusiasm, body language, tone of voice. **Social**	**Feedback using field PIES:** **What has changed?** **What is it like now?** **What is troubling you?** Feed back what is hear to the client. **Areas of focus:** Talk about a success or something positive you were looking forward to. **What is great about the coachee?** Making good progress. **Motivational.** Strong, beautiful, hardworking. **Ignore the gremlin** (the inner critic).

(Continued)

TABLE 7.12 ■ Coaching for Leadership—cont'd

Coaching at work: coaching topics:

Use coaching skills in the workplace with staff.
Meet deadlines/time management.
Conflict resolution.
Improve relationship in a team.
Effective management styles.
Reviewing performance: managing objectives.
Career development/progression.
Motivational speaking.
Decision-making, handling pressure.
Work-life-balance, influencing skills.

Coaching reality:

Questions relating to reality to resolve the issue which has been identified.
What do you feel you are missing with the method?
Encouraging: what steps might the client take to address the issue identified?
Are there any options the client have not tried?
What methods have the client tried?
How is the client getting on with that methods tried.?
What other options have the client tried?
What would the client preference be?

Coaching actions:

What would the client like to do now?
How? Where? What?
When can the client do them by?
Focus on resolving options, obstacles, decisions and commitments.

Supporting (skills of leadership):

Encouragement: in line with what is perceived as reasonable.
Brainstorming.
Enthusiasm.
Offering opinion.
Storytelling.
Relating your experience.
Offering analysis.
Recommendation regarding a particular belief.
Providing resources of my own.
Offering a model or paradigm.
360-degree feedback: register and use.

Coaching plan:

Ensuring that the client's **emotional connection** to the **vision** and **purpose** persists through the planning.
Inspiration: emotional connection to the vision.
Motivation: emotional connection to resources.
Optimism: planning to build resources and achieve goals.
Focus on **options, obstacles, commitment, decision**
Coaching plan questions:
What must be done next?
What is needed to get to the next level of the career or issue being discussed?
What are the barriers to arrive at the next level?
How can the client overcome these barriers?
How far have the client advanced?
What further information does the client need?

Summarised session and action:

Acknowledge great work.
Support.
Enthusiasm.

In addition to Table 7.12 on coaching for leadership, refer to Table 7.13 on coaching session note documentation on vision/reality/plan/action; and Section 5.2.5.9 for additional details on coaching. The coaching skills for managers testimonial in Box 7.7 indicates feedback on the benefits of leadership coaching for managers.

7.10 Mentor Portfolio of Evidence for Staff

The mentor portfolio for nurses, midwives and other staff is important. Various tools and resources can provide support, such as recognition of mentoring skills, and a guidance and mapping framework for stage 2 mentors. This tool is based on the Nursing and Midwifery Council (2008) Standards to Support Learning and Assessment in Practice and can be completed for personal professional portfolios as evidence of continuing development as a mentor.

TABLE 7.13 ■ Coaching Session Note Documentation on Vision/Reality/Plan/Action

The client refers to the person being coached.

What is the client leadership vision?	What is the client natural leadership style?	What is required to acquire, develop or alter?
What do the client want to achieve?	Where is the client now?	What is between where the client is now, and where they want to go?
What do the client want to create?	Who is the client now?	What has the client created so far?
Where do the client want to go?	What do the client have now?	What might the client do to get to where they want to go?
What do the client want to become?		What will the client do next to progress the actions identified?
What is great about the client?		

Vision	Reality	Plan and action
Examples include:	Examples include:	Examples include:
Work items to discuss in coaching session:	**Learn** from others to undertake activities the client is not familiar with.	How to work with different personalities?
1. **Prioritising:** ask for help, delegate.	**Be self-aware:** try to get know themself.	Confidence in self: put things in writing.
2. **Change mindset:** complete activities straight away.	**Leadership style:** reflect and take action on reflection.	Managing expectations.
3. **Confidence** and belief in own abilities.	**Be upfront:** ask for help when needed.	Share list of progress with actions undertaken.
4. **Challenges:** does some work at home; difficult to challenge colleagues.	Gain support and calm from managers / peers.	Plan duties in a diary.
5. **Vision:** equal workload with meaningful contribution to leadership.	Use coping mechanisms when working alone.	**Personality assessment traits:**
Speaking vision: Write your vision in a 30-second speech here:	Aim to do a good job.	Use online resources to assess personality.
	How does the client see themself?	Ask HR, learning and development (L&D) and leadership team for tools which was be used for personality assessment.
	Others may see the client as a team player. Is this correct?	Plan: prioritise three duties and take action, feedback on these at coaching sessions.
	Use evidence of how others undertake duties and roles the client intends to undertake.	

BOX 7.7	Coaching Skills for Managers Testimonial

Feedback from previous delegates of coaching courses states that attendees have increased confidence in coaching skills, as well as these coaching sessions being a good use of their time.

Ward manager

The **mentor and preceptor portfolio** include the following key domains:
- Establishing effective working relationships.
- Facilitating learning.
- Assessment and accountability.
- Evaluation of learning.
- Creating an environment for learning.
- Context of practice.

- Evidenced based practice.
- Leadership.

(University of Hertfordshire, 2023).

Staff can register for mentoring on the NHS Leadership Academy (2023d) website. Additional details on mentoring can be found in Section 5.3.7 on mentoring and Section 7.10 on the mentor portfolio of evidence for staff.

7.11 Job Applications, Curricula Vitae, Cover Letters and Interviews

Key elements of applying for jobs are summarised in Fig. 7.1, providing a sample supporting statement/cover letter; Fig. 7.2, providing a sample CV; and Box 7.8, providing supporting statement tips. In looking for a new role, applying for jobs, writing CVs and cover letters, and undertaking interviews might seem daunting, and will require as much support and preparation as possible. Box 7.9 provides an example of using advice, support and tools to help with interview preparation; Box 7.10, provides an example of a work situation that did not end very well; and Box 7.11, provides an example interview question answer. Section 2.2.7 provides additional information on applying for jobs from overseas to work in the UK.

7.11.1 TIPS FOR COMPLETING APPLICATION FORMS AND CVS

The first step in convincing potential employers to select individuals for a post in their organisation and in healthcare is completing an effective job application form and/or writing a winning CV.

7.11.2 WRITING A WINNING CV

A CV serves as a personal marketing tool to show employers that candidates have the necessary skills and professional, educational and personal experience to undertake the role being applied for.

CVs can be used for the following:

- When responding to a job advertisement, by applying in writing.
- As an additional submission to completing a standard job application form.
- When the employer's standard application form does not cover all points that the applicant wants to raise, in addition to the fully completed employers' application form.
- In speculative job applications aimed at interviewing for posts of interest that have not been advertised.

7.11.3 PREPARING TO WRITE A CV

Applicants should start by making a list of their experience and posts held, commencing with the most recent experience. For all posts held, dates of employment, name of employer, job titles, responsibilities and achievements in the role should be listed.

The next steps should include gathering and listing the following:

- All educational certificates, staring with the most recent.
- Courses undertaken and qualifications gained, including dates and names of educational organisations.

Sample supporting statement or cover letter for a newly qualified nurse applying for a post on a surgical ward.

I am applying for a post on Jasmine surgical ward because I have a strong commitment to meeting the needs of patients, families, carers and service users following surgery.
I developed an interest in this speciality following a 5-week management placement on a surgical ward, where I particularly enjoyed teaching patients how to manage their wound and check for signs and symptoms of infections after surgery.
I have completed a case study on a patient undertaking self-management following surgery. I also gained excellent feedback from my mentor and other staff on the unit and really enjoyed working with the multi-disciplinary team. I believe that I meet the requirements described in the job description and person specification as follows.

Qualifications and experience:

I am an NMC registered nurse, who has recently completed degree level pre-registration education, with an overall grade of upper second class. The course provided a strong emphasis on evidence-based practice and I completed an extended essay on the impact of pre-operative patient preparation prior to surgery as per NICE guidelines.

Skills and knowledge:

I believe I have excellent communication skills and have always been able to deal with challenging situations such as when a relative became angry about the treatment of their mother. I was able to allay the relative's anxiety by listening to and empathising with their concerns and arranging for them to discuss their mother's care with the senior nurse in charge. I have also developed teaching and mentoring skills when supervising the work of health care support workers and junior students. I am keen to pursue a mentorship course as soon as possible. I have taught students skills such as how to admit patients, perform dressings, use the Patient Administration System and monitor blood glucose levels. I always refer learners to relevant resources, such as teaching packs, and check the student's understanding of the topic by asking questions, supervising their practice and giving constructive feedback. I also enjoy promoting patients' health and teaching about the importance of healthy eating and smoking cessation. I have learnt how to prioritise a busy workload and during my management placement I managed the care of nine patients and the work of three health care support workers. On a very busy shift, I had to deal with two emergency admissions, arrange three discharges and initiate life support for a patient suffering respiratory arrest. I learnt the importance of affective delegation, communication, team work and referring to other health care professionals and senior staff when appropriate. I am aware of the importance of key documents such as the Standards of Care and have assisted in the auditing of nutrition and hygiene benchmarks during a placement nursing patient following surgery.

Personal qualities:

I believe that I am a cheerful, flexible and enthusiastic nurse who tries to be approachable at all times. I try to be respectful towards all individuals, from a variety of backgrounds and strictly adhere to all policies, including health and safety, infection prevention and control and confidentiality. I hope you will agree that I meet the requirements for the post and look forward to hearing from you.

Fig. 7.1 Sample supporting statement/cover letter. (With permission from Royal College of Nursing. (2023n). *Job applications and supporting statements*. https://www.rcn.org.uk/Professional-Development/Your-career/Job-applications. Accessed 22 October 2023.)

(September 2003–January 2009)
Nurse 2 Forest Road, Bedlington,
Bedlingshire, BSZ 4AA

Telephone: (05432) 65X XXX (Home)
Email: Jasmine.Nurse@hospital.nhs.uk

Date: 1 October

An enthusiastic registered nurse with over 5 years' experience of providing expert nursing care in surgical and medical settings. A conscientious professional committed to improving standards of care through evaluation of practice, knowledge of research and lifelong learning. Keen to explore options in community care.

KEY ACHIEVEMENTS AND SKILLS

• Promoted to senior staff nurse after 3 years' post registration experience.
• Gained expertise in nursing patients with various conditions requiring medical and surgical interventions.
• Awarded 120 diploma level points through the Bedlington University and working towards a BSc Health and Social Care.
• Consolidated recent completion of return to practice course with regular bank work in various settings.

EXPERIENCE

BEDLINGTON NHS TRUST – NHS Professionals
Bank nurse (band 5 - mainly medical nursing) - April 2009 – present

• Undertaking at least two shifts per week whilst completing diploma level studies in welfare, community health and working with children and families.
• Plan, implement and evaluate patient care using a range of recognised nursing models.
• Supervise and assess learning of care assistants and pre-registration students.

BENLINGTON UNIVERSITY
Return to practice course student (January 2009–April 2009)

• Completed placement on a 20-bed medical ward, including management of the unit.
• Awarded 20 academic credit points at level 2.
• Renewed competence in areas such as implementing models of care, medical assessment, record keeping, teaching, safe drug administration, catheterisation.
• Completed training and assessments in safe patient handling, medication administration, intravenous therapy and basic life support.

Career break – raising family (September 2003–January 2009)

• Ran a helpline for sufferers of prostate cancer (voluntary, part time), organised by the Prostate Cancer Awareness Group.
• Ran a youth group at my local church: organised a conference for 100 delegates, arranged speakers, venue and refreshments in December 2006. Regularly arrange social events for this group.

Fig. 7.2 Sample curriculum vitae (CV). (With permission from Royal College of Nursing. (2023n). *Job applications and supporting statements*. https://www.rcn.org.uk/Professional-Development/Your-career/Job-applications. Accessed 22 October 2023.)

BEDLINGTON NHS TRUST
Senior Staff Nurse – 24-bed surgical urology ward - May 2002 – September 2003

- Planned, implemented and evaluated the care of patients with various urological conditions.
- Led the nursing team and deputised for the ward manager on a regular basis.
- Managed the ward's stock control system.
- Contributed to ward managers' meetings on a regular basis. Organised staff rotas.
- Mentored qualified nurses and students.
- Wrote a comprehensive induction programme for new staff.
- Initiated and devised a nutritional status assessment tool in collaboration with the multi-disciplinary team.

Staff Nurse – 24-bed surgical urology ward - October 2001 – May 2002

- Managed the ward on a regular basis.
- Supervised, taught and assessed learning of pre-registration students.

BENLINGHAM NHS TRUST
Staff Nurse – 21-bed surgical ward - June 1999 – October 2001

- Planned, implemented and evaluated the care of patients preparing for and recovering from surgical procedures.

QUALIFICATIONS

120 diploma level points: Care, Welfare and Community, Working for Health, Working with Children and Families, Bedlington University - February 2010
Return to Practice (20 points, diploma level) - January 2009
ENB Urology course, Bedlington College of Nursing - January 2002
ENB Teaching and Assessing in Clinical Practice course, Bedlington College of Nursing - April 2001
Registered General Nurse, Bedlington College of Nursing
Pin No: 333333 (Expires 2010). Joined June 1999
2 A Levels and 8 GCSEs, Bedlington High School 1993 – 1995

PROFESSIONAL ACTIVITIES

Paper titled 'Principles of pain management after surgery' presented to the RCN Pain Forum conference in June 2000.

Fig. 7.2, Cont'd.

BOX 7.8   Supporting Statement Tips

My supporting statement included the following which assisted me in getting called for interview:
Why I wanted the job?
Why I was a good fit for the job?
Clarify any questions the recruiter may have, following speaking to them.
Showed the recruiter what I knew about the trust already.
I was innovative and creative in presenting my supporting statement.

Deputy director

BOX 7.9 Interview Preparation: Personal Testimony

As a new DON, I used the following to help me succeed at my interviews:

Talk to hiring manager, execs, CEO and senior staff about the role and what you can bring to the role – make an impression.

Go to visit and meet the trust staff as part of due diligence.

Find out their challenges and aspirations.

Tailor my skills to address the issues at the organisation.

Showed the best of me, what I am good at, and what I enjoy doing.

Prep before speaking on the phone or visiting.

Know the route to the interview.

Stay overnight before interview day for long journeys.

Practice presentation and mock questions before interview.

Take and review notes prior to the interview.

New Director of Nursing

BOX 7.10 Example of a Work Situation That Did Not End Very Well: Personal Testimony

As a new staff nurse, I didn't fully understand the importance of advocating for the patient. A doctor was trying to take blood from a patient and had difficulty in finding a vein. The patient was anxious and moving their arm about. The patient was clearly in a lot of pain and eventually the doctor had to give up and a more senior doctor took blood. I am now very experienced at venepuncture and can see that if the doctor had used a pillow to support the patient's arm, he would have had more success. I would now have no hesitation in taking the doctor aside to discuss training on venepuncture and to suggest more effective ways of taking blood. I would have intervened earlier to support the patient and halt the procedure.

New head of nursing

BOX 7.11 Example Interview Question Answer

I was shift co-ordinator, when two patients sharing a bay started arguing about one person's belongings taking up too much space. The discussion was becoming quite heated and I observed that other patients and relatives were looking anxious. To diffuse the tension, I suggested calmly we discuss the matter in a quiet area of the ward. I invited them to both to sit down and facilitated each to express their grievances.

To demonstrate I was listening, I summarised their grievances and conveyed how the other person's behaviour made them feel. I tactfully tried to help them see the situation from each other's point of view and to agree a way forward. The outcome was that one agreed to keep his belongings closer to his bed and the other apologised for 'flying off the handle', explaining he was having a 'bad day' as his stay in hospital would be longer than expected. This then gave me the opportunity to discuss these concerns with him later in the shift.

Staff nurse

- Professional activities and duties, including published articles and papers, conference presentations, membership in professional groups and voluntary duties.

7.11.4 CV FORMAT

There is no single format for a CV, but the format should be logical, clear and concise, should respond to the job description (JD) and person specification (PS) for the job being applied for, and should maximise focus on applicants' strengths.

A CV should include the following basic elements:

- **Personal details**: Include the applicant's name, address, contact telephone number and email.
- **Opening statement**: Write several sentences summarising personal and professional qualities. Applicants with extensive experience should include a bulleted list of approximately four major professional achievements.
- **Experience**: Applicants should start with their most recent role, listing dates, positions held and the name of the employer. Detail approximately four responsibilities at the most recent and senior post and four major achievements relevant to the post being applied for, ensuring relevance to the JD and the PS of the post being applied for.
- **Education**: Include details of professional qualifications and education to date.
- **Professional activities**: Include a list of published articles and papers, conference presentations, membership in professional groups and voluntary duties.
- **Personal**: Include additional information, such as interests and voluntary work undertaken with relevance to the job being applied for.

7.11.5 GENERAL CV TIPS

When writing a CV, follow the following general tips:

- The CV length should be no more than 2 to 4 pages, covering the most recent roles and job achievements, results and impact.
- Use action words, such as led, developed, coordinated, created, established, fulfilled, identified, implemented, improved, initiated, launched, managed, motivated, negotiated, organised, produced, undertook, completed and trained.
- Explain the reasons for any gaps in employment; any skills gained through that gap, such as from raising a family; and voluntary roles, such as school board governor.
- When detailing achievements, include numbers and data, for example, 'managed 40 staff and responsible for a budget of £800,000'.
- Minimise the number of pages of the CV. Individuals with extensive experience should summarise positions held more than 10 years prior. For published articles, list the most important and summarise the rest; for example, 'more than 30 articles published in many journals on various aspects of health and care, professional development, education and public health'.
- Use standard formatting, such as Arial font and 1.5 line spacing.
- Avoid using abbreviations.
- Include references and a cover letter highlighting the main points in the CV, relating them to the job being applied for.
- Have the CV proofread, obtain feedback and correct any errors.

7.12 Completing Job Application Forms

Currently, most job applications are completed electronically/online. Therefore, individuals can spell check their CV and cover letters; align the application to the job being applied for; and save electronic copies before submission. Ensure that the application is checked for the inclusion of all required information before pressing the 'send' or submit button.

7.12.1 COMPLETING HEALTH ASSESSMENT IN APPLICATION FORMS

Individuals are usually asked to complete a health questionnaire as part of the application. This form is confidential and is sent to the occupational health department for review by an occupational health nurse, to ensure that staff health and safety are not compromised by the role being applied for.

7.12.2 DECLARING ANY PREVIOUS CONVICTIONS

Application forms usually have a section for declaration of any previous convictions; this section should be completed accurately, as requested by the form. These forms are reviewed by the recruiting team and interview panel, taking account of the severity of the offence and whether it affects the role being applied for. Applicants undergo a Criminal Records Bureau (CRB) check and should discuss any related concerns with employers so that any potential issues can be addressed early.

7.12.3 SUPPORTING INFORMATION IN THE APPLICATION

The supporting information section is the most important part of the job application form. This section should match the skills and experience required for the role, as outlined in the job description (JD) and person specification (PS), by providing evidence of how the requirements are met by the applicant. This should also be aligned to any special requirements of the role. The JD and PS will also provide the knowledge and skills framework for the role and is outlined on job application sites such as NHS jobs and Indeed (Royal College of Nursing, 2023n). Box 7.8 provides tips on completing the supporting statement.

Fig. 7.1 provides a sample supporting statement and cover letter, to provide candidates with ideas for how to complete their own statement.

Fig. 7.2 provides a sample CV to give candidates ideas regarding how to complete their own CV.

7.13 Interview Skills Guide

Interview preparation overview:

An interview is essentially a performance whose success relies on careful preparation and practice. The following guidance offers advice, tips and examples for successful interviewing.

7.13.1 INTERVIEW PREPARATION

When preparing for an interview, applicants should perform the following:

- Review the person specification and job description, where available. Highlight all statements indicating the skills, experience and personal attributes required for the role being applied for. Reflect on the career to date and the state of how the applicant meets the requirements for the role. Prepare to expand on information provided in the application form or CV. Update the portfolio and have it ready to provide at the interview.
- Review the list of common interview questions (Section 7.13.6): practise answering these questions through mock interviews with a friend, relative, senior colleague, career adviser or coach. Obtain constructive feedback and practise several times. Rehearse the actual interview process (refer to the interview section).
- Prepare a list of questions to practice answering.
- Organise an informal visit, to talk to staff, assess whether the post and environment fit with the candidate's needs and obtain answers to questions.
- Be up to date with local and national initiatives in healthcare by searching relevant health websites or reading current healthcare and nursing journals.
- Plan the journey to the interview, including travel time, allowing time for delays such as traffic jams; become familiar with the journey route.
- Compile and prepare any documents requested by the organisation, such as certificates, passport and an up-to-date portfolio. Further guidance on compiling a portfolio is available from the Learning Zone on the Royal College of Nursing (RCN) website (Royal College of Nursing, 2023n).
- Dress: wear a smart, clean and comfortable suit for the interview.
- Get a good night's sleep the night before the interview. Ensure sufficient time to prepare on the day of the interview, including time to eat breakfast, get ready and perform a final mental rehearsal. Use relaxation techniques to help focus.

7.13.2 BREATHING EXERCISE TO HELP WITH RELAXATION BEFORE AN INTERVIEW

To allay nervousness, breathe more shallowly, using deep breathing techniques several minutes before the interview, to bring more oxygen to the brain.

To help with relaxation, follow these steps:

1. Stand up, where possible.
2. Inhale slowly to fill your lungs completely. Do this naturally, without excessive effort.
3. Count to three, then slowly exhale through the mouth.
4. Do not over- or hyperventilate. Take time to do the exercise gently for 3 or 4 minutes.

7.13.3 DURING THE INTERVIEW

- Smile when entering the room.
- Shake hands with members of the panel.

- Take some time to get comfortable.
- Ask the panel to repeat questions if more clarity is needed.
- Maintain good eye contact.
- Do not rush the answers.
- Ask questions at the end of the interview.

7.13.4 BODY LANGUAGE DURING THE INTERVIEW

Candidates should do the following:

- Smile to show friendliness and openness.
- Nod to demonstrate that you are paying attention.
- Make eye contact to show your sincerity and confidence, but do not stare.
- Do not cross your arms, to avoid appearing guarded.
- Sit well back in the chair, to show that you are relaxed and comfortable.
- Avoid hunching your shoulders.
- Avoid fumbling with jewellery or fidgeting; hold onto a pen.
- Hold your head up to avoid mumbling into your chest.
- Begin answers by looking at the person who asked the question, then direct it at the entire panel, by looking at each panel member.
- Make eye contact equally with each panel member.

7.13.5 AFTER THE INTERVIEW

If successful at an interview:

- Wait for confirmation in writing before resigning from any current post.
- Ensure that a contract and details of the terms and conditions of employment have been received.
- Clarify any concerns before accepting the job in writing.

If unsuccessful at an interview:

- Reflect on interview performance and write down what worked and what did not.
- Write down the most difficult questions. Think about potential responses for future interviews.
- Contact the interview panel lead and ask for constructive feedback on performance during the interview.
- If concerns exist regarding discrimination on the grounds of sex, race, age, sexuality, disability, marital status, gender reassignment status, religion or pregnancy, the RCN or other union should be contacted for support.

7.13.6 ANSWERING DIFFICULT INTERVIEW QUESTIONS

Example of answering difficult interview questions are outlined here.

7.13.6.1 Candidates' Weaknesses or Development Needs

Question: What are your weaknesses or development needs?

Answer: Think about ways of turning a negative into a positive.

For example, 'In the past, I have had a tendency to try to take on too much, but I have dealt with this by learning how to delegate responsibilities, prioritising by writing lists, planning my day in advance, and attending a time management course'.

Candidates may be new to the job being applied for and can arrange to discussion with the recruiting manager to explore possible support in adapting to the new job. This may include mentoring, a good induction programme, or a short course on skill development required for the role, for example, IV drug administration.

7.13.6.2 Example of a Work Situation That Did Not End Very Well

Question: Please give an example of a work situation that did not end very well:

Answer: Avoid dwelling on weaknesses; focus on the past rather than the present; and finish with what you learnt from the experience. Box 7.5 provides examples answer of a work situation that did not end very well.

7.13.6.3 Being the Only Qualified Nurse on Duty

Question: What would you do if you were the only qualified nurse on duty when:
- A patient falls of bed.
- A colleague is cut by broken glass.
- You observe that some drugs are missing.
- A patient complains of stolen belongings.

Answer: The interview panel will want to know that you would use basic principles, prioritising patient safety and wellbeing. Many similar scenarios would involve the following:
- Assessment of the situation.
- Taking appropriate action.
- Following procedures and guidelines.
- Appropriate communication.
- Record keeping.
- Evaluating and learning from the situation.

Other ways to answer interview questions include preparing examples from previous experience, to support the answers to the questions. Use the Situation Target Action Results (**STAR) interview technique** as a guide to provide as much detail as possible in each answer. Start by describing the **S**ituation; state the **T**arget to be achieved; and detail the **A**ctions taken and any end **R**esults achieved.**techniqueSTAR**

7.13.6.4 National Initiative in Nursing or Healthcare

Question: Tell us about a national initiative in nursing or healthcare:

Answer:
- Candidates are not required to have expertise in all aspects of healthcare development and policy. Read summary documents on current major initiatives.
- Browse through useful websites, such as those of the Health Departments in England (GOV.UK, 2023t), NHS Northern Ireland (2023), NHS Scotland (2023) and NHS Wales (2023).

7.13.6.5 Equality, Inclusion and Diversity at Work

Question: What do you understand about the term 'diversity' at work?

    Answer: Avoid saying 'treating everybody in the same way', which might appear overly simplistic. This question is usually about equality of access to services and resources and treating colleagues with support and respect; it is also about being aware of how each individual's own background, upbringing and culture might affect interactions with people belonging to different groups. Aim to obtain a copy of the organisation's equal opportunities or diversity statement, where available, and ensure general awareness of relevant legislation regarding sex, race, sexuality, age and disability discrimination. Refer to resources in this book.

7.13.6.6 Other Sample Interview Questions

Other sample interview questions include the following:
- Why do you want the job?
- What skills and experience would you bring to the role?
- Tell us about a recent situation in which you were required to use your own initiative.
- How do you cope with pressure/stress?
- What makes a good team player?
- What role do you play in a team environment?
- What motivates you as a nurse/midwife?
- Where do you see yourself in 2 to 5 years' time?
- How would you address a relative who was aggressive and verbally abusive?
- What would you do if a patient wants to make a complaint about the nursing and midwifery care on the ward/unit?
- Give example of a situation in which you have collaborated with the multidisciplinary team.
- How would you apply research findings to your practice?
- Describe any involvement in teaching and how this involvement would help create a learning environment.
- What are your strengths?
- How do you keep up to date with developments in nursing and midwifery practice?

More sample questions are available from the RCN Career Service website (Royal College of Nursing, 2023o).

7.13.6.7 Forms of Assessment Used by the Interview Panel

To ensure fairness, many interview panels use a points-based system to score the quality and detail of candidates' responses to each question. The panels usually add the scores for each applicant and award the job to the person with the most points. Following the tips above will maximise the ability to achieve a high score.

    Other forms of interviewer assessment may use include tests covering drug calculations or scenarios asking how to solve a problem or dilemma.

    The RCN Learning Zone (Royal College of Nursing, 2023p) includes a useful section on how to improve personal numeracy skills. The local organisation's or RCN resources library includes publications on drug calculations, which can help candidates become competent in these essential skills.

Some recruiters have used techniques from the business sector by holding an 'assessment centre' to recruit 'batches' of nurses for a pool of jobs, for example, newly qualified nurses, in specific areas such as NHS Direct, or candidates for senior manager positions. Some organisations use this tool for recruitment for all nursing and midwifery posts.

The assessment, or staff selection, day may include some or all of the following:

- Problem solving exercises.
- Group discussion of a scenario question.
- Roleplaying scenarios, for example, handling an NHS Direct call.
- A presentation.
- Arithmetic assessments.
- One-on-one interviews.
- Psychometric aptitude or personality tests (usually restricted to applicants for senior management roles).

The prospect of an assessment day might appear daunting but has the advantage of allowing candidates to make up for a weakness in one area with better performance in another type of assessment. Fact sheets are also available on presentation skills (Royal College of Nursing, 2023q).

7.13.6.8 Questions Candidates Can Ask at Interviews

At the end of a job interview, a good interviewer will offer candidates opportunities to ask questions. After answering the questions during the interview, candidates should have several questions ready for the interview panel. The interview is a two-way process giving candidates a chance to know whether a job is right for them. Questions to ask the panel may include those that help candidates better understand the organisation and impress the employer, including the following:

1. **What do you offer in terms of continuing professional development?**
   This question will show commitment to learning. The answer given may assist candidates in deciding whether they are being employed mainly to provide a 'set of hands' or whether the employer aims to assist with personal development and career progression.

2. **How would you describe the work culture in the organisation?**
   This question helps candidates determine whether the employer is committed to issues such as work/life balance.
   This question can also provide information about the team dynamics and whether the working environment will be positive. This question indicates candidates' keenness to work in a positive environment and to positively contribute.

3. **What are the main issues that the ward/unit/organisation will face over the coming months?**
   This question shows candidates' ability to see their role in a broader context. Candidates can also determine how the role might be affected by forthcoming changes or projects.

4. **I notice that you have recently introduced Shared Governance. How will this impact the ward/unit/organisation?**
   Similarly to the question above, this question demonstrates that candidates have taken the time to research the organisation.

5. **Do you have any doubts about employing me in this position?**

Candidates might feel nervous about asking this question, but it provides an opportunity to address any issues raised and also indicates a willingness to learn from constructive criticism.

7.14 Career Development Workbook

Career development is further supported by various workbooks covering the following:

Taking the next step; career paths; barriers; what panels look for; your support network; key stakeholders; CV and applications; interviews; and career planning (NHS Leadership Academy, 2023n).

7.15 Summary: Competencies and Tools for Use in Healthcare

This chapter covered competencies and tools for use in healthcare, including new induction tools; clinical supervision competencies; preceptorship competencies; clinical competencies; IPC, TVN, CVC and VAD specialist competencies; and urinary catheter care.

It also included orientation and competency for theatre support workers; the Core Competency Framework for Anaesthetic Practitioners; patient observations; fundamentals of care plans; skin care assessment; safety huddle records; and documentation. Cross-references were included for staff development/PDP competencies; leadership competencies; and coaching for leadership in other sections of this book. This chapter also covered the mentor portfolio of evidence for nurses; and preparation for job applications, including CVs, cover letters and interviews, with cross-reference to applying for jobs in Chapter 2. It is also cross-referenced to Chapters 4 and 5 on leadership competencies and Chapter 6 on staff development.

CHAPTER 8

Measurements, Abbreviations, Language and Terminologies

8.1 Introduction

This chapter covers some of the common measurements, abbreviations, language and terminology used in the United Kingdom (UK) health and care systems. Please refer to the glossary at the end of this book for linguistic phrases, terms and colloquialisms used in everyday practice.

Staff should be familiar with the information in this chapter as they progress through their daily duties.

8.2 Units of Measurements

Common units of measurements used in healthcare are listed in Table 8.1 (Royal College of Nursing, 2023d).

8.2.1 METRIC SYSTEM INTERNATIONAL (SI) UNITS

Use of metric units is vital for safety in clinical and other settings (Royal College of Nursing, 2023d). It is important to be careful when administering medicines to avoid serious errors and incidents. Refer to Table 8.1 for more information regarding how to convert metrics accurately and ensure the safety of patients (Royal College of Nursing, 2023d).

TABLE 8.1 ■ Metric SI Base Unit

Type of Measurement	Unit	Symbol
Volume	Litre	l or L
Length	Metre	m
Weight	Gram	g
Kilo = 1000 Times Greater Than the Base Unit (×1000)		
Length	Kilometre (1000 metres)	km
Weight	Kilogram (1000 grams)	kg
Milli = One Thousandth of the Base Unit (1/1000)		
Volume	Millilitre (one thousandth of a litre)	ml or mL
Length	Millimetre (one thousandth of a metre)	mm
Weight	Milligram (one thousandth of a gram)	mg
Micro = One Millionth of the Base Unit (1/1,000,000)		
Weight	Microgram (one millionth of a gram)	mcg (it is recommended that microgram be written in full)
Nano = One Billionth of the Base Unit (1/1,000,000,000)		
Weight	Nanogram (one billionth of a gram)	ng (it is recommended that nanogram be written in full)

From Royal College of Nursing (2023d). *Metric (SI) units*. https://www.rcn.org.uk/clinical-topics/Safety-in-numbers/Metric-units. Accessed 3 January 2023.
Note: Medication is usually administered to patients in small doses and prescriptions are commonly written in grams and milligrams. For infants, prescriptions in micrograms are common and nanograms are sometimes used. Great attention to detail is needed when administering medicines to avoid getting them mixed up; for example, avoid milligrams being confused with micrograms to prevent serious errors from occurring (Royal College of Nursing, 2023d).

Further information on medication calculations and metric units is available (Royal College of Nursing, 2023d), including:

- Converting between metric units
- Converting between very large and very small numbers
- Converting from imperial to metric units
- Examples of calculating units of measure

8.3 Abbreviations

Common medical abbreviations used in healthcare (and their meanings), which may be found in patients' health records, are listed here (National Health Service (NHS), 2023cc).

LIST OF ABBREVIATIONS

Abbreviation	Meaning
#	Broken bone (fracture)
A&E	Accident and emergency
a.c.	Before meals
a.m., am, AM	Morning
AF	Atrial fibrillation
AMHP	Approved mental health professional
APTT	Activated partial thromboplastin time (a measure of how long it takes blood to clot)
ASQ	Ages and Stages Questionnaire (a set of questions about children's development)
b.d.s., bds, BDS	Two times a day
b.i.d., bid, bd	Twice a day/twice daily/2 times daily
BMI	Body mass index
BNO	Bowels not open
BO	Bowels open
BP	Blood pressure
c/c	Chief complaint
CMHN	Community mental health nurse
CPN	Community psychiatric nurse
CSF	Cerebrospinal fluid
CSU	Catheter stream urine
CT	Computerised tomography scan
CVP	Central venous pressure
CXR	Chest X-ray
DNACPR	Do not attempt cardiopulmonary resuscitation
DNAR	Do not attempt resuscitation
DNR	Do not resuscitate
Dr	Doctor
DVT	Deep vein thrombosis
Dx	Diagnosis
ECG	Electrocardiogram
ED	Emergency department
EEG	Electroencephalogram
EMU	Early morning urine sample
ESR	Erythrocyte sedimentation rate (a blood parameter used to help diagnose conditions associated with inflammation)
EUA	Examination under anaesthetic
FBC	Full blood count (a type of blood test)
FY1 FY2	Foundation year doctor
GA	General anaesthetic
gtt., gtt	Drop(s)
h., h	Hour
h/o	History of
Hb	Haemoglobin (a substance in red blood cells that moves oxygen around the body)
HCA	Healthcare assistant

(Continued)

Abbreviation	Meaning
HCSW	Healthcare support worker
HDL	High-density lipoprotein (a type of cholesterol)
HRT	Hormone replacement therapy
Ht	Height
Hx	History
i	One tablet
ii	Two tablets
iii	Three tablets
i.m., IM	Intramuscular (injection into a muscle)
i.v., IV	Intravenous (injection directly into a vein)
INR	International normalised ratio (a measure of how long blood takes to clot)
IVI	Intravenous infusion
IVP	Intravenous pyelogram (an X-ray of the urinary tract)
Ix	Investigations
LA	Local anaesthetic
LDL	Low-density lipoprotein (a type of cholesterol)
LFT	Liver function test (a type of blood test measuring enzymes and proteins in the liver)
LMP	Last menstrual period
M/R	Modified release
MRI	Magnetic resonance imaging
MRSA	Methicillin-resistant *Staphylococcus aureus*
MSU	Mid-stream urine sample
n.p.o., npo, NPO	Nothing by mouth/not by oral administration
NAD	Nothing abnormal discovered
NAI	Nonaccidental injury
NBM	Nil by mouth
NG	Nasogastric (running between the nose and stomach)
nocte	Every night
NoF	Neck of femur
NSAID	Nonsteroidal antiinflammatory drug
o.d., od, OD	Once a day
o/e	On examination
OT	Occupational therapist
p.c.	After food
p.m., pm, PM	Afternoon or evening
p.o., po, PO	Orally/by mouth/oral administration
p.r., pr, PR	Rectally
p.r.n., prn, PRN	As needed
p/c	Presenting complaint
physio	Physiotherapist
POP	Plaster of Paris
PTT	Partial thromboplastin time (a measure of how quickly the blood clots)
PU	Passed urine
q.	Every

Abbreviation	Meaning
q.1.d., q1d	Every day
q.1.h., q1h	Every hour
q.2.h., q2h	Every 2 hours
q.4.h., q4h	Every 4 hours
q.6.h., q6h	Every 6 hours
q.8.h., q8h	Every 8 hours
q.d., qd	Every day/daily
q.d.s., qds, QDS	Four times a day
q.h., qh	Every hour, hourly
q.i.d., qid	Four times a day
q.o.d., qod	Every other day/alternate days
q.s., qs	Sufficient quantity (enough)
RN	Registered nurse
RNLD	Learning disability nurse
ROSC	Return of spontaneous circulation
RTA	Road traffic accident
Rx	Treatment
s.c., SC	Subcutaneous (injection under the skin)
S/R	Sustained release
SLT	Speech and language therapist
SpR	Specialist registrar
stat.	Immediately, with no delay, now
STEMI	ST segment elevation myocardial infarction
t.d.s., tds, TDS	Three times a day
t.i.d., tid	Three times a day
TCI	To come in
TFT	Thyroid function test
TPN	Total parenteral nutrition
TPR	Temperature, pulse and respiration
TTA	To take away
TTO	To take out
U&E	Urea and electrolytes
u.d., ud	As directed
UCC	Urgent care centre
UTI	Urinary tract infection
VLDL	Very low-density lipoprotein (a type of cholesterol)
VTE	Venous thromboembolism (a blood clot that forms in a vein)
Wt	Weight
(NHS, 2023cc)	

8.4 Languages Used in the UK

Hundreds of languages and accents are used in the UK, including in health and care systems. Efforts should be taken to work collaboratively with colleagues who speak these languages as part of endeavours to deliver effective healthcare across the nation. Additionally, as mentioned in Section 2.5 on NMC exams and processes: IELTs and OSCE exams, internationally recruited staff must pass the International English

Language Testing System (IELTS) exam and objective structured clinical examination (OSCE) prior to being registered to practice in the UK. However, appreciating the languages spoken by others is also important.

8.5 Linguistic Phrases, Terms and Colloquialisms (NHS, 2023dd)

8.5.1 COLLOQUIALISMS FOR LANGUAGES USED IN NURSING AND HEALTHCARE

Colloquial expressions (Case, 2023) for healthcare staff are idiomatic forms of technical medical terms that help staff understand and communicate with patients, carers and service users via simple language. The first list (Section 8.5.1.1) provides idiomatic forms of medical terminology. The second list (Section 8.5.1.2) explains what patients mean when they use non-specialist terms in medical situations. Refer to the glossary (NHS, 2023dd) at the end of the book further on medical terminology and non-specialist terms.

8.5.1.1 List of Colloquial Expressions for Medical Terms (Case, 2023)

This list (Section 8.5.1.1) gives actual medical words and their more everyday terms, which are easier for patients to understand. To the right of the slash, italics denote particularly idiomatic forms, such as slang and rude words, which medical staff might hear but will probably want to avoid using.

ACTUAL MEDICAL TERMS/EVERYDAY TERMS

Abdomen/belly or tummy
Abdominal muscles/abs, six-pack or stomach muscles
Abdominal pain/stomach cramps
Abdominoplasty/tummy tuck
Abrasion/graze or scratch or scrapes or skinned knees
Acne vulgaris/whitehead
Acne/pimples, spots, teenage spots or zits
Attention-deficit hyperactivity disorder (ADHD)/hyper or won't settle down
Adverse effect/side effect
Alopecia/going bald, going thin on top or hair loss
Amnesia/blackout or memory loss
Amniotic fluid/waters
Amphetamines/speed
Anaemia/iron deficiency
Anal sphincter/arse ring or sphincter
Analgesic/painkiller
Ankle sprain/twisted ankle
Anorexia/loss of appetite
Appendectomy/have your appendix out

Arthritis/stiff joints
Asphyxiation/suffocation
Avian influenza/bird flu
Axilla/armpit
Become infected/catch something
Bladder/waterworks
Bowel movement/number two or poo
Breast augmentation/boob job
Breast mass/lump in the breast
Breasts/boobs, bosoms or chest
Bruxism/grinding your teeth
Bulla/blister
Candida albicans/thrush
Carbohydrates/carbs
Caries/rotten teeth
Chemotherapy/chemo
Chronic pain/persistent pain
Cicatrix/scar
Clitoris/clit
Closed comedone/whitehead
Coma/persistent vegetative state
Common cold/sniffle
Complex carbohydrates/carbs
Conception/getting knocked up

Conjunctivitis/pink eye
Contusion/bruise
Cosmetic surgery/plastic surgery
Deciduous teeth/baby teeth or milk teeth
Defecate/do a number two
Delirium tremens/the shakes
Delirium/feverishness
Dementia/confusion
Dental caries/rotten tooth
Dental pain/toothache
Dental plaque/plaque
Dental restoration/filling
Dental scaling/tooth scraping
Dependent/hooked (on something)
Depressed/feeling down or feeling blue
Dermis/skin
Dry eye syndrome (DES)/dry eyes
Desquamation/peeling skin
Diarrhoea/dodgy tummy or the runs
Doctor/doc
Dry vomiting/dry heaving
Dysmenorrhoea/period pains
Dyspepsia/indigestion
Dysphagia/difficulty swallowing
Dyspnoea/breathlessness, difficulty breathing or out of breath/ dyspnoea
Dysuria/burning sensation when peeing, difficulty peeing, having to squeeze it out or pain when peeing
Embryo/baby in your tummy
Emergency birth control (EBC) pill/ morning after pill
Emesis/barfing, can't keep food down, hurling, spewing or throwing up
Epidermis/skin
Epistaxis/nosebleed
Eructation/belch or burp
Erythrocyte/red blood cells
Evacuate/have a number two or have a poo
Excise something/have something out
Excoriation/scrape or scratch
Facial plasty/face lift
Faeces/number two or poo
Febrile/burning up or feverish

Faecal incontinence/doing a boo-boo, an accident, pooing your pants or soiling yourself
Flatulence/passing gas or wind
Furuncle/boil
Gastroenteritis/tummy bug
Genital herpes/herpes
Genitals or genitalia/down there, privates or private parts
Gingival atrophy or recession/receding gums
Gingivitis/gum disease
Globus hystericus/feeling like you have a lump in your throat
Globus pharyngeus/feeling like something is stuck in your throat
Globus sensation/feeling like something is stuck in your throat
Grand mal/attack, episode or fit
Haemoptysis/coughing up blood or spitting up blood
Haemorrhage/heavy bleeding or gushing
Haemorrhoids/piles
Halitosis/bad breath
Hallucinating/seeing things
Hand tremors/shaking hands
Head lice/nits
Heart/ticker
Heat stroke/sunstroke
Hematemesis/vomiting up blood
Herniated disk/slipped disk
Herpes simplex/herpes
Herpes zoster/chickenpox
High-density lipoprotein (HDL)/good cholesterol
Hirsutism/hairiness
Hyperpyrexia/heat stroke
Hypertension/high blood pressure
Hypotension/low blood pressure
Immunisation/jabs
In vitro fertilisation/test tube baby
Indication/side effect
Infected/caught something
Infectious/catching
Influenza/flu
Inhaler/puffer
Injection/jab
Inoculations/jabs

(Continued)

Intestine/gut
Intoxicated/drunk, high or tipsy
Intrauterine (contraceptive) device/coil
Intravenous drip/drip
Intrauterine contraceptive device (IUCD) or intrauterine device (IUD)/ coil
Intravenous (IV) drip/drip
In vitro fertilisation (IVF)/test tube baby
Juvenile/correction facility for kids
Keratoconjunctivitis sicca (KCS)/dry eyes
Kyphosis/hunchback, humpback or hump
Larynx/voice box
Laxative/something to loosen me up
Low-density lipoprotein (LDL)/bad cholesterol
Learning difficulties or disabilities/not all there, simple or special
Lethargy/tiredness
Leukocytes/white blood cells
Libido/sex drive
Limb length discrepancy or inequality/ one leg longer than the other
Liposuction/lipo
Lose consciousness/faint, pass out or swoon
Low-density lipoprotein/bad cholesterol
Lumbago/lower back pain
Magnesium hydroxide/milk of magnesia
Male infertility/shooting blanks
Malocclusion/crooked teeth
Mandible/lower jaw
Melanoma/skin cancer
Menstruation/time of the month
Menstrual cramps/period pains
Mental health issues/mentally ill
Mentally disabled/not all there, simple or special
Migraine/throbbing head
Miliaria/heat rash or prickly heat
Molar teeth/back teeth
Movement/number two or poo
Multiple personality disorder/schizo
Myalgia/muscle pain
Myopic/short sighted
Naris/nostril
Nasal congestion/blocked up, bunged up or stuffed up nose

Nasal haemorrhage/nosebleed
Nasal mucus/snot
Nausea/feeling sick
Nausea gravidarum/morning sickness
Navel/belly button
Neonatal/newborn
Nerve entrapment syndrome/pinched nerve or trapped nerve
Nitrous oxide/laughing gas
Nonprescription medicine/over-the-counter drug or remedy
Obese/carrying extra weight, chubby, fat, overweight or podgy
Obesity/chubbiness, excess weight, fatness or podiness
Oedema/swelling
Oesophageal obstruction/something stuck in your throat
Onychocryptosis/ingrown toenail
Open comedone/blackhead
Oral contraceptive/the pill
Oral herpes/cold sore
Over-the-counter (OTC) drug/over-the-counter remedy
Ovum/egg
Palate/top of the mouth
Patella/kneecap
Pectoral muscles/pecs
Pellets/rabbit poo
Pelvic pain/pain down there
Pelvic region/down there, private parts, privates or unmentionables
Periodontitis/gum disease
Perspiration/sweat
Petit mal/(a bit of an) attack, episode or fit
Pharmacist/chemist
Pharyngitis/sore throat
Pharynx/(back of the) throat
Photopsia/seeing stars
Physician/doc/doctor
Pregnant/expecting or in the family way
Pressure ulcers/bedsores
Pruritus/itchy
Psychiatrist or psychologist/head doctor
Pyretic/burning up or feverish
Radiotherapy/zap something
Red blood cells/RBCs or erythrocytes
Recover/get better or get over something
Reduced mobility/stiff joints

Regurgitation/can't keep food down, hurling, puking up, spewing or throwing up

Reproductive organs/bits

Respiration/breathing

Restless sleep/tossing and turning

Resuscitation/mouth to mouth

Rheum/sleep in your eyes

Rheumatism/stiff joints

Rhinoplasty/nose job

Rhinorrhoea/runny nose

Rigidity/stiffness

Rubella/German measles

Rupture of membranes/waters breaking

Saliva/gob or spit

Sanitary pad/panty liner

Scapula/shoulder blade

Schizoid or schizophrenic/schizo

Sclera/whites of your eyes

Scoliosis/twisted spine

Scrotum/ball bag, ball sack or sack

Seborrheic dermatitis/dandruff

See a psychiatrist or psychologist/have your head examined

Semen/come

Senile lentigo/liver spots

Sexually transmitted disease/catch something

Solar lentigo/freckles (from the sun)

Somnambulism/sleepwalking

Somniloquy/talking in your sleep

Spinal curvature/curved spine

Sporadic/one-off

Sternum/breastbone

Sexually transmitted infection (STI)/catch something

Stool/number two or poo

Strain/pulled muscle or torn muscle

Sudden infant death syndrome/cot death or crib death

Suffering from hearing loss/hard of hearing

Suppository/up the arse, up the rear end or up there

Suppurate/ooze

Surgery/have something done or have an operation

Sutures/stitches

Tachycardia/racing heart beat

Tampon/Tampax

Testicles/gonads

Thoracic back pain/upper back pain

Thoracic cage/rib cage

Thrombosis/blood clot

Tibia/shin (bone)

Tinea pedis/athlete's foot

Tonsillectomy/have your tonsils out

Trachea/windpipe

Tussis/cough or coughing

Tympanic membrane/eardrum

Tympanum/eardrum

Ultrasonography/ultrasound

Umbilicus/belly button

Unguis incarnates/ingrown toenail

Unsteadiness/unsteady on your feet

Urinal/the bottle

Urinary incontinence/having an accident, having a little accident or peeing yourself

Urinate/have a pee, relieve yourself, spend a penny or wee

Urine/number one, pee or wee

Uterus/womb

Vaccinations/jabs

Vaginal thrush/thrush

Valium/mother's little helper

Varicella (zoster)/chickenpox

Varicosities/varicose veins

Vasectomy/the snip

Ventilator/puffer

Verruca/wart

Vertigo/dizziness or feeling like your head is turning around

Vesicle/blister

Virus/bug

Volvulus/twisted bowel

Xeroderma/dry skin

Xerophthalmia/dry eyes

(Case, 2023)

(Continued)

8.5.1.2 List of Everyday Medical Expressions With Proper Medical Terms (Case, 2023)

This list (Section 8.5.1.2) gives colloquial terms that are more easily understood by patients with their equivalent more technical medical terms.

COLLOQUIAL TERMS/TECHNICAL MEDICAL TERMS

Abortion/termination
Abs/abdominal muscles
Anorexia/anorexia nervosa
Armpit/axilla
Arse ring/anal sphincter
Athlete's foot/tinea pedis
Attack/grand mal or petit mal
Baby in your tummy/embryo
Baby teeth/deciduous teeth
Back of the throat/pharynx
Back teeth/molar teeth
Bad breath/halitosis
Ball bag or ball sack/scrotum or
  testicles
Barfing/emesis or regurgitation
Bedsores/pressure ulcers
Belch/eructation
Belly button/navel or umbilicus
Belly/abdomen
Bird flu/avian influenza
Bits/reproductive organs
Blackhead/open comedone
Blackout/amnesia
Blister/vesicle or bulla
Blocked-up nose/nasal congestion
Blood clot/thrombosis
Blow off/flatulence
Blue/depressed
Boil/furuncle
Boob job/breast augmentation
Breaking wind/flatulence
Breastbone/sternum
Breathing/respiration
Breathlessness, difficulty breathing or
  out of breath/dyspnoea
Bruise/contusion
Bug/virus
Bunged up nose/nasal congestion
Burning sensation when peeing/dysuria
Burning up/febrile or pyretic

Burp/eructation
Can't keep food down/emesis
  or regurgitation
Carbs/(complex) carbohydrates
Catch something/become infected
Catching/infectious
Chemist/pharmacist
Chemo/chemotherapy
Chest/breasts
Chickenpox/herpes zoster, varicella or
  varicella zoster
Chubby/obese
Chucking up/emesis or regurgitation
Cold sore/oral herpes
Confusion/dementia
Cot or crib death/sudden infant death
  syndrome (SIDS)
Cough/tussis
Coughing up blood/haemoptysis
Crooked teeth/malocclusion
Curved spine/spinal curvature
Dandruff/seborrheic dermatitis
Difficulty breathing/dyspnoea
Difficulty peeing/dysuria
Difficulty swallowing/dysphagia
Dizziness/vertigo
Doc/doctor or physician
Dodgy tummy/diarrhoea
Doing a boo-boo/faecal incontinence
Down/depressed
Down there/pelvic region
Drunk/intoxicated
Dry heaving/dry vomiting
Dry skin/xeroderma
Eardrum/tympanic membrane or
  tympanum
Eating for two/pregnant
Egg/ovum
Episode/grand mal or petit mal
Expecting/pregnant

Face lift/facial plasty
Faint/lose consciousness
Fat/obese
Feeling like your head is turning around/vertigo
Feeling like you have a lump in your throat/globus hystericus
Feeling blue/depressed
Feeling down/depressed
Feeling sick/nausea
Feels like something is stuck in my throat/globus pharyngeus or globus sensation
Feverish/febrile or pyretic
Feverishness/delirium
Filling/dental restoration
Fit/grand mal or petit mal
Flu/influenza
For kids/juvenile
Freckles (from the sun)/solar lentigo
Gas/flatulence
German measles/rubella
Get better/recover
Get over something/recover
Gob/saliva
Going bald/alopecia
Going thin on top/alopecia
Gonads/testicles
Graze/abrasion
Grinding your teeth/bruxism
Gum disease/gingivitis or periodontitis
Guts/intestine
Hair loss/alopecia
Hairiness/hirsutism
Hard of hearing/suffering from hearing loss
Have a number two/defecate or evacuate
Have a pee/urinate
Have a poo/defecate or evacuate
Have a wee/urinate
Have an accident or have a little accident/(faecal or urinary) incontinence
Have something done/have an operation or have surgery
Have something out/excise something
Have your appendix out/appendectomy

Have your head examined/see a psychologist or psychiatrist
Have your tonsils out/tonsillectomy
Having to squeeze it out/dysuria
Head doctor/psychiatrist or psychologist
Heart rate monitor/electrocardiograph
Heat rash/miliaria
Heat stroke/hyperpyrexia
Heavy bleeding/haemorrhage
Herpes/genital herpes or herpes simplex
High blood pressure/hypertension
High/intoxicated
Hooked on/dependent
Human vegetable/persistent vegetative state
Hunchback/kyphosis
Hurling/emesis or regurgitation
In the family way/pregnant
Indigestion/dyspepsia
Ingrown toenail/onychocryptosis or unguis incarnates
Iron deficiency/anaemia
Itchy/pruritus
Jab/injection
Jabs/inoculations, vaccinations or immunisation
Kneecap/patella
Kyphosis/hunchback, humpback or hump
Lady parts/pelvic region
Laughing gas/nitrous oxide
Lipo/liposuction
Liver spots/senile lentigo
Loose stool/diarrhoea
Loss of appetite/anorexia
Low blood pressure/hypotension
Lower back pain/lumbago
Lower jaw/mandible
Lump in the breast/breast mass
Memory loss/amnesia
Milk of magnesia/magnesium hydroxide
Milk teeth/deciduous teeth
Morning sickness/nausea gravidarum
Mother's little helper/Valium
Mouth to mouth/resuscitation
Muscle pain/myalgia
Newborn/neonatal
Nits/head lice

(Continued)

Nosebleed/epistaxis or nasal haemorrhage
Nose job/rhinoplasty
Nostril/naris
Not all there/mentally disabled, learning difficulties or learning disabilities
Number one/urine
Number two/bowel movement or faeces or movement or stool
Obese/carrying extra weight or chubby or fat or overweight or podgy
Obesity/chubbiness or excess weight or fatness or podginess
One leg longer than the other/limb length inequality or limb length discrepancy
One-off/sporadic
Ooze/suppurate
Out of breath/dyspnoea
Over-the-counter drug or over-the-counter remedy/nonprescription medicine or OTC
Overweight/obese
Pain down there/pelvic pain
Pain when peeing/dysuria
Painkiller/analgesic
Panty liner/sanitary pad
Pass out/lose consciousness
Passing gas or wind/flatulence
Pecs/pectoral muscles
Pee/urine
Peeing yourself/urinary incontinence
Peeling skin/desquamation
Period pains/dysmenorrhoea or menstrual cramps
Persistent pain/chronic pain
Piles/haemorrhoids
Pimples/acne
Pinched nerve/nerve entrapment syndrome
Pink eye/conjunctivitis
Plaque/dental plaque
Plastic surgery/cosmetic surgery
Podgy/obese
Poo/bowel movement or faeces or movement or stool
Pooing your pants or yourself/faecal incontinence
Poop/bowel movement
Prickly heat/miliaria

Private parts/genitals or genitalia
Privates/genitals or genitalia
Puffer/inhaler or ventilator
Puking up/emesis or regurgitation
Pulled muscle or torn muscle/strain
Rabbit poo/rabbit stool or pellets
Racing heart beat/tachycardia
Receding gums/gingival recession or gingival atrophy
Relieve yourself/urinate
Rib cage/thoracic cage
Rotten tooth/caries or dental caries
Runny nose/rhinorrhoea
Scar/cicatrix
Schizo/schizoid, schizophrenic or suffering from multiple personality disorder
Scrape or scratch/abrasion or excoriation
Seeing stars/photopsia
Seeing things/hallucinating
Shaking hands/hand tremors
Shin (bone)/tibia
Short sighted/myopic
Shoulder blade/scapula
Side effect/adverse effect or indication
Simple/mentally disabled, learning difficulties or learning disabilities
Six-pack/abdominal muscles
Skin/dermis or epidermis
Skin cancer/melanoma
Skinned knees/abrasion
Sleep in your eyes/rheum
Sleepwalking/somnambulism
Slipped disk/herniated disk
Sniffle/(minor) common cold
Snot/nasal mucus
Soiling yourself/faecal incontinence
Something stuck in your throat/oesophageal obstruction
Something to loosen me up/laxative
Sore throat/pharyngitis
Special/mentally disabled, learning difficulties or disabilities
Speed/amphetamines
Spewing/emesis or regurgitation
Sphincter/anal sphincter
Spit/saliva
Spitting up blood/haemoptysis

Stiff joints/joint with reduced mobility, arthritis or rheumatism
Stiffness/rigidity
Stitches/sutures
Stomach cramps/abdominal pain
Stomach muscles/abdominal muscles
Stuffed up nose/nasal congestion
Suffocation/asphyxiation
Sunstroke/heat stroke
Sweat/perspiration
Swelling/oedema
Swoon/lose consciousness
Talking in your sleep/somniloquy
Tampax/tampon
Teenage spots/acne
The bottle/urinal
The pill/oral contraceptive
The runs/diarrhoea
The shakes/delirium tremens
The snip/vasectomy
The trots/diarrhoea
Throat/pharynx
Throbbing head/migraine
Throwing up/emesis or regurgitation
Thrush/candida albicans or vaginal thrush
Ticker/heart
Time of the month/menstruation
Tipsy/intoxicated
Tiredness/lethargy
Tooth scraping/dental scaling
Toothache/dental pain
Top of the mouth/palate
Tossing and turning/restless sleep
Trapped nerve/nerve entrapment syndrome

Tummy/abdomen
Tummy bug/gastroenteritis
Tummy tuck/abdominoplasty
Turd/bowel movement, faeces or stool/ defecate or evacuate
Tussis/cough or coughing
Twisted ankle/ankle sprain
Twisted bowel/volvulus
Twisted spine/scoliosis
Ultrasound/ultrasonography
Unmentionables/pelvic region
Unsteady on your feet/unsteadiness
Up the rear end/suppository
Up there/suppository
Upper back pain/thoracic back pain
Varicose veins/varicosities
Voice box/larynx
Vomiting up blood/hematemesis
Wart/verruca
Wasted/intoxicated
Waters/amniotic fluid
Waters breaking/rupture of membranes
Waterworks/bladder
Wee/urinate or urine
White blood cells/leukocytes
Whitehead/acne vulgaris or closed comedone
Whites of your eyes/sclera
Wind/flatulence
Windpipe/trachea
Womb/uterus
Zap something/radiotherapy
Zits/acne
(Case, 2023)

8.6 Summary: Measurements, Abbreviations, Language and Terminologies

Elements and processes regarding measurements, abbreviations, terminologies and language were covered in this chapter. Understanding the common abbreviations, terminologies and language used in the UK helps international staff to adapt to the working processes of new organisations quickly. The use of measurements for ensuring safe healthcare delivery is important. This chapter also provided a list of phrases, terms and colloquialisms used in everyday practice, knowledge of which helps staff navigate their way around systems and processes in daily health and care practices.

CHAPTER 9

Conclusion and Recommendations

9.1 Recapping

This book, written by Annesha Archyangelio, a practising director of nursing, has been highly anticipated by many for some time. It provides comprehensive information to support internationally recruited staff to live, work and thrive in the United Kingdom (UK). It has the significant advantage of supplementing other information already available to support internationally recruited staff. The author contributes to supporting an extensive network of internationally trained nurses, midwives, care staff and allied health professionals (AHPs), including through the numerous nursing associations in the UK, which are sources of international nurses. This book will be helpful not only for staff recruitment to the UK but also to other countries such as the United States, which has been recruiting international staff for many years now. It is hoped that you enjoy this book and experience great success in your personal and work life in the UK and further afield.

This book provides resources, information and steps that internationally recruited staff can take, including how to use the book in their role. It also outlines how to use it as part of their professional development plan, which includes having conversations with their managers regarding their needs and aspirations in their role as internationally recruited staff who are working as part of the healthcare in the UK.

The broad themes covered in Chapters 1–8 of this book include: (1) preparing internationally recruited staff for successful completion of the recruitment process; (2) giving internationally recruited staff strategies for coping with and flourishing in their role; (3) cultural competency and (4) accelerating staff development and progression in the workplace, including reflections from the author.

These four areas covered in this book which were presented across Chapters 1–8 are summarised here.

This includes preparing the internationally recruited (IR) healthcare staff for successful completion of the recruitment process, including exams preparation, sitting and progression; onboarding; and adjusting to their new working environment, community setting and home life.

There was an introduction to professional organisations, healthcare registration bodies and trade unions, like the Nursing and Midwifery Council (NMC), Royal College of Nursing (RCN), Health and Care Professions Council (HCPC) and other professional bodies. There was an outline of a guide to the National Health Service (NHS) structure, including introduction to NHS England, the Care Quality Commission (CQC), and other regulatory organisations and bodies.

There was also information and introduction on the history and milestone of the wider NHS, its structure, and the wider health and social care service.

This book provided information on the organisation and regulation of healthcare for nurses, midwives, AHPs and healthcare support staff in the UK. There are also elements regarding nursing and other healthcare processes, which are required to ensure delivery of best practice. Information on nursing, midwifery and AHPs; adaptation and assessment programmes; career support and development; and current models of nursing, healthcare and service delivery was also outlined in this book.

Strategies for working and flourishing in their role as an internationally recruited staff was outlined in this book, including advice on the pathways of development into senior roles and information on where to access funded, non-funded and freely available training and development.

The processes for accelerating development and progression in the workplace for the internationally recruited staff is detailed, including any additional study or training, which may be needed to top up in addition to original programmes of study, including to convert some qualifications to UK awards. This is then followed by any additional development required for progression in the workplace.

There is a section on cultural competency, highlighting the strategies to address communication challenges and general cultural competency dimension, which are aimed at all nurses, midwives, AHPs and care staff in the health and care workplace.

Communication challenges and solutions were also covered, including commonly used everyday healthcare related terminologies to communicate with staff, patients, families and carers who may be unfamiliar with the cultures of individuals from another countries. This includes communication specific to nursing and the wider health and care practice.

There were also elements regarding documentation and recording in nursing which are required to ensure delivery of best practice.

Chapters towards the end of this book included useful information on reflection from the author; languages used in the UK; competencies and tools used in healthcare; applying for jobs; units of measurements; abbreviations; and further information, reading, resources, links and other sources. I hope you enjoy using this book, as you live, work and thrive in the UK.

Act Academy (2023). QSIR practitioner programme: Change concepts. The improvement guide 2nd Edition Lanley et al. (2009), pages 357–408.

Adams, R. (Ed.) (2017). *Nursing degree applications slump after NHS bursaries abolished*. The Guardian. Available at: https://www.theguardian.com/education/2017/feb/02/nursing-degree-applications-slump-after-nhs-bursaries-abolished, Accessed 7 July 2024.

AHSN Network (2023). Quality improvement (QI) resource pack. Available at: https://www.ahsnnetwork.com/wp-content/uploads/2023/06/QI-PSC-resource-pack-final_updated-22-may.pdf. Accessed 31 October 2023.

Al-Sawai, A. (2013). Leadership of healthcare professionals: Where do we stand? *Oman Medical Journal, 28*(4), 285–287.

AQUA (2023). Quality, service improvement and redesign (QSIR). Available at: https://aqua.nhs.uk/qsir/. Accessed 31 October 2023.

Association for Perioperative Practice (AfPP) (2023). Core competencies for adult day surgery. Available at: https://www.afpp.org.uk/news/Core-Competencies-for-the-Day-Surgery-Team. Accessed 31 October 2023.

Aston Organisational Development (2023). Aston Team Performance Inventory (ATPI). Available at: https://abeyanttraining.files.wordpress.com/2010/09/atpi.pdf. Accessed 31 October 2023.

Axelos (2023). *Prince2 Certification | Qualifications and Exams – Axelos*. Available at: https://www.axelos.com/certifications/propath/prince2-project-management/. Accessed 20 August 2023.

Bailey, T. (2022). *Nye Bevan: 7 quotations that define Aneurin Bevan*. Available at: https://radicalte-atowel.co.uk/blog/7-quotations-that-define-aneurin-bevan. Accessed 23 May 2022.

British Dental Association (BDA) (2023). Advice. Available at: https://bda.org/advice. Accessed 31 October 2023.

British Federation of Women Graduates (BFWG) (2023). The British Federation of Women Graduates. Available at: https://bfwg.org.uk/bfwg2/. Accessed 31 October 2023.

British Medical Association (BMA) (2023). BMA – Home | British Medical Association. Available at: https://www.bma.org.uk/. Accessed 31 October 2023.

British Society of Interventional Radiology (2023). Central venous access. Available at: https://www.bsir.org/. Accessed 13 October 2023.

Buckinghamshire New University (2023). BSc (Hons) Nursing (Adult) with NMC Registration. Available at: https://www.bucks.ac.uk/courses/undergraduate/bsc-hons-nursing-adult-nmc-registration. Accessed 31 October 2023.

Burgess, A., McGregor, D., & Mellis, C. (2014). Applying guidelines in a systematic review of team-based learning in medical schools. *Academic Medicine, 89*(4), 678–688.

Burgess, A., van Diggele, C., & Mellis, C. (2018). Mentorship in the health professions: A review. *The Clinical Teacher, 14*, 1–6.

Buswell, G. (2023). Healthcare in the UK—A guide to the NHS. Available at: https://www.expatica.com/uk/healthcare/healthcare-basics/the-national-health-service-and-health-insur-ance-in-the-uk-1092057/. Accessed 27 March 2023.

Byrman, A. (2006). Leadership in organisations. In S. R. Clegg, C. Harvey, & W. R. Nord (Eds.), *Handbook of organisational studies*. London: Sage.

Care Quality Commission (CQC) (2023). We're CQC, the independent regulator of health and social care in England. Available at: https://www.cqc.org.uk/. Accessed 29 October 2023.

Carers UK (2023). Care regulations—Care standards. Available at: https://www.carersuk.org/help-and-advice/. Accessed 29 October 2023.

Case, A. (2023). Colloquial expressions for medical terms. Available at: https://www.usingenglish. com/teachers/articles/colloquial-expressions-for-medical-terms.html. Accessed 21 March 2023.

Cavell Nurses' Trust (2023). Supporting the nursing and midwifery family through tough times. Available at: https://cavell.org.uk/. Accessed 31 October 2023.

Charity Choice (2023). Browse this sector for health charities. Available at: https://www.charity-choice.co.uk/charities/health. Accessed 29 October 2023.

Citizens Advice (2023). Welcome to Citizens Advice. Available at: https://www.citizensadvice. org.uk/. Accessed 29 October 2023.

Clarke, J. (2015). Clinical Leadership and Engagement: No Longer an Optional Extra. In S. Patole (Ed.), *Management and leadership – A guide for clinical professionals*. Switzerland: Springer International Publishing.

Department of Health (2013). NHS and social care structures from April 2013. Available at: https://richmondcvs.org.uk/community-involvement-nhs-and-social-care-map/. Accessed 29 October 2023.

Department of Health and Social Care (2023a). Applying for health and social care jobs in the UK from abroad. Available at: https://www.gov.uk/government/publications/applying-for-health-and-social-care-jobs-in-the-uk-from-abroad/applying-for-health-and-social-care-jobs-in-the-uk-from-abroad. Accessed 28 October 2023.

Department of Health and Social Care (2023b). Working for DHSC. Available at: https://www. gov.uk/government/organisations/department-of-health-and-social-care/about/recruitment. Accessed 28 October 2023.

Equality Act (2010). Available at: https://www.legislation.gov.uk/ukpga/2010/15. Accessed 31 October 2023.

European Centre for Disease Prevention and Control (ECDC) (2023). Core competencies for infection control and hospital hygiene professionals in the European Union. Available at: https://www.ecdc.europa.eu/en/publications-data/core-competencies-infection-control-and-hospital-hygiene-professionals-european. Accessed 13 September 2023.

European Commission (2023). Top tips for onboarding new international employees. Available at: https://eures.ec.europa.eu/top-tips-onboarding-new-international-employees-2020-11-27-0_ en. Accessed 29 October 2023.

Evolution (2021). 7 key elements of effective communication. Available at: https://evolutionjobs. com/exchange/7-key-elements-of-effective-communication/. Accessed 29 July 2021.

Faculty of Public Health (FPH) (2023). What is public health? Available at: https://www.fph.org. uk/. Accessed 29 October 2023.

Federation of Holistic Therapists (FHT) (2023). About us. Available at: https://www.fht.org.uk/ about-us. Accessed 29 October 2023.

Florence Nightingale Foundation (FNF) (2023a). Leadership programmes. Available at: https:// florence-nightingale-foundation.org.uk/academy/leadership-scholarship-2022/. Accessed 31 October 2023.

Florence Nightingale Foundation (FNF) (2023b). Scholarships for midwives and health visitors. Available at: https://maternityandmidwifery.co.uk/florence-nightingale-foundation-scholar-ships-midwives/. Accessed 31 October 2023.

Fukada, M. (2018). Nursing competency: Definition, structure and development. *Yonago Acta Medica, 61*(1), 1–7.

General Medical Council (GMC) (2023). Get to know good medical practice 2024. Available at: https://www.gmc-uk.org/. Accessed 29 October 2023.

Glover, T. S., Abbott, C., Oswalk, A., & Frank, J. R. (2015). *CanMEDS teaching and assessment tools guide*. Canada: Royal College of Physicians and Surgeons.

GOV.UK (2022). Health and Social Care Act 2008: Code of practice on the pre-vention and control of infections. Available at: https://www.gov.uk/government/

publications/the-health-and-social-care-act-2008-code-of-practice-on-the-prevention-and-control-of-infections-and-related-guidance. Accessed 13 December 2022.

GOV.UK (2023a). Life in the UK test. Available at: https://www.gov.uk/life-in-the-uk-test. Accessed 28 October 2023.

GOV.UK (2023b). Apply for citizenship if you have indefinite leave to remain or 'settled status'. Available at: https://www.gov.uk/apply-citizenship-indefinite-leave-to-remain/how-to-apply. Accessed 28 October 2023.

GOV.UK (2023c). Family visas: Apply, extend or switch. Available at: https://www.gov.uk/uk-family-visa. Accessed 28 October 2023.

GOV.UK (2023d). Apply to the EU Settlement Scheme (settled and pre-settled status). Available at: https://www.gov.uk/settled-status-eu-citizens-families/family-member-eligible-person-from-northern-ireland. Accessed 28 October 2023.

GOV.UK (2023f). UK visas and immigration. Available at: https://www.gov.uk/government/organisations/uk-visas-and-immigration. Accessed 28 October 2023.

GOV.UK (2023g). New immigration system: What you need to know. Available at: https://www.gov.uk/guidance/new-immigration-system-what-you-need-to-know. Accessed 28 October 2023.

GOV.UK (2023h). Health and care worker visa. Available at: https://www.gov.uk/health-care-worker-visa. Accessed 28 October 2023.

GOV.UK (2023i). Skilled worker visa: Shortage occupations. Available at: https://www.gov.uk/government/publications/skilled-worker-visa-shortage-occupations. Accessed 28 October 2023.

GOV.UK (2023j). Apply to the EU Settlement Scheme (settled and pre-settled status). Available at: https://www.gov.uk/settled-status-eu-citizens-families. Accessed 28 October 2023.

GOV.UK (2023k). Biometric residence permits (BRPs). Available at: https://www.gov.uk/biometric-residence-permits. Accessed 28 October 2023.

GOV.UK (2023l). View and prove your immigration status: Get a share code. Available at: https://www.gov.uk/view-prove-immigration-status. Accessed 28 October 2023.

GOV.UK (2023m). Graduate visa. Available at: https://www.gov.uk/graduate-visa. Accessed 28 October 2023.

GOV.UK (2023n). Guidance: New employee coming to work from abroad. Available at: https://www.gov.uk/guidance/new-employee-coming-to-work-from-abroad. Accessed 29 October 2023.

GOV.UK (2023o). Medicines and Healthcare products Regulatory Agency (MHRA). Available at: https://www.gov.uk/government/organisations/medicines-and-healthcare-products-regulatory-agency. Accessed 29 October 2023.

GOV.UK (2023p). Find a Sure Start Children's Centre. Available at: https://www.gov.uk/find-sure-start-childrens-centre. Accessed 29 October 2023.

GOV.UK (2023q). International Nurses Day: Celebrating our values, strengths and ambition. Available at: https://socialcare.blog.gov.uk/2023/05/12/international-nurses-day-celebrating-our-values-strengths-and-ambition/. Accessed 31 October 2023.

GOV.UK (2023r). COVID-19. Available at: https://www.gov.uk/coronavirus#:~:text=There%20are%20no%20coronavirus%20. Accessed 31 October 2023.

GOV.UK (2023s). COVID-19: Personal protective equipment uses for non-aerosol generating procedures guidance. Available at: https://www.gov.uk/government/publications/covid-19-personal-protective-equipment-use-for-non-aerosol-generating-procedures. Accessed 31 October 2023.

GOV.UK (2023t). Department of Health and Social Care. Available at: https://www.gov.uk/government/organisations/department-of-health-and-social-care. Accessed 31 October 2023.

Handtke, O., Schilgen, B., & Mösko, M. (2019). Culturally competent healthcare – A scoping review of strategies implemented in healthcare organizations and a model of culturally competent healthcare provision. *PLoS ONE, 14*(7), e0219971.

Health and Care Professions Council (HCPC) (2023). Regulating health and care professionals. Available at: https://www.hcpc-uk.org/. Accessed 29 October 2023.

Health Education England (HEE) (2023a). Building understanding of international recruitment through lived experience. Available at: https://www.hee.nhs.uk/our-work/allied-health-professions/increase-capacity/supporting-international-recruitment-ahp%E2%80%99s/building-understanding-international-recruitment-0. Accessed 29 October 2023.

Health Education England (HEE) (2023b). Maternity. Available at: https://www.hee.nhs.uk/our-work/maternity. Accessed 31 October 2023.

Health Education England (HEE) (2023c). Nursing associates. Available at: https://www.hee.nhs.uk/our-work/nursing-associates. Accessed 31 October 2023.

Health Education England (HEE) (2023d). Training and development—Nursing associates. Available at: https://nursing-associates.hee.nhs.uk/about-the-role/training-and-development/. Accessed 31 October 2023.

Health Education England (HEE) (2023e). Career framework: The Capital Nurse Digital Career Framework tool. Available at: https://www.hee.nhs.uk/our-work/capitalnurse/workstreams/career-framework. Accessed 31 October 2023.

Health Education England (HEE) (2023f). Work experience and work-related learning activity. Available at: https://www.hee.nhs.uk/our-work/work-experience-pre-employment-activity. Accessed 31 October 2023.

Health Foundation (2023). Regulation in the NHS and other high-risk industries. Available at: https://www.health.org.uk/research-projects/regulation-in-the-nhs-and-other-high-risk-industries. Accessed 29 October 2023.

Health and Safety Executive (HSE) (2023). Who regulates health and social care. Available at: https://www.hse.gov.uk/healthservices/arrangements.htm#:~:text=HSE%20is%20the%20national%20independent,care%20settings%20in%20Great%20Britain. Accessed 29 October 2023.

Healthcare Financial Management Association (HFMA) (2023). HFMA helps healthcare financial management professionals and their organizations succeed. Available at: https://www.hfma.org/. Accessed 29 October 2023.

Healthcare Quality Improvement Partnership (HQIP) (2023). A guide to quality improvement tools. Available at: https://www.hqip.org.uk/resource/guide-to-quality-improvement-methods/. Accessed 7 July 2024.

Hecimovich, M. D. (2009). National Institutes of Health. Available at: https://www.ncbi.nlm.nih.gov. Accessed 1 March 2023.

Hector, D., (2009). A retrospective analysis of nursing documentation in the intensive care units of an academic hospital in the Western Cape. Available at: https://www.researchgate.net/figure/Illustration-showing-the-nursing-process-Illustration-by-author_fig4_45635377. Accessed 19 May 2023.

Human Fertilisation and Embryology Authority (HEFA) (2023). HFEA: UK fertility regulator. Available at: https://www.hfea.gov.uk/. Accessed 29 October 2023.

HM Government (2024). Prevent duty guidance. Available at: https://www.legislation.gov.uk/ukdsi/2015/9780111133309/pdfs/ukdsiod_9780111133309_en.pdf. Accessed 8 June 2024.

IEEE Awards (2023). IEEE Biomedical Engineering Award. Available at: https://corporate-awards.ieee.org/award/ieee-biomedical-field-engineering-award/. Accessed 31 October 2023.

Indeed (2022a). Indeed Career Guide. Available at: https://www.indeed.com/career-advice. Accessed 25 June 2022.

Indeed (2022b). Career development: 12 Characteristics for effective leadership in health care. Available at: https://www.indeed.com/career-advice/career-development/leadership-in-health-care. Accessed 25 June 2022.

Indeed (2022c). The five steps in the ADPIE nursing process (with benefits). Available at: https://uk.indeed.com/career-advice/career-development/adpie#:~:text=ADPIEs. Accessed 16 May 2023.

Indeed (2022d). What is health care management. Available at: https://www.indeed.com/career-advice/finding-a-job/what-is-healthcare-management. Accessed 16 May 2023.

Infection Prevention Society (IPS) (2022). IPS Competencies framework. Available at: https://www.ips.uk.net/ips-competencies-framework. Accessed 13 September 2022.

Infection Prevention Society (IPS) (2023). Infection Prevention Society (IPS). Available at: https://www.ips.uk.net/. Accessed 10 October 2023.

Institute for Healthcare Improvement (IHI) (2023). IHI Open School Quality Improvement Courses. Available at: https://www.ihi.org/education/ihi-open-school/ihi-open-school-quality-improvement-courses. Accessed 30 October 2023.

Institute of Health Visiting (IHV) (2023a). Becoming a health visitor. Available at: https://ihv.org.uk/for-health-visitors/becoming-a-hv/. Accessed 30 October 2023.

Institute of Health Visiting (IHV) (2023b). Fellowship of the Institute of Health Visiting (FiHV) award. Available at: https://ihv.org.uk/about-us/fellows/. Accessed 30 October 2023.

International Council of Nurses (ICN) (2023). The global voice of nursing. Available at: https://www.icn.ch/. Accessed 10 August 2023.

International English Language Testing System (IELTS) (2023). Preparation resources. Available at: https://ielts.org/take-a-test/preparation-resources. Accessed 28 October 2023.

Joy, G. V., Alomari, A. M. A., Singh, K., Hassan, N., Mannethodi, K., Kunjavara, J., l., A., & Lenjawi, B. (2023). Nurses' self-esteem, self-compassion and psychological resilience during COVID-19 pandemic. *Nursing Open*, *00*, 1–9.

King's Fund (2021). How funding flows in the NHS. Available at: https://www.kingsfund.org.uk/audio-video/how-is-nhs-structured-funding-flow. Accessed 21 February 2021.

King's Fund (2023a). The King's Fund: Ideas that change health and care. Available at: https://www.kingsfund.org.uk. Accessed 21 February 2023.

King's Fund (2023b). How to build effective teams in general practice. Available at: https://www.kingsfund.org.uk. Accessed 21 February 2023.

King's Fund (2023c). Health and Care Act 2022. Available at: https://www.kingsfund.org.uk. Accessed 20 January 2023.

King's Fund (2023d). Integrated care systems: How will they work under the Health and Care Act? Available at: https://www.kingsfund.org.uk/audio-video/integrated-care-systems-health-and-care-act. Accessed 20 January 2023.

King's Fund (2023f). How does the NHS in England work and how is it changing? Available at: https://www.kingsfund.org.uk/audio-video/how-does-nhs-in-england-work. Accessed 29 October 2023.

King's Fund (2023g). Integrated care systems: how will they work under the Health and Care Act? Available at: https://www.kingsfund.org.uk/insight-and-analysis/data-and-charts/integrated-care-systems-health-and-care-act. Accessed 29 October 2023.

King's Fund (2023h). The Health and Care Act: Six key questions? Available at: https://www.kingsfund.org.uk/publications/health-and-care-act-key-questions. Accessed 29 October 2023.

Langley, G. L., Moen, R., Nolan, K. M., Nolan, T. W., Norman, C. L., Provost, L. P. (2009). *Institute for Healthcare Improvement: The Improvement Guide* (2nd ed.; pp. 357–408). San Francisco: Jossey-Bass Publishers. Available at: https://www.ihi.org/resources/publications/improvement-guide-practical-approach-enhancing-organizational-performance. Accessed 31 October 2023.

Levi, D. (2011). *Group dynamics for teams*. Thousand Oaks, CA: Sage.

Local Government Association (2023). Better Care Fund – Local Government Association. Available at: https://www.local.gov.uk/better-care-fund. Accessed 31 October 2023.

London Business School (2023). Senior executive programme. Available at: https://www.london.edu/executive-education/general-management/senior-executive-programme. Accessed 31 October 2023.

Managers in Partnership (MIP) (2023). The union for health and care managers. Available at: https://www.miphealth.org.uk/. Accessed 31 October 2023.

Matthews, J. H., Morley, G. L., Crossley, E., & Bhanderi, S. (2017). Teaching leadership: The medical student society model. *The Clinical Teacher*, *15*, 2.

McKimm, J., & Swanwick, T. (2011). Leadership development for clinicians: What are we trying to achieve? *Clin. Teach*, *8*, 181–185.

Mind (2023). Mind helplines. Available at: https://www.mind.org.uk/information-support/helplines/. Accessed 31 October 2023.

Morris, D., & Morris, A. (2021). Cultural awareness and overseas assignments. Available at: https://www.davidsonmorris.com. Accessed 8 August 2021.

Mytime Active (2023). Health Services. Available at: https://www.mytimeactive.co.uk/activities/health-services. Accessed 29 October 2023.

Nair, L., & Adetayo, O. A. (2019). Cultural competence and ethnic diversity in healthcare. *Plastic and Reconstructive Surgery Global Open*, *7*(5), e2219. May 16.

National Association of Primary Care (NAPC) (2023). Ahead of the game: Leading neighbourhood care, population health and integrated working. Available at: https://napc.co.uk/. Accessed 31 October 2023.

National Care Forum (NCF) (2023). Pastoral care guide for international recruitment in social care. Available at: https://www.nationalcareforum.org.uk/projects/pastoral-care-guide-for-international-recruitment-in-social-care/. Accessed 31 October 2023.

National Careers Service (2023). Explore healthcare careers. Available at: https://nationalcareers.service.gov.uk/job-categories/healthcare. Accessed 31 October 2023.

National Institutes for Health and Care Research (NIHR) (2023a). UK clinical academic training for nurses, midwives, AHPs and other health and care professionals: Principles and obligations. Available at: https://www.nihr.ac.uk/documents/uk-clinical-academic-training-for-nurses-midwives-and-other-professionals-allied-to-medicine-principles-and-obligations/27109?pr=. Accessed 22 October 2023.

National Institutes for Health and Care Research (NIHR) (2023b). Doctoral Awards: Oxford Biomedical Research Centre. Available at: https://oxfordbrc.nihr.ac.uk/training-hub/doctoral-awards/. Accessed 31 October 2023.

National Institutes of Health (2023). Keeping good nursing records: A guide. Available at: https://www.ncbi.nlm.nih.gov. Accessed 22 April 2023.

NHS (2021). *Chief nurse, director of nursing, director of midwifery career pathway summary key finding*. London: NHS England.

NHS (2022a). National Community Nursing Plan 2021–2026 Engagement Document. Available at: https://future.nhs.uk/system/login?nextURL=%2Fconnect%2Eti%2FNationalCommunityNursing%2Fview%3FobjectId%3D117401317. Accessed 2 March 2022.

NHS (2022b). HR framework for developing Integrated Care Boards. Available at: https://www.england.nhs.uk/wp-content/uploads/2021/06/B1427-Human-resources-framework-for-developing-integrated-care-boards-version-2-March-2022.pdf. Accessed 2 August 2022.

NHS (2022c). Career framework competency-based job descriptions. Available at: https://www.england.nhs.uk/wp-content/uploads/2018/03/career-framework-competency-based-job-descriptions-sfh-7-9.pdf. Accessed 2 September 2022.

NHS (2022d). Nursing associate. Available at: https://www.healthcareers.nhs.uk/explore-roles/nursing/roles-nursing/nursing-associate. Accessed 2 September 2022.

NHS (2022e). Skills development strategy for Kent, Surrey, and Sussex. Available at: https://www.bsuh.nhs.uk/wp-content/uploads/sites/5/2016/09/Health-Education-KSS-Skills-Development-Leaflet.pdf. Accessed 31 December 2022.

NHS (2022f). How to become an allied health professional. Available at: https://www.healthca-reers.nhs.uk/explore-roles/allied-health-professionals/studying-be-allied-health-professional. Accessed 31 October 2022.

NHS (2022g). Training and development (human resources management). Available at: https://www.healthcareers.nhs.uk/career-planning/resources. Accessed 31 November 2022.

NHS (2022h). Healthcare support worker overview. Available at: https://www.healthcareers.nhs.uk/we-are-the-nhs/healthcare-support-worker. Accessed 31 November 2022.

NHS (2022i). Working in health. Available at: https://www.healthcareers.nhs.uk/working-health. Accessed 2 September 2022.

NHS (2022j). 350 careers, one NHS, your future. Available at: https://www.healthcareers.nhs.uk/career-planning/resources/350-careers-one-nhs-your-future-print-ready-pdf. Accessed 24 October 2022.

NHS (2022k). New Digital Leadership Scholarships for nurses and midwives. Available at: https://digital-transformation.hee.nhs.uk/news/new-digital-leadership-scholarships-for-nurses-and-midwives. Accessed 12 October 2022.

NHS (2022l). NHS Interim Management and Support (NHS IMAS). Available at: https://www.nhsimas.nhs.uk/home/. Accessed 12 December 2022.

NHS (2022m). Theatre support worker. Available at: https://www.healthcareers.nhs.uk/explore-roles/wider-healthcare-team/roles-wider-healthcare-team/clinical-support-staff/theatre-sup-port-worker. Accessed 17 October 2022.

NHS (2022n). Children's health. Available at: https://www.nhs.uk/common-health-questions/childrens-health/. Accessed 31 October 2022.

NHS (2022o). Children and young people. Available at: https://www.england.nhs.uk/get-involved/cyp/. Accessed 31 October 2022.

NHS (2022p). NHS Scientist Training Programme. Available at: https://www.healthcareers.nhs.uk/career-planning/study-and-training/graduate-training-opportunities/nhs-scientist-train-ing-programme. Accessed 31 October 2022.

NHS (2022q). Physical sciences and biomedical engineering. Available at: https://www.healthca-reers.nhs.uk/explore-roles/healthcare-science/roles-healthcare-science/physical-sciences-and-biomedical-engineering. Accessed 31 October 2022.

NHS (2023a). NHS pay and benefits. Available at: https://www.healthcareers.nhs.uk/working-health/working-nhs/nhs-pay-and-benefits. Accessed 28 October 2023.

NHS (2023b). How to register with a GP surgery. Available at: https://www.nhs.uk/nhs-services/gps/how-to-register-with-a-gp-surgery/. Accessed 28 October 2023.

NHS (2023c). What is an NHS number. Available at: https://www.nhs.uk/using-the-nhs/about-the-nhs/what-is-an-nhs-number/. Accessed 28 October 2023.

NHS (2023d). Moving to England from EU countries or Norway, Iceland, Liechtenstein or Switzerland. Available at: https://www.nhs.uk/nhs-services/visiting-or-moving-to-england/moving-to-england-from-eu-countries-or-norway-iceland-liectenstein-or-switzerland/. Accessed 28 October 2023.

NHS (2023e). Overseas health professionals. Available at: https://www.healthcareers.nhs.uk/working-health/overseas-health-professionals. Accessed 28 October 2023.

NHS (2023f). Working in health. Available at: https://www.healthcareers.nhs.uk/working-health. Accessed 28 October 2023.

NHS (2023h). Information for overseas allied health professionals. Available at: https://www.healthcareers.nhs.uk/explore-roles/allied-health-professionals/information-overseas-allied-health-professionals. Accessed 28 October 2023.

NHS (2023i). Information for overseas dentists. Available at: https://www.healthcareers.nhs.uk/explore-roles/dental-team%20/information-overseas-dentists. Accessed 28 October 2023.

NHS (2023j). Information for overseas doctors. Available at: https://www.healthcareers.nhs.uk/explore-roles/doctors/information-overseas-doctors. Accessed 28 October 2023.

NHS (2023k). Information for overseas healthcare scientists. Available at: https://www.health-careers.nhs.uk/Explore-roles/healthcare-science/information-overseas-healthcare-scientists. Accessed 28 October 2023.

NHS (2023l). Information for overseas midwives. Available at: https://www.healthcareers.nhs.uk/explore-roles/midwifery/information-overseas-midwives. Accessed 28 October 2023.

NHS (2023m). We are nurses. We are the NHS. Available at: https://www.healthcareers.nhs.uk/we-are-the-nhs/nursing-careers/international-recruitment. Accessed 28 October 2023.

NHS (2023n). Information for overseas pharmacists. We are the NHS. Available at: https://www.healthcareers.nhs.uk/explore-roles/explore-roles/pharmacy/pharmacy/information-overseas-pharmacists. Accessed 28 October 2023.

NHS (2023o). We're here for you: Helping you take control of your health and wellbeing. Available at: https://www.nhs.uk/. Accessed 29 October 2023.

NHS (2023p). Visitors who do not need to pay for NHS treatment. Available at: https://www.nhs.uk/nhs-services/visiting-or-moving-to-england/visitors-who-do-not-need-to-pay-for-nhs-treatment/. Accessed 29 October 2023.

NHS (2023q). Understanding NHS dental charges. Available at: https://www.nhs.uk/nhs-services/dentists/dental-costs/understanding-nhs-dental-charges/. Accessed 29 October 2023.

NHS (2023r). NHS prescription charges. Available at: https://www.nhs.uk/nhs-services/prescriptions-and-pharmacies/nhs-prescription-charges/. Accessed 29 October 2023.

NHS (2023s). Family doctor services registration GMS1 form. Available at: https://assets.publishing.service.gov.uk/government/uploads/system/uploads/attachment_data/file/1017019/GMS1-family-doctor-services-registration-form.pdf. Accessed 29 October 2023.

NHS (2023t). 111 online: Get help for your symptoms. Available at: https://111.nhs.uk/. Accessed 29 October 2023.

NHS (2023u). Women's health. Available at: https://www.nhs.uk/womens-health/. Accessed 29 October 2023.

NHS (2023v). Choice and personalised care in maternity services. Available at: https://www.england.nhs.uk/mat-transformation/choice-and-personalisation/. Accessed 29 October 2023.

NHS (2023w). Paediatrics. Available at: https://www.healthcareers.nhs.uk/explore-roles/doctors/roles-doctors/paediatrics. Accessed 29 October 2023.

NHS (2023x). Vaccinations. Available at: https://www.nhs.uk/conditions/vaccinations/. Accessed 29 October 2023.

NHS (2023y). NHS emergency dentist: UK NHS dentistry online resources, news and public information. Available at: https://www.nhsemergencydentist.co.uk/. Accessed 29 October 2023.

NHS (2023z). Urgent treatment centres. Available at: https://www.england.nhs.uk/urgent-emergency-care/urgent-treatment-centres/. Accessed 29 October 2023.

NHS (2023aa). COVID-19 advice and services. Available at: https://www.nhs.uk/covid-19-advice-and-services/. Accessed 29 October 2023.

NHS (2023bb). When to call 999. Available at: https://www.nhs.uk/nhs-services/urgent-and-emergency-care-services/when-to-call-999/. Accessed 29 October 2023.

NHS (2023cc). Abbreviations you may find in your health records. Available at: https://www.nhs.uk/nhs-app/nhs-app-help-and-support/health-records-in-the-nhs-app/abbreviations-commonly-found-in-medical-records/. Accessed 30 October 2023.

NHS (2023dd). Glossary – NHS Health Careers. Available at: https://www.nmc.org.uk/about-us/our-role/. Accessed 22 February 2023.

NHS Business Services Authority (2023). NHS pensions. Available at: https://www.nhsbsa.nhs.uk/member-hub/your-options-flexible-retirement. Accessed 28 October 2023.

NHS Confederation (2019). Chairs and non-executives in the NHS: The need for diverse leadership. Available at: https://www.nhsconfed.org/system/files/media/Chairs-and-non-executives-NHS-diverse-leadership.pdf. Accessed 26 August 2023.

NHS Confederation (2023). Aspiring Mental Health Nurse Directors Programme. Available at: https://www.nhsconfed.org/leadership-support/aspiring-mental-health-nurse-directors-programme. Accessed 26 August 2023.

NHS Employers (2022). Routes into the NHS infographic. Available at: https://www.nhsemployers.org/articles/routes-nhs-infographic. Accessed 7 October 2022.

NHS Employers (2023a). The future of nursing careers. Available at: https://www.nhsemployers.org/articles/your-future-nurses. Accessed 24 March 2023.

NHS Employers (2023b). Quick guide: Code of Practice for International Recruitment. Available at: https://www.nhsemployers.org/publications/quick-guide-code-practice-international-recruitment. Accessed 28 October 2023.

NHS Employers (2023c). Code of Practice for International Recruitment – March 2023. Available at: https://www.nhsemployers.org/articles/code-practice-international-recruitment-march-2023. Accessed 29 October 2023.

NHS Employers (2023d). Preceptorships for newly qualified staff. Available at: https://www.nhsemployers.org/articles/preceptorships-newly-qualified-staff. Accessed 31 October 2023.

NHS Employers (2023e). Return to practice for healthcare professionals. Available at: https://www.nhsemployers.org/articles/return-practice-healthcare-professionals. Accessed 31 October 2023.

NHS Employers (2023f). Calendar of national campaigns. Available at: https://www.nhsemployers.org/events/calendar-national-campaigns. Accessed 31 October 2023.

NHS England (2016). Leading change, adding value: A framework for nursing, midwifery and care staff. Available at: https://www.england.nhs.uk/wp-content/uploads/2016/05/nursing-framework.pdf. Accessed 11 September 2023.

NHS England (2018). The Queen's Nursing Institute: General practice nursing induction template. Available at: https://www.qni.org.uk/wp-content/uploads/2019/05/General-Practice-Nursing-Induction-Template.pdf. Accessed 3 September 2023.

NHS England (2019a). General practice – Developing confidence, capability, and capacity: A 10-point action plan for general practice nursing, milestone report. Available at: https://www.england.nhs.uk/wp-content/uploads/2018/01/general-practice-nursing-ten-point-plan-v17.pdf. Accessed 3 August 2023.

NHS England (2019b). Maternity workforce strategy – Transforming the maternity workforce. Available at: https://www.hee.nhs.uk/sites/default/files/document/MWS_Report_Web.pdf. Accessed 3 August 2023.

NHS England (2020). A fair experience for all. Available at: https://www.england.nhs.uk/about/equality/equality-hub/workforce-equality-data-standards/equality-standard/fair-experience/. Accessed 30 October 2023.

NHS England (2021). We are the NHS: People Plan for 2020/2021 – Action for us all. Available at: https://www.england.nhs.uk/publication/we-are-the-nhs-people-plan-for-2020-21-action-for-us-all/. Accessed 9 March 2021.

NHS England (2022a). NHS Long Term Plan. Available at: https://www.england.nhs.uk/long-term-plan/. Accessed 29 December 2022.

NHS England (2022b). Shared Governance: Collective Leadership programme. Available at: https://www.england.nhs.uk/nursingmidwifery/shared-governance-and-collective-leadership/. Accessed 7 October 2023.

NHS England (2022c). Priorities and operational planning guidance 2022/23, NHS operating plan deliverables. Available at: https://www.england.nhs.uk/wp-content/uploads/2022/02/20211223-B1160-2022-23-priorities-and-operational-planning-guidance-v3.2.pdf. Accessed 29 December 2022.

NHS England (2022d). National preceptorship framework for nursing. Available at: https://www.england.nhs.uk/long-read/national-preceptorship-framework-for-nursing/. Accessed 31 December 2022.

NHS England (2022e). Guidance, publications and resources. Available at: https://www.england.nhs.uk/ahp/implementing-ahp-action/. Accessed 1 October 2022.

NHS England (2022f). Developing allied health professional leaders – An interactive guide for clinicians and trust boards. Available at: https://www.england.nhs.uk/ahp/implementing-ahp-action/developing-allied-health-professional-leaders-an-interactive-guide-for-clinicians-and-trust-boards/. Accessed 1 November 2022.

NHS England (2022g). HCSW2020 Accelerated Care Certificate: NHS England. Available at: https://www.e-lfh.org.uk/programmes/hcsw2020-accelerated-care-certificate/. Accessed 1 December 2022.

NHS England (2022h). CSO's Excellence in Healthcare Science Lifetime Achievement award winner. Available at: https://nshcs.hee.nhs.uk/csos-2022-excellence-in-healthcare-science-lifetime-achievement-award-winner/#:~:text=We%20are%20ecstatic%20to%20announce,month%20at%20the%20annual%20CSO. Accessed 10 December 2022.

NHS England (2022i). Clinical networks and senate. Available at: https://www.england.nhs.uk/contact-us/privacy-notice/how-we-use-your-information/public-and-partners/clincal-networks-and-senate/. Accessed 10 December 2022.

NHS England (2022j). Events and news. Available at: https://www.england.nhs.uk/nhsbirthday/events-and-news/. Accessed 10 December 2022.

NHS England (2022k). About the Cultural Competence programme. Available at: https://www.e-lfh.org.uk/programmes/cultural-competence/. Accessed 10 December 2022.

NHS England (2022l). Community health services two-hour urgent community response standard. Available at: https://www.england.nhs.uk/wp-content/uploads/2021/07/B1406-community-health-services-two-hour-urgent-community-response-standard.pdf. Accessed 28 May 2024.

NHS England (2022m). Chief allied health professional's handbook. Available at: https://www.england.nhs.uk/publication/chief-allied-health-professionals-handbook/. Accessed 31 October 2022.

NHS England (2023a). NHS history: Milestones of the NHS. Available at: https://www.england.nhs.uk/nhsbirthday/about-the-nhs-birthday/nhs-history/. Accessed 18 May 2023.

NHS England (2023b). An introduction to the NHS. Available at: https://www.england.nhs.uk/get-involved/nhs/. Accessed 22 March 2023.

NHS England (2023c). Our approach to reducing healthcare inequalities. Available at: https://www.england.nhs.uk. Accessed 31 October 2023

NHS England (2023d). What are integrated care systems? Available at: https://www.england.nhs.uk/integratedcare/what-is-integrated-care/. Accessed 27 June 2023.

NHS England (2023e). Nursing workforce – International recruitment. Available at: https://www.england.nhs.uk/nursingmidwifery/international-recruitment/. Accessed 29 October 2023.

NHS England (2023f). We lead the NHS in England to deliver high quality services for all. Available at: https://www.england.nhs.uk/. Accessed 29 October 2023.

NHS England (2023g). The equality and health inequalities hub. Available at: https://www.england.nhs.uk/about/equality/equality-hub/. Accessed 29 October 2023.

NHS England (2023h). NHS Workforce Race Equality Standard. Available at: https://www.england.nhs.uk/about/equality/equality-hub/workforce-equality-data-standards/equality-standard/. Accessed 29 October 2023.

NHS England (2023i). NHS England and NHS Confederation launch expert research centre on health inequalities. Available at: https://www.england.nhs.uk/2020/05/nhs-england-and-nhs-confederation-launch-expert-research-centre-on-health-inequalities/. Accessed 29 October 2023.

NHS England (2023j). National infection prevention and control manual (NIPCM) for England. Available at: https://www.england.nhs.uk/national-infection-prevention-and-control-manual-nipcm-for-england/. Accessed 29 October 2023.

NHS England (2023k). NHS provider directory. Available at: https://www.england.nhs.uk/publication/nhs-provider-directory/. Accessed 29 October 2023.

NHS England (2023l). Find services near you. Available at: https://www.nhs.uk/nhs-services/services-near-you/. Accessed 29 October 2023.

NHS England (2023m). Find a pharmacy. Available at: https://www.nhs.uk/service-search/pharmacy/find-a-pharmacy. Accessed 29 October 2023.

NHS England (2023n). Mental health. Available at: https://www.england.nhs.uk/five-year-forward-view/next-steps-on-the-nhs-five-year-forward-view/mental-health/. Accessed 29 October 2023.

NHS England (2023o). Example induction checklist template for multidisciplinary team staff in general practice. Available at: https://view.officeapps.live.com/op/view.aspx?src=https%3A%2F%2Fwww.england.nhs.uk%2Fwp-content%2Fuploads%2F2023%2F05%2FPRN00057i-example-induction-checklist-template-mdt-general-practice.docx&wdOrigin=BROWSELINK. Accessed 29 October 2023.

NHS England (2023p). A Model Employer: Increasing Black and minority ethnic representation at senior levels across the NHS. Available at: https://www.england.nhs.uk/publication/a-model-employer/. Accessed 29 October 2023.

NHS England (2023q). Freedom to speak up. Available at: https://www.england.nhs.uk/our-work/freedom-to-speak-up/. Accessed 30 October 2023.

NHS England (2023r). Staff networks. Available at: https://www.england.nhs.uk/about/working-for/staff-networks/. Accessed 30 October 2023.

NHS England (2023s). E-Learning for Health resources: National School of Healthcare Science. Available at: https://nshcs.hee.nhs.uk/about/equality-diversity-and-inclusion/e-learning-for-health-resources/. Accessed 30 October 2023.

NHS England (2023t). Freedom to Speak Up in Healthcare in England programme, e-learning for healthcare. Available at: https://www.e-lfh.org.uk/programmes/freedom-to-speak-up/. Accessed 30 October 2023.

NHS England (2023u). A just culture guide. Available at: https://www.england.nhs.uk/patient-safety/a-just-culture-guide/. Accessed 8 October 2023.

NHS England (2023v). Patient Safety Incident Response Framework. Available at: https://www.england.nhs.uk/patient-safety/incident-response-framework/. Accessed 8 October 2023.

NHS England (2023w). Directory of board level learning and development opportunities. Available at: https://www.england.nhs.uk/long-read/directory-of-board-level-learning-and-development-opportunities/. Accessed 2 August 2023.

NHS England (2023x). Primary care networks. Available at: https://www.england.nhs.uk/primary-care/primary-care-networks/. Accessed 31 August 2023.

NHS England (2023y). NHS IMPACT. Available at: https://www.england.nhs.uk/nhsimpact/. Accessed 1 October 2023.

NHS England (2023z). Nursing and Midwifery Matters. Available at: https://www.england.nhs.uk/email-bulletins/cno-bulletin/. Accessed 31 October 2023.

NHS England (2023aa). NHS Five Year Forward View. Available at: https://www.england.nhs.uk/five-year-forward-view/. Accessed 31 October 2023.

NHS England (2023bb). Types of nursing. Available at: https://www.healthcareers.nhs.uk/explore-roles/nursing/roles-nursing. Accessed 31 October 2023.

NHS England (2024). Learning disability and autism. Available at: https://www.longtermplan.nhs.uk/areas-of-work/learning-disability-autism/. Accessed 28 May 2024.

NHS Graduate Management Training Scheme (2023). NHS Graduate Management Training Scheme (GMTS) applications. Available at: https://graduates.nhs.uk/. Accessed 26 October 2023.

NHS Jobs (2023). Apply on NHS jobs. Available at: https://www.jobs.nhs.uk/candidate. Accessed 28 October 2023.

NHS Leadership Academy (2023a). Talent Management Hub. Available at: https://www.leadershipacademy.nhs.uk/talent-management-hub/. Accessed 6 October 2023.

NHS Leadership Academy (2023b). Talent Management Toolkit. Available at: https://www.leadershipacademy.nhs.uk/talent-management-hub/talent-management-toolkit-home-page/. Accessed 6 October 2023.

NHS Leadership Academy (2023c). Apprenticeships to help you develop as a leader. Available at: https://www.leadershipacademy.nhs.uk/programmes/apprenticeships/. Accessed 26 October 2023.

NHS Leadership Academy (2023d). Programmes to help you grow as a leader. Available at: https://www.leadershipacademy.nhs.uk/programmes/. Accessed 31 October 2023.

NHS Leadership Academy (2023e). Coaching and mentoring. Available at: https://www.leadershipacademy.nhs.uk/programmes/coaching-and-mentoring/. Accessed 31 October 2023.

NHS Leadership Academy (2023f). Development support for clinical leaders. Available at: https://www.leadershipacademy.nhs.uk/programmes/clinical-leadership-development/. Accessed 31 October 2023.

NHS Leadership Academy (2023g). Executive Director Pathway (EDP). Available at: https://www.leadershipacademy.nhs.uk/senior-leadership-support-and-development/executive-directors-and-aspiring-leaders-2/executive-director-pathway-2/. Accessed 31 October 2023.

NHS Leadership Academy (2023h) Aspiring Chief Executive programme. Available at: https://www.leadershipacademy.nhs.uk/aspiring-chief-executive-programme/. Accessed 31 October 2023.

NHS Leadership Academy (2023i). Chief Executive Development Network. Available at: https://www.leadershipacademy.nhs.uk/senior-leadership-support-and-development/chief-executive-officers/chief-exec-development/. Accessed 31 October 2023.

NHS Leadership Academy (2023j). Aspiring and current executive directors. Available at: https://www.leadershipacademy.nhs.uk/senior-leadership-support-and-development/executive-directors-and-aspiring-leaders-2/. Accessed 31 October 2023.

NHS Leadership Academy (2023k). Develop your career connect with peers grow as a leader. Available at: https://www.leadershipacademy.nhs.uk/. Accessed 31 October 2023.

NHS Leadership Academy (2023l). Review and career conversations. Available at: https://www.leadershipacademy.nhs.uk/toolkit/identifying-managing-and-retaining-talent/review-and-career-conversations/. Accessed 31 October 2023.

NHS Leadership Academy (2023m). Developing outstanding leadership in primary care. Available at: https://www.leadershipacademy.nhs.uk/wp-content/uploads/dlm_uploads/2019/05/Primary-care-leadership-eBook-May-2019.pdf. Accessed 31 August 2023.

NHS Leadership Academy (2023n). Chief executive officers. Available at: https://www.leadershipacademy.nhs.uk/senior-leadership-support-and-development/chief-executive-officers/. Accessed 23 October 23.

NHS London Leadership Academy (2023). Talent Management Toolkit. Available at: https://london.leadershipacademy.nhs.uk/leadership-programmes/talent-management/. Accessed 19 October 2023.

NHS Northern Ireland (2023). Health and Social Care. Available at: https://online.hscni.net/. Accessed 31 October 2023.

NHS Professionals (2023a). NHS Staffing Pool Hub – Getting started – Having a career conversation. Available at: https://www.nhsprofessionals.nhs.uk/nhs-staffing-pool-hub/getting-started. Accessed 25 March 2023.

NHS Professionals (2023b). Developing cultural competence for leaders. Available at: https://www.nhsprofessionals.nhs.uk/partners/academy-courses/management-and-leadership-courses/developing-cultural-competence-for-leaders. Accessed 31 October 2023.

NHS Scotland (2023). Scotland's health on the web. Available at: https://www.scot.nhs.uk/. Accessed 31 October 2023.

NHS Wales (2023). NHS Wales website. Available at: https://www.nhs.wales/. Accessed 31 October 2023.

Northouse, P. (2011). *Leadership: Theory and practice* (6th ed.). London: Sage.

Nuffield Trust (2023). The history of the NHS. Available at: https://www.nuffieldtrust.org.uk/health-and-social-care-explained/the-history-of-the-nhs. Accessed 18 May 2023.

Nurse.org (2022). Nursing ranked as the most trusted profession for 21st year in a row. Available at: https://nurse.org/articles/nursing-ranked-most-honest-profession/. Accessed 21 December 2022.

Nursing and Midwifery Council (2008). The code: Standards of conduct, performance and ethics for nurses and midwives. Available at: https://www.nmc.org.uk/globalassets/sitedocuments/standards/nmc-old-code-2008.pdf. Accessed 31 October 2023.

Nursing and Midwifery Council (2021a). What is revalidation? Available at: https://www.nmc.org.uk/revalidation/overview/what-is-revalidation/. Accessed 26 July 2021.

Nursing and Midwifery Council (2021b). Keep records of all evidence and decisions. Available at: https://www.nmc.org.uk/employer-resource/local-investigation/guiding-principles/record-evidence-decisions/. Accessed 28 March 2021.

Nursing and Midwifery Council (2023a). Who we are and what we do. Available at: https://www.healthcareers.nhs.uk/glossary. Accessed 21 March 2023.

Nursing and Midwifery Council (2023b). Objective Structured Clinical Examination (OSCE). Available at: https://www.nmc.org.uk/registration/joining-the-register/toc/toc-2021/osce/. Accessed 28 October 2023.

Nursing and Midwifery Council (2023c). The Code: Professional standards of practice and behaviour for nurses, midwives and nursing associates. Available at: https://www.nmc.org.uk/standards/code/. Accessed 28 October 2023.

Nursing and Midwifery Council (2023d). Search the register – The Nursing and Midwifery Council. Available at: https://www.nmc.org.uk/registration/search-the-register/. Accessed 28 October 2023.

Nursing and Midwifery Council (2023e). Standards for competence for registered nurses. Available at: https://www.nmc.org.uk/standards/standards-for-nurses/pre-2018-standards/standards-for-competence-for-registered-nurses/. Accessed 28 October 2023.

Nursing and Midwifery Council (2023f). Accepted English language tests. Available at: https://www.nmc.org.uk/registration/joining-the-register/english-language-requirements/accepted-english-language-tests/#SIFE. Accessed 28 October 2023.

Nursing and Midwifery Council (2023g). Provide language evidence. Available at: https://www.nmc.org.uk/registration/joining-the-register/register-nurse-midwife/trained-outside-uk/how-to-guide/registration-application/language/. Accessed 28 October 2023.

Nursing and Midwifery Council (2023h). Test combining calculator. Available at: https://www.nmc.org.uk/registration/joining-the-register/english-language-requirements/accepted-english-language-tests/test-combining-calc/. Accessed 28 October 2023.

Nursing and Midwifery Council (2023i). Preparation materials. Available at: https://www.nmc.org.uk/registration/joining-the-register/toc/toc-2021/resources/. Accessed 28 October 2023.

Nursing and Midwifery Council (2023j). Standards for pre-registration nursing programmes. Available at: https://www.nmc.org.uk/standards/standards-for-nurses/standards-for-pre-registration-nursing-programmes/. Accessed 29 October 2023.

Nursing and Midwifery Council (2023k). Resources and templates. Available at: https://www.nmc.org.uk/revalidation/resources/. Accessed 29 October 2023.

Nursing and Midwifery Council (2023l). Revalidation stories. Available at: https://www.nmc.org.uk/revalidation/case-studies/. Accessed 29 October 2023.

Nursing and Midwifery Council (2023m). What you need to do. Available at: https://www.nmc.org.uk/revalidation/requirements/. Accessed 29 October 2023.

Nursing and Midwifery Council (2023n). Support to help you revalidate. Available at: https://www.nmc.org.uk/globalassets/sitedocuments/revalidation/support-to-help-you-revalidate.pdf. Accessed 29 October 2023.

Nursing and Midwifery Council (2023o). Enabling professionalism in nursing and midwifery practice. Available at: https://www.nmc.org.uk/globalassets/sitedocuments/other-publications/enabling-professionalism.pdf. Accessed 29 October 2023.

Nursing and Midwifery Council (2023p). Standards for nursing associates. Available at: https://www.nmc.org.uk/standards/standards-for-nursing-associates/. Accessed 29 October 2023.

Nursing and Midwifery Council (2023q). Standards of proficiency for registered nursing associates. Available at: https://www.nmc.org.uk/standards/standards-for-nursing-associates/standards-of-proficiency-for-nursing-associates/. Accessed 29 October 2023.

Nursing and Midwifery Council (2023r). Standards for student supervision and assessment. Available at: https://www.nmc.org.uk/standards-for-education-and-training/standards-for-student-supervision-and-assessment/. Accessed 27 July 2023.

Nursing and Midwifery Council (2024a). The code: Professional standards of practice and behaviour for nurses, midwives and nursing associates. Available at: https://www.nmc.org.uk/standards/code/. Accessed 9 June 2024.

Nursing and Midwifery Council (2024b). Standards of competence for registered midwives. Available at: https://www.nmc.org.uk/globalassets/sitedocuments/standards/nmc-standards-for-competence-for-registered-midwives.pdf. Accessed 9 July 2024.

Nursing Now Challenge (2023). Championing leadership development opportunities for student and early career nurses and midwives around the world. Available at: https://www.nursingnow.org/. Accessed 31 October 2023.

Nursing Times (2023). Journal Club. Available at: https://www.nursingtimes.net/learning-units-and-portfolio/journal-club-learning-units-and-portfolio/. Accessed 31 October 2023.

Occupational English Test (OET) (2021). Patient Safety Communication Whitepaper 2021. Available at: https://s3-prod.modernhealthcare.com/2021-05/OET-Patient-Safety-Communication-Whitepaper-2021.pdf. Accessed 31 August 2023.

Occupational English Test (OET) (2023a). The easiest choice for healthcare professionals. Available at: https://oet.com/. Accessed 28 October 2023.

Occupational English Test (OET) (2023b). The easiest choice for healthcare professionals. Available at: https://support.occupationalenglishtest.org/s/article/How-do-I-give-verification-institutions-permission-to-view-my-results. Accessed 28 October 2023.

Occupational English Test (OET) (2023c). Find the right test for you. Available at: https://ielts.org/take-a-test/test-types. Accessed 28 October 2023.

Occupational English Test (OET) (2023d). IELTS sample test questions. Available at: https://ielts.org/take-a-test/preparation-resources/sample-test-questions. Accessed 28 October 2023.

Occupational English Test (OET) (2023e). Preparation information. Available at: https://oet.com/learn/preparation-information. Accessed 29 October 2023.

Operation Black Vote (2023). Pathway to Success open for applications. Available at: https://www.magd.ox.ac.uk/news/pathway-to-success-open-for-applications/. Accessed 7 October 2023.

Parandeh, A., Khaghanizade, M., Mohammadi, E., & Mokhtari-Nouri, J. (2016). Nurses' human dignity in education and practice: An integrated literature review. *Iranian Journal of Nursing and Midwifery Research*, *21*(1), 1–8.

Parkinson, J., & Brooker, C. (2004). *Everyday English for international nurses: A guide working in the UK*. Milton Keynes: Churchill Livingstone.

Pearce, C. L., Manz, C. C., & Sims, H. P. (2009). Where do we go from here? Is shared leadership the key to team success? *Orgnisational Dynamics.*, *38*(3), 234–238.

Post Graduate Funding (2023). Royal College of Midwives (RCM). Available at: https://www.postgraduatefunding.com/provider-757/. Accessed 29 October 2023.

Prospects (2023). 5 routes to getting a Doctorate. Available at: https://www.prospects. ac.uk/postgraduate-study/phd-study/5-routes-to-getting-a-doctorate. Accessed 31 October 2023

Public and Commercial Services (PCS) (2023). Join PCS for security at work. Available at: https://www.pcs.org.uk/. Accessed 31 October 2023

Public Health England (2020c). Disparities in the risk and outcomes of Covid-19. Available at: https://assets.publishing.service.gov.uk/media/5f328354d3bf7f1b12a7023a/Disparities_in_the_ risk_and_outcomes_of_COVID_August_2020_update.pdf. Accessed 29 December 2022.

Public Service Consultants (PSC) (2023). National Mental Health Act Quality Improvement pro- gramme. Available at: https://thepsc.co.uk/page/national-mental-health-act-QI-programme. Accessed 29 October 2023.

Professional Standards Authority (PSA) (2023). We protect the public by overseeing the regula- tion and registration of healthcare professionals. Available at: https://www.professionalstan- dards.org.uk/home. Accessed 29 October 2023.

Queen's Nursing Institute (QNI) (2023a). QNI Awards. Available at: https://qni.org.uk/explore- qni/qni-awards/. Accessed 31 October 2023

Queen's Nursing Institute (QNI) (2023b). Queen's Nurse Leadership Programme. Available at: https://www.qni.org.uk/wp-content/uploads/2018/01/Queens-Nurse-Leadership-Programme- Poster.pdf. Accessed 31 October 2023

Ramalisa, R. J., du Plessis, E., & Koen, M. P. (2018). Increasing coping and strengthening resil- ience in nurses providing mental health care: Empirical qualitative research. *Health SA, 23*, 1094. 12.

Royal College of General Practitioners (RCGP) (2023). Quality improvement in general practice. Available at: https://www.rcgp.org.uk/learning-resources/quality-improvement. Accessed 29 October 2023.

Royal College of Midwives (RCM) (2023). About us. Available at: https://www.rcm.org.uk/ about-us/. Accessed 29 October 2023.

Royal College of Nursing (2021). Nursing workforce standards. Available at: https://www.rcn. org.uk/Professional-Development/publications/rcn-workforce-standards-uk-pub-009681. Accessed 7 October 2023.

Royal College of Nursing (2023a). Preparing for IELTS, OET and OSCE exams. Available at: https://www.rcn.org.uk/Get-Help/Member-support-services/Immigration-Advice-Service/ Preparing-for-IELTS-and-OSCE-exams. Accessed 19 October 2023.

Royal College of Nursing (2023b). We are the world's largest nursing union and professional body. Available at: https://www.rcn.org.uk/. Accessed 29 October 2023.

Royal College of Nursing (2023c). Executive nurse network. Available at: https://www.rcn.org. uk/Get-Involved/Forums/Executive-Nurse-Network. Accessed 29 October 2023.

Royal College of Nursing (2023d). Metric (SI) units. Available at: https://www.rcn.org.uk/clini- cal-topics/Safety-in-numbers/Metric-units. Accessed 3 January 2023.

Royal College of Nursing (2023e). Discipline. Available at: https://www.rcn.org.uk/Get-Help/ RCN-advice/discipline. Accessed 27 October 2023.

Royal College of Nursing (2023f). Guide to common English expressions. Available at: https:// www.rcn.org.uk/Get-Help/common-english-expressions. Accessed 27 October 2023.

Royal College of Nursing (2023g). Become a midwife: Advice on beginning your midwifery career. Available at: https://www.rcn.org.uk/Professional-Development/become-a-midwife. Accessed 14 August 2023.

Royal College of Nursing (2023h). Career paths for nursing support workers. Available at: https:// www.rcn.org.uk/Professional-Development/Your-career/HCA/Career-paths-for-HCAs. Accessed 31 August 2023.

Royal College of Nursing (2023i). Become a nursing associate. Available at: https://www.rcn. org.uk/Professional-Development/Nursing-Support-Workers/Become-a-nursing-associate. Accessed 31 August 2023.

Royal College of Nursing (2023j). Healthcare assistant overview. Available at: https://www.rcn. org.uk/professional-development/your-career/hca. Accessed 31 August 2023.

Royal College of Nursing (2023k). Careers: Step into the spotlight: What can nursing staff bring to leadership roles usually held by GPs? Available at: https://www.rcn.org.uk/magazines/ Career/2023/Aug/Clinical-director-leadership#:~:text=What%20is%20a%20clinical%20 director,the%20delivery%20of%20those%20services. Accessed 31 August 2023.

Royal College of Nursing (2023l). RCN Nursing Awards. Available at: https://rcni.com/nurse-awards. Accessed 31 October 2023.

Royal College of Nursing (2023m). RCN Fellows and Honorary Fellows. Available at: https:// www.rcn.org.uk/About-us/RCN-Fellows-and-Honorary-Fellows/How-to-nominate Accessed 31 October 2023.

Royal College of Nursing (2023n). Job applications and supporting statements. Available at: https://www.rcn.org.uk/Professional-Development/Your-career/Job-applications. Accessed 22 October 2023.

Royal College of Nursing (2023o). Interview skills RCN Career Service advice. Available at: https://studylib.net/doc/14174472/interview-skills-rcn-career-service-a-d-v-i-c-e.   Accessed 22 October 2023.

Royal College of Nursing (2023p). Nursing Support Workers' Day. Available at: https://www.rcn. org.uk/. Accessed 31 October 2023.

Royal College of Nursing (2023q). Presentation skills for nurses. Available at: https://www.rcn. org.uk/Professional-Development/Your-career/Nurse/Presentation-skills. Accessed 31 October 2023.

Royal College of Nursing Institute (RCNi) (2022). Record-keeping and documentation in nursing. Available at: https://rcni.com/nursing-standard/newsroom/analysis/record-keeping-and-documentation-nursing-how-to-get-it-right-189616. Accessed 6 April 2022.

Royal College of Nursing Institute (RCNi) (2023). Quality improvement. Available at: https:// rcni.com/keywords/quality-improvement. Accessed 31 October 2023.

Royal College of Paediatrics and Child Health (RCPCH) (2023). Quality improvement. Available at: https://www.rcpch.ac.uk/topic/quality-improvement. Accessed 31 October 2023.

Royal College of Physicians Quality Improvement (RCPQI) (2023). RCP Quality Improvement (RCPQI). Available at: https://www.rcplondon.ac.uk/projects/rcp-quality-improvement-rcpqi. Accessed 31 October 2023.

Royal College of Psychiatrists (RCP) (2023). Using quality improvement. Available at: https:// www.rcpsych.ac.uk/improving-care/using-quality-improvement. Accessed 31 October 2023.

Samaritans (2023). We're waiting for your call. Available at: https://www.samaritans.org/. Accessed 30 September 2023.

Scullion, H., & Collings, D. G. (Eds.). (2006). *Global staffing* (1st ed.). London: Routledge.

Shepherd, S. M., Willis-Esqueda, C., Newton, D., Sivasubramaniam, D., & Paradies, Y. (2019). The challenge of cultural competence in the workplace: Perspectives of healthcare providers. *BMC Health Service Res, 19*(1), 135. Feb 26.

Sherman, R. O., & Eggenberger, T. (2008). Transitioning internationally recruited nurses into clinical settings. *The Journal of Continuing Education in Nursing, 12*, 535–544. 39.

Siwicki, B. (2020). Business Intelligence: Here are the major issues facing healthcare in 2021, according to PwC. Available at: https://www.healthcareitnews.com/news/here-are-major-issues-facing-healthcare-2021-according-pwc. Accessed 16 December 2020.

Skills for Care (2023a). Care Certificate. Available at: https://www.skillsforcare.org.uk/Developing-your-workforce/Care-Certificate/Care-Certificate.aspx?gclid=CjwKCAjw7oeqBhBwEiwAL yHLM7uYqIyLuHugkzyhB1Cq0ryJBduWHikalaMoSTCEZBCwjLPNgtHzHBoCONIQ AvD_BwE. Accessed 31 October 2023.

Skills for Care (2023b). The Care Certificate Framework. Available at: https://www.skillsforcare.org.uk/resources/documents/Developing-your-workforce/Care-Certificate/The-Care-Certificate-Framework.pdf. Accessed 31 October 2023.

Skills for Care (2023c). Code of conduct for healthcare support workers and adult social care workers in England. Available at: https://www.skillsforcare.org.uk/resources/documents/Support-for-leaders-and-managers/Managing-people/Code-of-conduct/Code-of-Conduct.pdf. Accessed 31 October 2023.

Skills for Care (2023d). The Care Certificate Standards. Available at: https://www.skillsforcare.org.uk/resources/documents/Developing-your-workforce/Care-Certificate/The-Care-Certificate-Standards.pdf. Accessed 31 October 2023.

Skills for Care (2023e). Skills for Care: Supporting the adult social care sector. Available at: https://www.skillsforcare.org.uk/Home.aspx. Accessed 31 October 2023.

Swanwick, T., & McKimm, J. (2011). What is clinical leadership and why is it important. *Clin. Teach*, *8*, 22–26.

The Honours System of the United Kingdom (2023). Nominate today. Available at: https://honours.cabinetoffice.gov.uk/. Accessed 30 October 2023.

The Myers-Briggs Company (2023). Myers-Briggs Type Indicator® (MBTI®). Available at: https://www.themyersbriggs.com/en-US/Products-and-Services/Myers-Briggs. Accessed 31 October 2023.

Myers-Briggs Foundation (2023). The 16 MBTI® Personality Types. Available at: https://www.myersbriggs.org/my-mbti-personality-type/the-16-mbti-personality-types/. Accessed 3 October 2023.

The University of Manchester (2023). Jobs at The University of Manchester. Available at: https://www.jobs.manchester.ac.uk/Home/Job. Accessed 31 October 2023.

Thomas, B. G. (2016). *A brief history of nursing in the U.K.* London: Memories of nursing.

Triggle, N., (2017). EU nurse applicants drop by 96% since Brexit vote 23 June 2016. BBC News. Available at: https://www.bbc.co.uk/news/health-40248366. Accessed 31 October 2023.

UK Health Security Agency (UKHSA) (2023a). One You: A step towards better health and more sustainable services. Available at: https://ukhsa.blog.gov.uk/2016/03/07/one-you-a-step-towards-better-health-and-more-sustainable-services/. Accessed 30 October 2023.

UK Health Security Agency (UKHSA) (2023b). Practice examples. Available at: https://ukhsalibrary.koha-ptfs.co.uk/practice-examples-2/. Accessed 31 October 2023.

UK Parliament (2023). Backbench Business Committee. Available at: https://committees.parliament.uk/committee/202/backbench-business-committee/. Accessed 30 October 2023.

UNISON (2023). Unison – the public service union. Available at: https://www.unison.org.uk/. Accessed 31 October 2023.

Unite The Union (2023). Unite for a Workers' Economy. Available at: https://www.unitetheunion.org/campaigns. Accessed 30 October 2023.

United Nations (UN) Careers (2023). Young Professionals Programme. Available at: https://careers.un.org/lbw/home.aspx?viewtype=nce. Accessed 30 October 2023.

University of Hertfordshire (2023). Mentor portfolio of evidence for nurses: Recognition of mentorship skills, guidance and mapping. Framework for Stage 2 mentors. Available at: https://www.herts.ac.uk/__data/assets/pdf_file/0020/28325/stage2_healtcare_mentor_mapping_tool.pdf. Accessed 17 August 2023.

Van Diggele, C., Burgess, A., Roberts, C., et al. (2020). Leadership in healthcare education. *BMC Medical Education*, *vol 20*(Suppl 2), 456.

Walsall Healthcare NHS Trust (2023). Research and clinical education: Professional development. Available at: https://www.walsallhealthcare.nhs.uk/professionals/research-and-clinical-education/professional-development/. Accessed 3 April 2023.

Waring, J., Bishop, S., Clarke, J., Exworthy, M., Fulop, N. J., Hartley, J., & Ramsay, A. I. G. (2018). Healthcare leadership with political astuteness (HeLPA): A qualitative study of how service leaders understand and mediate the informal 'power and politics' of major health system change. *BMC Health Services Research*, *vol. 18*, 918.

Wayne, G., (2023). The Nursing Process: A Comprehensive Guide. Available at: https://nurs-eslabs.com/nursing-process/. Accessed 7 July 2024.

Willis, P. (2012). *Quality with compassion: The future of nursing education. Report of the Willis Commission on Nursing Education.* London: Royal College of Nursing.

World Bank (2023). The World Bank Group Young Professionals Programme. Available at: https://www.worldbank.org/en/about/careers/programs-and-internships/young-professionals-program. Accessed 31 October 2023

World Health Organization (WHO) (2016). Core components for IPC. Available at: https://www.who.int/teams/integrated-health-services/infection-prevention-control/core-components. Accessed 4 May 2023.

World Health Organization (WHO) (2023a). Nursing now campaign. Available at: https://www.who.int/news/item/27-02-2018-nursing-now-campaign. Accessed 31 October 2023

World Health Organization (WHO) (2023b). Collaborating centres. Available at: https://www.who.int/about/collaboration/collaborating-centres. Accessed 31 October 2023

World Trade Organization (WTO) (2023). Young Professionals Programme. Available at: https://www.wto.org/english/thewto_e/vacan_e/ypp_e.htm. Accessed 31 October 2023

This section includes useful reading, resources guidance, links, sources and general websites on health and care services across the UK, which staff can access to gain support.

Chapter 2: Preparing Internationally Recruited Staff for Successful Completion of the International Recruitment Process

UK PAY RATES AND SCALES

Agenda for Change NHS Pay Bands 2023/24
https://nursingnotes.co.uk/agenda-for-change-nhs-pay-bands/ (Accessed 31 October 2023)

Chapter 3: Basic Guide to the National Health Service Structures

3.3 HEALTHCARE ORGANISATIONS IN THE UK (ACCESSED 31 OCTOBER 2023)

National Health System
https://www.nhs.uk/ (NHS, 2023o)
NHS England
https://www.england.nhs.uk/ (NHS England, 2023f)
NHS Scotland
https://www.scot.nhs.uk/ (NHS Scotland, 2023)
NHS Wales
https://www.nhs.wales/ (NHS Wales, 2023)
NHS Northern Ireland Health and Social Care
https://online.hscni.net/ (NHS Northern Ireland, 2023)
Department of Health and Social Care (gov.uk, 2023t) and (NHS, 2023a)

3.5.11 CHILDREN'S HEALTHCARE IN THE UK

Raising a Child in the UK

Childcare and parenting: gov.uk
https://www.gov.uk/browse/childcare-parenting (Accessed 31 October 2023)

Schools for Children in the UK

Types of school: Overview: gov.uk
https://www.gov.uk/types-of-school (Accessed 31 October 2023)

Lists of schools in England
https://en.wikipedia.org/wiki/Lists_of_schools_in_England (Accessed 31 October 2023)

3.7 MODELS OF NURSING CARE DELIVERY IN THE UK

Roles in nursing: NHS health careers
https://www.healthcareers.nhs.uk/explore-roles/nursing/roles-nursing (Accessed 31 October 2023)

Chapter 4: Cultural Competency

4.2 CULTURAL COMPETENCY TO SUPPORT INTERNATIONALLY RECRUITED STAFF

BAME and other international and diverse groups staff networks:
https://www.england.nhs.uk/about/working-for/staff-networks/ (Accessed 31 October 2023)
We are the NHS: People Plan for 2020/21 – action for us all
https://www.england.nhs.uk/publication/we-are-the-nhs-people-plan-for-2020-21-action-for-us-all/ (Accessed 31 October 2023)

Chapter 5: Strategies for Coping With and Flourishing in Your Healthcare Staff Role

Royal College of Nursing (RCN): Nursing careers resource | Professional development
https://www.rcn.org.uk/Professional-Development/Nursing-careers-resource (Accessed 31 October 2023)
Nursing and Midwifery Council (NMC): Continuing professional development
https://www.nmc.org.uk/revalidation/requirements/cpd/ (Accessed 31 October 2023)
NHS England: Career development and pathways
https://www.england.nhs.uk/nursingmidwifery/healthcare-support-worker-programme/summary-of-best-practice/career-development-and-pathways/ (Accessed 31 October 2023)
Career development
https://www.leadershipacademy.nhs.uk/career-development/ (Accessed 31 October 2023)
Health and Care Professions Council (HCPC): Continuing professional development (CPD):
https://www.hcpc-uk.org/cpd/ (Accessed 31 October 2023)
Ward leader's handbook
https://webarchive.nationalarchives.gov.uk/ukgwa/20200501113105mp_/https://improvement.nhs.uk/documents/3359/Ward_leaders_handbook.pdf (Accessed 31 October 2023)

Matron's handbook

https://www.england.nhs.uk/mat-transformation/matrons-handbook/ (Accessed 31 October 2023)

Continuing professional development (CPD): NHS healthcare careers

https://www.healthcareers.nhs.uk/career-planning/career-planning/developing-your-health-career/continuing-professional-development-cpd (Accessed 31 October 2023)

Career development

https://www.skillsyouneed.com/ps/continuing-professional-development.html (Accessed 31 October 2023)

Allied health professionals

https://www.healthcareers.nhs.uk/explore-roles/allied-health-professionals/roles-allied-health-professions/roles-allied-health-professions (Accessed 31 October 2023)

5.2.2 CHIEF NURSE/DIRECTOR OF NURSING/DIRECTOR OF MIDWIFERY CAREER PATHWAY/DEVELOPMENT

Florence Nightingale Foundation (FNF): leadership programmes

https://florence-nightingale-foundation.org.uk/academy/leadership-development/leadership-programmes/ (Accessed 31 October 2023)

The Aspiring Mental Health Nurse Directors Programme (NHS Confederation, 2023)

https://www.nhsconfed.org/leadership-support/aspiring-mental-health-nurse-directors-programme#:~:text=Run%20by%20the%20Mental%20Health,next%20step%20in%20their%20career (Accessed 31 October 2023)

Becoming a NED: New NED and chair competencies and appraisals: NHS senior leadership onboarding and support

https://www.cgi.org.uk/knowledge/governance-and-compliance/careers/november-2016-becoming-a-ned

Chief allied health professional's handbook

https://www.england.nhs.uk/publication/chief-allied-health-professionals-handbook/ (Accessed 31 October 2023)

5.2.6 MID-CAREER LEADERSHIP PROGRAMMES

Clinical Leadership Competency Framework

https://www.leadershipacademy.nhs.uk/wp-content/uploads/2012/11/NHSLeadership-Leadership-Framework-Clinical-Leadership-Competency-Framework-CLCF.pdf (Accessed 31 October 2023)

Leadership and organisational development

https://www.kingsfund.org.uk/courses (Accessed 31 October 2023)

5.2.12 STUDY PATHWAYS FOR NURSES, MIDWIVES, NURSING ASSOCIATES AND AHPS

List of Nursing PhD/MSc/PGDip/PGCert

378 MSc degrees in nursing
https://www.postgraduatesearch.com/pgs/search?course=nursing&qualification=msc (Accessed 31 October 2023)

Postgraduate courses in nursing courses
https://www.postgrad.com/courses/nursing/ (Accessed 31 October 2023)

Best 21 nursing PhD programmes in the UK in 2023
https://www.phdportal.com/study-options/268927089/nursing-united-kingdom.html (Accessed 31 October 2023)

5.2.5 MANAGEMENT DEVELOPMENT AND BESPOKE PROGRAMME

NHS careers (NHS, 2022j)
www.nhscareers.nhs.uk//nhs

Healthcare careers (National Careers Service, 2023)
https://nationalcareers.service.gov.uk/job-categories/healthcare

5.3.1 MANAGEMENT VERSUS LEADERSHIP

Management and leadership courses: NHS Professionals
https://www.nhsprofessionals.nhs.uk/en/partners/academy-courses/management-and-leadership-courses (Accessed 31 October 2023)

5.4 CAREER CONVERSATIONS AND REVIEWS

Talent management toolkit
https://www.leadershipacademy.nhs.uk/toolkit/ (Accessed 31 October 2023)

Enabling a culture of talent management
https://www.leadershipacademy.nhs.uk/toolkit/enabling-a-culture-of-talent-management-page/ (Accessed 31 October 2023)

Equality, diversity and inclusion in talent management
https://www.leadershipacademy.nhs.uk/toolkit/equality-diversity-and-inclusion-in-talent-management/ (Accessed 31 October 2023)

Identifying, managing and retaining talent
https://www.leadershipacademy.nhs.uk/talent-management-hub/ (Accessed 31 October 2023)

Developing and mobilising talent
https://www.leadershipacademy.nhs.uk/toolkit/developing-and-mobilising-talent/ (Accessed 31 October 2023)

Connecting talent interventions across local systems
https://www.leadershipacademy.nhs.uk/toolkit/connecting-talent-interventions-across-local-systems/ (Accessed 31 October 2023)

Diagnostic toolkit
  https://www.leadershipacademy.nhs.uk/toolkit/access-the-diagnostic-tool/
    (Accessed 31 October 2023)
Talent management toolkit (Leadership Academy 2023)
  https://www.leadershipacademy.nhs.uk/toolkit/ (Accessed 31 October 2023)
  What are apprenticeships? (Accessed 31 October 2023)
  https://www.nhsprofessionals.nhs.uk/en/nhs-staffing-pool-hub/apprenticeships
  www.instituteforapprenticeships.org
  www.healthcareers.nhs.uk
  www.findapprenticeship.service.gov.uk
  www.ucas.com

Skills for Health
  https://www.skillsforhealth.org.uk/
  e-learning for healthcare:
  https://www.e-lfh.org.uk/

Workforce, training and education
  https://www.hee.nhs.uk/our-work/capitalnurse/workstreams/career-framework
    (Accessed 31 October 2023)

Resources to Support NHS Staff

Support available for our NHS people
  https://www.england.nhs.uk/supporting-our-nhs-people/support-now/
    (Accessed 31 October 2023)
Inspire, Attract and Recruit toolkit: NHS Employers
  https://www.nhsemployers.org/inspire-attract-and-recruit (Accessed 31 October
    2023)

Chapter 6: Accelerating Staff Development and Progression in the Workplace

Three obstacles hindering women's career advancement
  https://www.forbes.com/sites/forbesnycouncil/2018/04/18/three-obstacles-
    hindering-womens-career-advancement/?sh=6ee40de799e9 (Accessed 31
    October 2023)

6.4.18 STRATEGIES OF PROGRESSING INTO CURRENT ROLE

Volunteering in the NHS
  https://www.england.nhs.uk/get-involved/get-involved/volunteering/ (Accessed
    31 October 2023)
Becoming a hospital volunteer
  https://www.royalvoluntaryservice.org.uk/volunteering/volunteering-in-hospi-
    tals/ (Accessed 31 October 2023)
The British Red Cross
  https://www.redcross.org.uk/ (Accessed 31 October 2023)

NHS Cadets youth volunteering programme
> https://www.england.nhs.uk/ourwork/nhs-cadets-youth-volunteering-pro-
> gramme/ (Accessed 31 October 2023)

6.5.4.1 RCN AND ROYAL COLLEGE OF NURSING INSTITUTE (RCNI) AWARDS

> https://www.rcn.org.uk/Get-Involved/RCN-awards (Accessed 31 October 2023)

RCN Awards
> https://www.rcn.org.uk/Get-Involved/RCN-awards/RCN-award-of-merit
> (Accessed 31 October 2023)

6.5.4.2 RCN FELLOWSHIP

How to nominate RCN Fellows
> https://www.rcn.org.uk/About-us/RCN-Fellows-and-Honorary-Fellows/How-
> to-nominate (Accessed 31 October 2023)

6.5.4.3 QUEENS NURSE AWARD

Queen's Nursing Institute (QNI) Awards
> https://qni.org.uk/explore-qni/qni-awards/

Queen's Nurses
> https://qni.org.uk/nursing-in-the-community/queens-nurses/queens_nurses_
> hero-1/ (Accessed 31 October 2023)

6.5.4.4 QNI GRANTS

Queen's Nurse Leadership Programme
Educational grants for community nurses
> https://qni.org.uk/support-for-nurses/educational-grants/
> - Educational grants: QNI
> - Community Nurse Executive Network (CNEN)
> - Executive Nurse Leadership Programme
> (Accessed 31 October 2023)

6.5.4.5 FELLOWSHIP OF THE INSTITUTE OF HEALTH VISITING (FIHV)

Fellows: FiHV
> https://ihv.org.uk/about-us/fellows/ (Accessed 31 October 2023)

6.5.4.6 ADDITIONAL NURSING AWARDS THAT STAFF CAN APPLY FOR

NHS Parliamentary Awards
> https://www.england.nhs.uk/nhs-parliamentary-awards/ (Accessed 31 October
> 2023)

Health Service Journal (HSJ) Awards
https://awards.hsj.co.uk/ (Accessed 31 October 2023)
Nursing Times Awards
https://awards.nursingtimes.net/ntaw23/en/page/home (Accessed 31 October
2023)
Health awards and social care awards
https://awards-list.co.uk/uk-awards/health-awards-and-social-care-awards/
(Accessed 31 October 2023)

6.5.4.7 DOCTORAL AWARDS

**Doctoral Awards | National Institute for Health and Care Research (NIHR),
Oxford Biomedical Research Centre**
https://oxfordbrc.nihr.ac.uk/training-hub/doctoral-awards/

6.5.4.8 THE BRITISH FEDERATION OF WOMEN GRADUATES (BFWG)

https://bfwg.org.uk/bfwg2/ (Accessed 31 October 2023)
Routes to getting a doctorate
https://www.prospects.ac.uk/postgraduate-study/
phd-study/5-routes-to-getting-a-doctorate
(Accessed 31 October 2023)

6.5.4.10 EXCELLENCE IN HEALTHCARE SCIENCE AWARDS

**Chief Scientific Officer's (CSO's) 2022 Excellence in Healthcare Science
Lifetime Achievement award**
https://nshcs.hee.nhs.uk/csos-2022-excellence-in-healthcare-science-lifetime-
achievement-award-winner (Accessed 31 October 2023)

6.5.4.11 INSTITUTE OF ELECTRICAL AND ELECTRONICS ENGINEERS (IEEE) BIOMEDICAL ENGINEERING AWARD

https://corporate-awards.ieee.org/award/ieee-biomedical-field-engineering-award/
(Accessed 31 October 2023)

6.5.5 CLINICAL NETWORKS AND CLINICAL SENATES

https://www.england.nhs.uk/contact-us/privacy-notice/how-we-use-your-
information/public-and-partners/clincal-networks-and-senate/ (Accessed 31
October 2023)

6.5.6 NHS EVENTS AND NEWS

https://www.england.nhs.uk/nhsbirthday/events-and-news/ (Accessed 31 October
2023)

6.5.7 CALENDAR OF NATIONAL CAMPAIGNS

https://www.nhsemployers.org/events/calendar-national-campaigns (Accessed 31 October 2023)

6.5.8 INTERNATIONAL NURSES' DAY: 12 MAY

https://socialcare.blog.gov.uk/2023/05/12/international-nurses-day-celebrating-our-values-strengths-and-ambition/ (Accessed 31 October 2023)

6.5.8.1 INTERNATIONAL DAY OF THE MIDWIVES

https://www.who.int/europe/event/international-day-of-the-midwife (Accessed 9 July 2024)

6.5.9 SETTING UP A JOURNAL CLUB

https://www.nursingtimes.net/learning-units-and-portfolio/journal-club-learning-units-and-portfolio/ (Accessed 31 October 2023)

Top Nursing, Midwifery, AHP and Care Staff Journals

British Journal of Midwifery (BJM)
https://www.markallengroup.com/brands/british-journal-of-midwifery/ (Accessed 31 October 2023)
Nursing Standard: RCNi
https://journals.rcni.com/nursing-standard (Accessed 31 October 2023)
Nursing Times: Resources for the Nursing Profession
https://www.nursingtimes.net/ (Accessed 31 October 2023)

Support for Nurses

Supporting health and wellbeing
https://www.england.nhs.uk/nursingmidwifery/shared-governance-and-collec-tive-leadership/nursing-covid-19-catalogue-of-change/supporting-health-and-wellbeing/ (Accessed 31 October 2023)

6.5.10 BULLETINS AND NEWSLETTERS

https://www.england.nhs.uk/email-bulletins/cno-bulletin/ (Accessed 31 October 2023)

Staff Networks

Digital Nurse Network
https://www.england.nhs.uk/ournhspeople/people-stories/digital-nurse-net-work-supporting-nurses-across-the-nhs-to-use-and-promote-digital-services/ (Accessed 31 October 2023)

Primary care networks

https://www.england.nhs.uk/primary-care/primary-care-networks/ (Accessed 31 October 2023)

Community Nurse Executive Network (CNEN)

https://qni.org.uk/explore-qni/community-nurse-executive-network/ (Accessed 31 October 2023)

Conferences for Nursing, Midwifery, AHP and Care Staff

Infection Prevention Society (IPS) conference

https://www.ips.uk.net/conference-2022 (Accessed 31 October 2023)

RCN Congress

https://www.rcn.org.uk/congress/ (Accessed 31 October 2023)

AHP International Conference

https://www.ahp.org/events/international-conference (Accessed 31 October 2023)

Nursing Times Workforce Summit

https://10times.com/nursing-times-workforce-summit-london (Accessed 31 October 2023)

Nursing Summit

https://www.england.nhs.uk/cno-summit/about-the-summit/ (Accessed 31 October 2023)

International Council of Nurses (ICN) Congress

https://www.icn.ch/events/icn-congress-2023-montreal (Accessed 31 October 2023)

European Public Health Conference 2023

https://eurohealthnet.eu/publication/european-public-health-conference-2023/ (Accessed 31 October 2023)

UK healthcare conferences

https://www.healthcareconferencesuk.co.uk/ (Accessed 31 October 2023)

Special Roles for Staff

RCN representatives

https://www.rcn.org.uk/Get-Involved/rcn-reps (Accessed 31 October 2023)

Resources for BAME staff

International nursing and midwifery associations

https://www.england.nhs.uk/nursingmidwifery/international-recruitment/international-nursing-and-midwifery-associations/ (Accessed 31 October 2023)

International retention toolkit

https://www.nhsemployers.org/publications/international-retention-toolkit (Accessed 31 October 2023)

Improving through inclusion

https://www.england.nhs.uk/wp-content/uploads/2017/08/inclusion-report-aug-2017.pdf (Accessed 31 October 2023)

Nursing workforce: International recruitment
https://www.england.nhs.uk/nursingmidwifery/international-recruitment/ (Accessed 31 October 2023)

Small grants for International Nursing and Midwifery Associations (INMA) in England
https://florence-nightingale-foundation.org.uk/academy/leadership-development/leadership-programmes/current-programmes/small-grants-for-inma-england/ (Accessed 31 October 2023)

Professional associations: Nursing, midwifery and palliative care
https://libguides.kcl.ac.uk/nmpccollections/professionalassocs (Accessed 31 October 2023)

Refugee healthcare professionals
https://www.nhsemployers.org/articles/refugee-healthcare-professionals (Accessed 31 October 2023)

Wellbeing support for Black, Asian and Minority Ethnic staff
https://nshcs.hee.nhs.uk/training-support/wellbeing-support-for-bame-nhs-staff/ (Accessed 31 October 2023)

Infection Prevention and Control (IPC) Resources

Communicable disease outbreak management: Operational guidance
https://www.gov.uk/government/publications/communicable-disease-outbreak-management-operational-guidance (Accessed 31 October 2023)

Epic3: National evidence-based guidelines for preventing healthcare-associated infections (HCAIs) in NHS hospitals in England
https://www.journalofhospitalinfection.com/article/s0195-6701(13)60012-2/fulltext (9.7.24)

Health and Social Care Act 2008: Code of practice on the prevention and control of infections
https://www.gov.uk/government/publications/the-health-and-social-care-act-2008-code-of-practice-on-the-prevention-and-control-of-infections-and-related-guidance (Accessed 31 October 2023)

National Standards of Healthcare Cleanliness 2021
https://www.england.nhs.uk/publication/national-standards-of-healthcare-cleanliness-2021/ (Accessed 31 October 2023)

NICE guidance on surgical site infections: Prevention and treatment
https://www.nice.org.uk/guidance/ng125 (Accessed 31 October 2023)

RCN: Understanding aseptic techniques
https://www.rcn.org.uk/professional-development/publications/pub-007928 (Accessed 31 October 2023)

UK 20-year vision for antimicrobial resistance
https://www.gov.uk/government/publications/uk-20-year-vision-for-antimicrobial-resistance (Accessed 31 October 2023)

UK 5-year action plan for antimicrobial resistance 2019 to 2024

https://www.gov.uk/government/publications/uk-5-year-action-plan-for-antimicrobial-resistance-2019-to-2024 (Accessed 31 October 2023)

World Health Organization (WHO): Global strategy on infection prevention and control

https://apps.who.int/gb/ebwha/pdf_files/WHA75/A75_ACONF5-en.pdf (Accessed 31 October 2023)

WHO guidelines on hand hygiene in healthcare

https://www.who.int/publications/i/item/9789241597906 (Accessed 31 October 2023)

COVID-19: Personal protective equipment use for non-aerosol generating procedures

www.gov.uk/government/publications/covid-19-personal-protective-equipment-use-for-non-aerosol-generating-procedures (Accessed 31 October 2023)

Chapter 7: Competencies and Tools for Use in the Healthcare Setting

Standards of proficiency for registered nurses

Standards of proficiency for registered nurses: The NMC (Accessed 31 October 2023)

https://www.nmc.org.uk/standards/standards-for-nurses/standards-of-proficiency-for-registered-nurses/ (7.7.24)

Standards framework for nursing and midwifery education

https://www.nmc.org.uk/standards-for-education-and-training/standards-framework-for-nursing-and-midwifery-education/ (Accessed 31 October 2023)

NMC Code

https://www.nmc.org.uk/standards/code/ (Accessed 31 October 2023)

The code: Professional standards of practice and behaviour for nurses, midwives and nursing associates

https://www.nmc.org.uk/globalassets/sitedocuments/nmc-publications/nmc-code.pdf (Accessed 31 October 2023)

Standards of proficiency for registered nurses

https://www.nmc.org.uk/standards (Accessed 31 October 2023)

A&E   Accident and emergency.

Acute medical unit   The first area of entry into hospital for patients who are referred as emergencies by their general practitioner (GP) or who require admission from the A&E department.

ADHD   Attention-deficit hyperactivity disorder.

Agenda for Change (AfC)   The main pay system for NHS staff, except doctors, dentists and senior managers.

Agenda for Change (AfC)   is also known as NHS Terms and Conditions of Service.

Aneurysm   Caused by dilation of a blood vessel and can lead to rupture and death.

Angioedema   Swelling of the deeper layers of the skin caused by a build-up of fluid.

Aorta   The largest artery in the body.

Aspiration   The drawing off of fluid from a cavity by means of suction.

Autoimmune disease   Disease causing a problem with the body's immune system where it starts to attack healthy cells, tissues and organs, such as lupus and rheumatoid arthritis.

Bariatric surgery   Surgery for weight loss, such as gastric bypass surgery or gastric band.

Biopsy   A sample of cells or tissue that is removed from the body and tested to exclude or establish diagnoses such as cancer.

Brachytherapy   A cancer treatment whereby radioactive material is inserted directly into the tumour.

Bronchoscopy   Examination of the airways using a bronchoscope (a flexible or rigid tube with a small camera and light at the end).

Cardiac arrest   Cessation of the normal regular muscular contractions of the heart, meaning blood cannot be pumped around the body.

Cardiopulmonary resuscitation (CPR)   Involves the administration of lifesaving chest compressions to someone who is not breathing or who has suffered a cardiac arrest.

Cardiovascular   Concerning the heart and blood vessels.

Catheter   A flexible tube that is inserted into the body to remove or introduce fluids. Catheters also have other uses, such as widening obstructed blood vessels.

Certificate of completion of training (CCT)   The CCT confirms that a doctor has completed an approved training programme in the UK and is eligible for entry onto the GP register or the specialist register. The Certificate of Eligibility for Specialist Registration (CESR) provides an alternative route to the specialist register for those doctors who have not followed a traditional training programme but who may have gained the same skills as CCT holders.

Chemotherapy   Treatment for cancer patients with drugs that destroy cancer cells.

Chartered Institute for Environmental Health (CIEH)   An independent organisation representing the interests of the environmental health profession.

Clinical audit   A process that has been defined as 'a quality improvement' (QI) process that seeks to improve patient care and outcomes through systematic review of care against explicit criteria and the implementation of change.

Clinical commissioning group (CCG)   A group of GPs responsible for designing local health services in England.

Clinical effectiveness   A measure of the extent to which a particular treatment or intervention works.

Cognitive behavioural therapy (CBT)   A talking therapy that can help people manage their problems by changing the way they think and behave.

Colonoscopy   A procedure allowing examination of the colon using a thin flexible tube with a light and camera at one end (known as an endoscope).

Colorectal   Relating to the colon or rectum.

Competition ratio   Competition ratios tell you how many applications were received relative to the number of places available.

Core medical training   Core medical training was replaced by internal medicine training.

Corporate governance   A system that incorporates processes to minimise all risks in an organisation.

Corticosteroids   A class of steroid hormones that are produced in the adrenal cortex of vertebrates, as well as the synthetic analogues of these hormones.

Corticosteroid drugs   Similar to corticosteroid hormones that are produced by the adrenal glands, which are small glands at the top of the kidney. Often known as steroids, they are prescribed for a variety of conditions as tablets, injections, inhalers, creams and so on.

Croup   A common condition in babies and young children resulting in narrowing and inflammation of the airways that causes hoarseness, noisy breathing and a cough. It is usually viral.

Computerised tomography (CT) scans   Uses X-rays and a computer to create detailed images of the inside of the body. Sometimes referred to as a computerised axial tomography (CAT) scan or computed tomography scan.

Cyclotron   A particle accelerator that accelerates charged particles in a spiralling motion, which are then extracted from the accelerator to be used for many different purposes in medical or research activities.

Data mining   The process of extracting information from a set of data and putting it into a format that can be easily understood for further use.

Developmental language disorder   A lifelong condition that significantly affects how someone understands what is said to them and/or how they express themselves.

Differential diagnosis   A series of potential diagnoses that could explain the symptoms a patient is experiencing, which can then potentially lead to the correct diagnosis.

Deoxyribonucleic acid (DNA)   The hereditary material in humans and almost all other organisms.

Doppler   The Doppler effect (or the Doppler shift) is the change in frequency or wavelength of a wave.

Elective   A period of time (often 6 to 12 weeks) spent away from a medical degree on a placement, often overseas. A wide range of other health-related degree courses can also include an elective programme.

Electroconvulsive therapy   A standard psychiatric treatment in which seizures are electrically induced in patients to provide relief from psychiatric illnesses. Formerly known as electroshock therapy.

Electrocardiograms   A test that checks for problems with the electrical activity of the heart.

Electroencephalogram (EEG)   A test to record the electrical activity of the brain used for the diagnosis and monitoring of certain conditions that affect the brain.

Endocrine system   The endocrine system includes eight major glands throughout the body, such as the thyroid gland, pituitary gland, adrenal gland and pancreas.

Endometrial ablation   A medical procedure that is used to remove (ablate) or destroy the endometrial lining of the uterus.

Endoscope   A flexible or rigid tube with a small camera and light at the end used for examination, photography, biopsy and surgery/treatment. Light is carried along the tube by very fine glass fibres.

Endoscopy   Examination of a body cavity using an endoscope, which is a flexible or rigid tube with a small camera and light. Operations can also sometimes be carried out by passing instruments into the endoscope.

Endotracheal intubation   A medical procedure in which a tube is placed into the windpipe (trachea) through the mouth or nose.

Endovascular   Using wires, catheters, balloons, stents and devices to treat arterial disease in a minimally invasive way.

Epidemiology   The study of patterns of health and disease in populations.

Epidural   This is the injection of local anaesthetic or other pain-relieving medicines into a space that surrounds the spinal cord. It temporarily numbs the nerves.

Endoscopic retrograde cholangiopancreatography (ERCP)   A technique where a thin flexible tube with a light and camera is inserted via the mouth. It is mainly used to diagnose and treat bile duct and pancreatic duct conditions.

Fissure sealant   Fissure sealants are plastic coatings that are painted onto the grooves of the back teeth.

Flexible sigmoidoscopy   An endoscopic procedure that allows examination of the lining of the rectum and the lower part of the colon. A long flexible tube that has a camera and light at one end (known as an endoscope) is inserted.

Foundation training   Part of a doctor's training that takes place after the completion of a medical degree at university. It comprises a series of rotations in different specialties within hospitals or in the community. The first year of training is known as FY1 and the second year as FY2. Foundation training precedes specialist training in medicine or surgery.

General Certificate of Secondary Education (GCSE) at grades A–C   Results for GCSE subjects in England are graded U to 9, with grades 4 to 9 being equivalent to GCSE grade C and above.

Genetics   The branch of science that deals with how you inherit physical and behavioural characteristics, including medical conditions.

Genomics   A discipline in genetics that looks at the function and structure of genomes (the complete set of DNA within a single cell of an organism).

General Osteopathic Council (GOC)   The regulatory body for osteopaths in the UK.

Grades A-C   Results for GCSE subjects in England are graded U to 9, with grades 4 to 9 being equivalent to GCSE grades C and above.

Haemodialysis   A method of removing waste products from the blood using a dialyser or artificial kidney.

Harvesting veins   Removal of healthy veins to be used elsewhere in the body.

Health and Care Professions Council (HCPC)   A regulatory body that maintains a register of a number of healthcare professions.

Heart murmurs   Abnormal sounds caused by turbulent blood flow within the heart.

Holistic   Relating to the whole thing rather than just a part. In a health setting this means having a concern for the whole person, where body and mind are linked.

NHS Higher Specialist Scientific Training (HSST)   Training for registered clinical scientists to enable them to practise at consultant healthcare scientist level.

Human Genome Project   A project to gain a better understanding of how certain traits and characteristics are passed on from parents to children.

Hypertension   Abnormally high blood pressure.

Hysteroscopy   A procedure used to examine the inside of the uterus (womb).

In vitro   Techniques conducted in a laboratory setting, where a glass dish or test tube is used for observations made outside the body. A well-known example is in vitro fertilisation, where sperm and egg are fertilised outside the body.

Informatics   The science of computer information systems. As an academic field it involves the practice of information processing, and the engineering of information systems.

Intensive care   The care of seriously ill people.

Intrauterine contraceptives   A small T-shaped device made from plastic and copper that is fitted into the uterus to prevent pregnancy. Also called a coil.

Intubate   The insertion of a tube into a part of the body, often a breathing tube into the trachea (breathing passages). This enables mechanical ventilation, for example during surgery or as an emergency procedure.

Laryngeal   Pertaining to the larynx.

Linear accelerator (LINAC)   A device used for external beam radiation treatments for patients with cancer.

Lipid disorders   Metabolic disorders that result in abnormal amounts of fatty substances that are insoluble in water (lipids), which may lead to serious illnesses.

Local area network (LAN)   A computer network that connects computers within a limited area such as a home, hospital or office building using network media.

Lumbar puncture   The insertion of a hollow needle into the spinal canal, to inject drugs or other substances or to withdraw cerebrospinal fluid.

Magnetic resonance imaging (MRI)   An imaging technique that uses powerful magnetic fields and radio waves to provide detailed cross-sectional or three-dimensional images of the body.

Metabolic   The processes, both physical and chemical, by which the living body is built up and maintained, and by which molecules are broken down to make energy available to the organism.

MHRA   Medicines and Healthcare Products Regulatory Agency.

Microvascular   Small arteries or veins.

Mitral valve   Valve with two tapered cusps located between the left atrium and the left ventricle of the heart. Also called the bicuspid valve.

MRCP   Membership of the Royal College of Physicians (RCP).

Multimorbidity   Multiple long-term, chronic health conditions.

Multidisciplinary team meeting (MDT)   Different professionals meet to discuss the diagnosis and treatment of patients. They include doctors from different specialties, nurses and many other professionals such as physiotherapists and occupational therapists.

Nanotechnology   Enables scientists to examine molecules and atoms at the smallest possible microscopic level. Measurements are made in nanometers, which is a billionth of a metre.

Nebuliser   A device used to administer drugs including corticosteroids for conditions such as asthma.

Neonatal   The period of time following a baby's birth, up to 4 weeks after birth.

National Institute for Health and Care Excellence (NICE)   Provides national guidance and advice to improve health and social care.

NHS Constitution   Sets out the rights that patients, the public and staff are entitled to, and the pledges that the NHS is committed to fulfilling.

NHS Practitioner Training Programme (PTP)   An undergraduate route into healthcare science via an accredited BSc (Hons) in healthcare science.

NHS Scientist Training Programme (STP)   A graduate entry route to become a clinical scientist who would like to work in healthcare (NHS, 2022p).

Nursing and Midwifery Council (NMC)   A regulatory body that maintains a register of nurses, midwives and health visitors.

Objective structured clinical examination (OSCE)   A type of examination used in medicine and other health professions to test a broad range of clinical skills and other skills, such as communication. The examination takes place via a series of stations and usually lasts 5 to 10 minutes, and the student progresses from station to station with a different examiner each time. Actors may be used in place of real patients.

Oedema   A build-up of fluid in the body, causing the affected tissue to become swollen.

On-call   Where a member of staff is available to be called for work, usually outside normal working hours. This can involve answering enquiries over the phone or physically attending the workplace. It can also sometimes involve sleeping at the workplace to be available to deal with emergencies.

Oncology   The branch of medicine that deals with the study and treatment of tumours, particularly cancerous tumours.

Orthoses   Devices worn in shoes either to change the way the foot works while walking or to provide support. They are used to relieve pain outside the foot such as in the ankle, knee, hip or back.

Paracentesis   Puncture of the wall of a body cavity by a hollow needle to draw off excess fluid or obtain diagnostic material (e.g. abdomen or chest).

Parenteral   The administration of drugs or other fluids into the body by any route except via the gastrointestinal tract (e.g. by intravenous or intramuscular injection or infusion).

Parenteral nutrition   The provision of carbohydrate, fat and proteins via intravenous administration (feeding).

Perioperative   The time before and after an operation.

Perioperative care   The goal of perioperative care is to provide better conditions for patients before, during and after the operation.

Personal development plan   An action plan based on self-awareness, values, reflection, goal-setting and planning for career development. Abbreviated to PDP.

Physical sciences and biomedical engineering   Healthcare science and biomedical engineering staff in this area develop methods of measuring what is happening in the body, devise new ways of diagnosing and treating disease and ensure that equipment is functioning safely and effectively (NHS, 2022q).

Physiology   The science of the functions of living organisms.

Pleural aspiration   A small needle is inserted into the space between the lungs and the chest wall to remove fluid that has accumulated around the lung.

Plexus blocks   Regional anaesthesia techniques that are sometimes employed as an alternative to general anaesthesia for surgery of the shoulder, arm, forearm, wrist and hand.

Polypharmacy   The administration of different drugs taken together, which increases the likelihood of side effects from drug interactions.

Primary care   Care provided by GP practices, dental practices, community pharmacies and high street optometrists. It is many people's first (primary) point of contact with the NHS. Around 90% of patient interaction is with primary care services.

Prostheses   Plural of prosthesis. An artificial device that replaces a missing body part that may have been lost through trauma, disease or congenital conditions.

Public Health England (PHE)   PHE was an executive agency of the Department of Health and Social Care, established in April 2013 and functioning up to April 2023 to 'protect the public from hazards, deal with public health emergencies like coronavirus, improve the nation's health and wellbeing and reduce health inequalities'. PHE was replaced by the UK Health Security Agency (UKHSA).

Pulmonary embolism   A blood clot in the pulmonary artery or in the lung.

Quality and Outcomes Framework (QOF)   The annual reward and incentive programme that measures the achievements of GP practices.

Quality assurance   A way of preventing mistakes or defects in products and avoiding problems in customer service.

Radiotherapy   Treatment of cancer patients with X-rays or other radiation.

Red flag   Symptoms that indicate a potentially serious disease and warrant prompt investigation and treatment.

Respiratory   Related to the respiratory (breathing) system, which includes the nose, throat (pharynx), larynx, windpipe (trachea), lungs and diaphragm.

Royal College of Physicians (RCP)   An independent, patient-centred and clinically led organisation that drives improvements in health and care through advocacy, education and research to improve to the diagnosis of disease, the care of individual patients and the health of the population in the UK and across the globe.

Run through   Some medical trainee pathway posts are structured such that, once the trainee starts a pathway and provided they meet the Annual Review of Competence Programme (ARCP), they will continue on that pathway until they reach the end of their training.

Secondary care   Relates to services provided by specialist doctors or other health professionals who generally do not have the first contact with the patient but are referred by primary care (often by a GP). Secondary care services are usually provided in a hospital or clinic.

Sepsis   A life-threatening condition that arises when the body's response to an infection injures its own tissues and organs.

Sickle cell disease   A serious inherited blood disorder where the red blood cells develop abnormally.

Spinal block   This is an alternative to general anaesthesia when the surgical site is located on the lower extremities, perineum (e.g. surgery on the genitalia or anus), or lower abdominal area.

Stroke   Caused when there is interruption of the blood supply to the brain, which is often the result of a blood clot in a cerebral (brain) artery (ischaemic stroke). It may also be caused by the rupturing of a blood vessel in or near the brain (haemorrhagic stroke).

Subdermal contraceptive implants   A type of birth control. A small flexible tube measuring about 40 mm in length is inserted under the skin.

Suture   A stitch or series of stitches used to close a wound.

T levels   T Levels are new 2-year, technical-based qualifications in England that will follow GCSEs and are equivalent to three A Levels. They will offer students a mixture of classroom learning and 'on-the-job' experience during an industry placement of at least 45 days.

Tertiary care   Treatment given in a large regional hospital that provides highly specialised care, such as cardiac surgery or oncology.

Thrombosis   The formation of a blood clot in the blood vessels or heart.

Tinnitus   Noises heard in the ear without an external cause, such as buzzing or ringing.

Topical fluoride   Professionally applied topical fluorides include higher-strength rinses, gels, foams and fluoride varnishes.

Topologies   Plural of topology, an area of mathematics concerned with the properties of space.

Tracheostomies   Plural of tracheostomy, an opening created at the front of the neck so a tube can be inserted into the windpipe (trachea) to aid breathing.

Transient ischaemic attack (TIA)   Also known as a 'ministroke', this occurs when there is a brief interruption of the blood supply to the brain, causing symptoms similar to those of a stroke. The symptoms typically last less than 1 hour and are completely resolved within 24 hours.

Trauma and orthopaedic (T&O)   Covers injuries and conditions relating to bones, joints, ligaments, tendons, muscles and nerves.

UK Health Security Agency (UKHSA)   Responsible for protecting every member of every community from the impact of infectious diseases, chemical, biological, radiological and nuclear incidents and other health threats.

Ultrasound   A procedure that uses high-frequency sound waves to produce images of body structures. Can also be used to provide treatment or assist with the healing process.

United Kingdom Public Health Register (UKPHR) (previously PHE)   A register providing public assurance for the provision of a competent workforce that contributes to a high-quality public health service.

Urticaria   A raised, itchy rash on the skin. Also known as hives, welts or nettle rash.

Wide area networks   A network covering a broad area, i.e. any telecommunications network that links regional, national or international boundaries using leased telecommunications.

Working Time Directive   Gives European Union (EU) workers the right to a minimum number of holidays each year, rest breaks and rest of at least 11 hours in any 24 hours; restricts excessive night work; gives a day off after a week's work; and provides the right to work no more than 48 hours per week.

INDEX

Note: Page numbers followed by '*f*' indicate figures, '*t*' indicate tables and '*b*' indicate boxes.